SPLINTERED REFLECTIONS

SPLINTERED REFLECTIONS

Images of the Body in Trauma

JEAN GOODWIN
AND REINA ATTIAS

BASIC
BOOKS

A Member of the Perseus Books Group

Copyright © 1999 by Basic Books, A Member of the Perseus Books Group

A CIP catalog record for this book is available from the Library of Congress
ISBN: 0-465-09544-5

99 01 02 03 ❖/RRD   10   9   8   7   6   5   4   3   2   1

FIRST EDITION

This work is dedicated to our patients,
whose courage and profound generosity make it possible
for all of us to learn.

Contents

Introduction:
How to Use This Book

For more than fifteen years we have spent many hours of each working day listening to our patients describe tragic moments from childhood and strange, inexplicable bodily symptoms and experiences. This book represents our efforts to discuss and connect these phenomena in conversation with our patients, so as to open pathways to symptom reduction and the resumption of previously blocked development in the areas of self-perception and mastery. This has been a long struggle to wrest the beginnings of a language from symptoms created to express experiences beyond language.

How can we convey this new language to readers? This Introduction is the first of five editorial segments describing the stages in the intellectual voyage that brought us to our present approaches to this material. In the Editors' Comments on Part I, "The Body Speaks," we describe the strange bodily symptoms in traumatized individuals that first drew our attention to these problems and quote directly from our patients as they have tried to convey to us their experiences in this inarticulate realm. In "The Body Silenced" (Part II), we share some of the reading and historical research into which we were propelled as we tried to answer our own and our patients' questions about the traumatized body, questions already asked in detail in the nineteenth century. The societal silencing of certain aspects of these questions and their answers comes into clear focus when we look at Jean-Martin Charcot and his students in the Salpêtrière, but it is a tendency toward silence that we are still struggling with a century later. Part III's Editors' Comments, "The Body in the Mirror," recounts theoretical and clinical aspects of our quest, as we explored psychoanalytic, trauma and attachment theories for concepts that would express and illuminate the intrapsychic experience that links the traumatic moment to the bodily symptom and that further links bodily experiences to the capacity to function effectively in the world. Certain images kept recurring as we tried to decipher this language of the body: mirrors, trees, houses, paper. In the last Editors' Comments section, "The Body Finds Its Voice," we explain our present clinical stance and how we approach messages from the traumatized body now both in dialogue with patients and with ourselves and our culture as we confront the body-mind split that is so endemic in the present technological zeitgeist.

The book is organized into four parts. Part I, "Symptoms: Body Responses to Trauma," reviews the body's acute responses to overwhelming trauma and the long-term bodily symptoms reported in traumatized individuals. Part II, "Experiences: Body Image in Trauma," introduces the powerful concept of body image and discusses its manifestations, the impacts produced on it by psychological trauma or bodily damage and the consequences of distorted body image in terms of symptoms and ego functioning. Part III, "Psychotherapy: The Traumatized Body in Treatment," further explores concepts of body-ego functioning and effectiveness in the light of attachment theory and gives clinical examples from psychotherapeutic encounters in which these are addressed. Part IV, "Reflections: Body and Self in Dialogue," continues this theme into the rehabilitation phase of psychotherapy, when symptoms are contained, the traumatic distortions of body image are understood and the task is to bring body and self into dialogue so that problems of living can be solved in a more integrated way.

Readers may choose to (1) read sequentially, (2) focus first on the subjective editorial thread, or (3) focus on a particular section emphasizing body symptoms, body-image distortions, body-ego functioning or developments in the late, or outcome, phase of treatment.

The first three parts are organized as follows: The first chapter in each part describes research and introduces a simple research tool; the second chapter focuses on the major theoretical concept addressed in that section; the third chapter describes a clinical application; and the last chapter presents a literary or historical application of the concepts. This organization offers readers the additional option of focusing either on research, theory, clinical applications or models drawn from history or literature.

Working in this way, researchers can turn from Bruce Perry's elegant physiological use of the pulse as an indicator of the state of the traumatized body (Chapter 1), to Armsworth, Stronck and Carlson's use of psychological instruments for measuring body-image damage and body-ego function (Chapter 5), and then to Cohen and Mills's discussion of drawings as tools to assess the presence of dissociative ego defenses and distorted body image (Chapter 9). Theoreticians can go from trauma theory's predictions about bodily involvement (Chapter 2) to a discussion of psychoanalytic concepts of body image (Chapter 6) to an analysis of how the attachment disturbances of the traumatized child lead to bodily symptoms (Chapter 10). Clinicians would begin with Loewenstein and Goodwin's review of the bodily symptoms that have been reported in traumatized individuals (Chapter 3), then go on to our suggestions about how psychotherapy techniques can be used to explore body image and body ego (Chapter 7), and end with Kluft's clinical discussion of the body-image and body-ego changes that occur as dissociated alters are integrated (Chapter 11).

The applied analytic chapters begin with Nijenhuis and van der Hart's work demonstrating Pierre Janet's systematization of nineteenth-century ideas about hysteria by applying them to a contemporary case (Chapter 4). Sinason uses the Greek god Hephaestus and Shakespeare's *Richard III* to describe the secondary body-image problems that can further inhibit ego functioning in children struggling with visible developmental disabilities (Chapter 8). Then we explore Franz Kafka's *Metamorphosis* in order to discuss in detail the devastating body-image and body-ego distortions that take place when the self escapes trauma by assuming animal form (Chapter 12).

We emphasize these multiple approaches to reading and rereading this book, because we have found this material extremely elusive and difficult and have ourselves needed to review and reconceptualize in many different ways as we began to approach these questions clinically.

The last chapter of the book is titled "A Place to Begin." Clinicians may choose to take the title as an invitation to begin at the end—the satisfying clinical interchanges documented in that last chapter may provide motivation for going back to the beginning of the book for a grounding in the fundamentals of brain functioning, trauma and psychoanalytic theory and previous clinical and population research that can facilitate similarly eloquent clinical dialogues in their own practices.

A few additional signposts: For readers who learn best from detailed cases, these can be found in Chapters 1, 4, 7 and 8. And readers who prefer to follow a single voice can begin with our five commentary sections and five chapters before branching out into the six chapters told by different voices.

Readers may note that we have used the terms "client" and "patient" somewhat interchangeably. We are not entirely happy with either term and envy the French analysts, who can swiftly and accurately describe a person engaged in rearranging psychic contents as "the one who is analyzing."

The references to each chapter will guide readers to the theoretical and clinical literature that informs our work: trauma theory, psychoanalytic theory, attachment theory and research on child abuse and adversity, combat trauma, the holocaust and refugees and minorities. We are aware that these theories and the research supporting them are not universally embraced and that our synthetic use of these building blocks carries this work into even more speculative realms. We have elected in this book not to go into the various debates and controversies about these viewpoints and data sets. The work of sequential conceptualization required of readers is already strenuous enough without our interrupting to ask new and different sets of questions.

Our understanding of the nineteenth-century experience with traumatized bodies leads us to believe that today's objections, debates and shocking headlines will be forgotten in a hundred years. What will remain are the clinical problems and multiple societal forces that prevent us from addressing respectfully and productively the layered biopsychosocial dilemmas that our patients bring to us. As grateful readers of Freud and Janet, we hope that the detailed clinical descriptions in this book will be recognizable and useful to clinicians who might pick up this volume a hundred years from now.

Acknowledgments

We are grateful to the contributors, who as we worked on this project invariably supplied, in addition to the requested chapters, more intricate gifts including clinical sharing, mutual consultations, long conversations over wonderful meals, scenic walks and many other manifestations of welcome and sustenance.

Our thanks go as well to the American Psychiatric Association for accepting as an Annual Meeting Symposium (New York City, May 1996) a presentation previewing early versions of Chapters 1, 3, 10 and 11. Early versions of Chapters 4 and 5 were presented in a symposium at the 1996 meeting of the International Society for the Study of Traumatic Stress (Jerusalem, June 1996). The Institute of Medical Humanities at the University of Texas Medical Branch sponsored a colloquium at which an early draft of Chapter 12 was reviewed. Chapters 6 and 7 are based on papers presented at annual meetings of the International Society for the Study of Dissociation (Chicago, 1994, and Orlando, Florida, 1995). Chapters 3 and 9 developed in part from presentations at the Eastern Regional Meetings on Trauma and Dissociation (Alexandria, Virginia, 1993, 1994).

Participants at those meetings and many others helped us absorb and digest this material and think about it more clearly. Olga Heijtmaier (Amsterdam) helped us understand the cross-cultural validity of the tree-drawing task (Chapter 9) and its value as a clue to the presence of cryptic forms of dissociation even when other clinical and psychological test indicators are absent. Brett Kahr (London) gave us his brilliant biography of D. W. Winnicott, which we deployed in the theoretical summaries in Chapter 10, and also introduced us to Valerie Sinason. Rudi Binion (Boston) reviewed Chapter 12, and in the preconceptualization phase of trying to write about metamorphosis, Teresita McCarty (Albuquerque) gave clarifying advice, as did all the members of the Advanced Candidates Class at the Houston-Galveston Psychoanalytic Institute. Bessel van der Kolk (Boston) brilliantly discussed the papers given at the New York symposium. Eric Vermetten (Netherlands) grounded us in the neurochemistry and neuroanatomy that underlie Chapters 1 and 3. Judy Herman (Boston) was, as always, supportive, steadying and clarifying whenever we discussed this material. Vera John-Steiner (Albuquerque) helped us to understand the problems of language acquisition in children undergoing trauma. Joan Buresch and Puenani Harvey helped us access Jungian insights and texts, especially concerning trees and fairy tales.

The places where we did bits and pieces of this thinking and writing— most often Santa Fe, New Mexico, and Galveston, Texas—have nurtured us in many ways. Memory will always connect particular fleeting insights to the landscapes of Disneyland, Chicago's Loop and Greenwich Village or with Amsterdam's canals or Jerusalem's Old City Walls. Kinko's computers in El Paso were the first to read the completed manuscript.

We are thankful to the many friends who listened and were supportive. And we are especially grateful to our husbands, John Menken and James Goodwin, who, in addition to going beyond tolerance in every dimension imaginable, read critically certain chapters, told us which books and myths to read, supplied quotations, found references, and made superb comments and coffee.

List of Contributors

Mary Taylor Armsworth, Ed.D.   Associate Professor, Department of Educational Psychology, Counseling Psychology Program, University of Houston, Houston, Texas

Reina Attias, Ph.D.   Private practice, Santa Fe, New Mexico

Coleen D. Carlson   Doctoral candidate, University of Houston College of Education, Houston, Texas

Barry M. Cohen, ATR-BC   Private practice, Art Therapy Services, Alexandria, Virginia

Jean M. Goodwin, M.D.   Clinical Professor of Psychiatry and Behavioral Sciences, University of Texas Medical Branch; Private practice, General and Forensic Psychiatry and Psychoanalysis, Galveston, Texas

Richard P. Kluft, M.D.   Clinical Professor of Psychiatry, Temple University School of Medicine; Private practice of Psychiatry and Psychoanalysis, Bala Cynwyd, Pennsylvania

Richard J. Loewenstein, M.D.   Medical Director, Trauma Disorders Program, Sheppard Pratt Health Systems, Baltimore, Maryland

Anne Mills, ATR-BC   Private practice, Art Therapy Services, Alexandria, Virginia

Ellert R. S. Nijenhuis   Psychologist and Psychotherapist, Outpatient Department, General Psychiatric Hospital, Drenthe, Assen, The Netherlands; Researcher, Cats-Polm Institute, Bilthoven, The Netherlands

Bruce D. Perry, M.D., Ph.D.   Senior Fellow, CIVITAS Initiative, Chicago, Illinois; Professor of Child Psychiatry and Vice-Chairman for Research, Department of Psychiatry and Behavioral Sciences, Baylor College of Medicine, Houston, Texas

Valerie Sinason, BA Hons, PGTC, MACP   Director, Clinic for Dissociative Studies, Consultant Research Psychotherapist, St. George's Hospital Medical School Psychiatry of Disability Department; Consultant Child Psychotherapist, Tavistock Clinic, London; Honorary Consultant Child Psychotherapist, University of Capetown Child Guidance Clinic, Capetown, South Africa

Karin Stronck, M. Ed.   Doctoral candidate, Counseling Psychology, Loyola University, Chicago, Illinois

Onno van der Hart, Ph.D.   Professor, Department of Psychology, Utrecht University, Utrecht, The Netherlands; Chief of Research, Cats-Polm Institute, Bilthoven, The Netherlands

PART I

Symptoms
Body Responses to Trauma

One of the first things I remember knowing was that my mother was hurting my brain. It was like she was burning my brain with a hot poker, branding it. Later I knew it would destroy my life.

Patient in psychotherapy, unpublished

Emotion, feeling and biological regulation all play a role in human reason. The lowly orders of our organism are in the loop of high reason.

A. R. Damasio (1994, xiii)

It is the intense pain that destroys a person's self and world . . . it is also language-destroying.

Elaine Scarry (1985, 35)

There are some deep-seated griefs so subtle and so pervasive that it is difficult to grasp whether they belong to our soul or our body. . . . Everything hurts me—memory, eyes, arms.

Fernando Pessoa (1991, 45)

I am a memory come alive. Hence also the inability to sleep.

Franz Kafka (1976, 392)

Sometimes I think my body is the only proof I have that it all happened.

Patient in psychotherapy, unpublished

The Body Speaks
Bodily Disturbances After Childhood Trauma

We have arrived at this place, authors and readers alike, because we have been called here by the bodily manifestations and vicissitudes, in imagination and reality, of childhood trauma. We have been called, often inarticulately, by traumatized bodies that stymied, provoked, puzzled, intrigued, harried, worried, beleaguered or rejected us in some way, conveying to us the need to become better and more attentive listeners.

One of us (J.G.) began to encounter traumatized children in the 1970s as a psychiatric consultant to a child protective agency. Medical training had prepared me for tangible bodies that could voice discomforts audibly and accurately through comprehensible and visible signs of illness. However, as I began meeting children and families living in a world of violence and neglect, I realized I was dealing with a much more problematic idea of the body.

Toddlers who said "I hurt" might not be referring to current pain in the body. Sometimes they meant that a loved person had hurt them emotionally or physically (Goodwin 1982). Even with older children, complaints about the body shifted interchangeably into complaints about their situations. Pediatricians became exasperated at times with adolescents who came to the clinic incessantly for "psychosomatic" stomach pain or "faked" seizures. Later, as adults, such patients have explained that they kept going back, again and again, hoping the doctor would finally ask the right question and their abuse would be revealed and halted and its implications discussed. One woman told me how her seizure diagnosis had begun at age eleven when her uncle pursued her from the dining table to the bathroom. There was no way for her to tell anyone at the family gathering that he was molesting her again, but she could fall to the ground in a dissociative faint (see Chapter 1), and that achieved her exit from the situation (Goodwin 1993).

In those days, before the rediscovery of childhood sexual abuse, the body provided almost the only exit. Children's disclosures were almost uniformly dismissed as fantasies, so it was the body finally that spoke; pregnancy and venereal disease were relatively common among the infrequent sexual abuse cases that were substantiated in that era (Goodwin 1989).

The self and the body often told different stories. I remember a family session in which all three children eloquently retracted their sexual abuse allegations, apologized to the father, and explained to everyone that they no longer needed to remain in foster placement. Impressed, we set about arranging for the parents to take the children home that day for a trial visit. When we got back to our vehicle, we found the children hiding in the backseat. Their tongues were pleading to return home, but their bodies were telling us, "No way." The body is often at its most eloquent when saying no.

There were other paradoxes. Sometimes at the very moment when the fact of abuse seemed most firmly established and undeniable, everything would shift, becoming once again murky, confused and evanescent. Here is another scene from those times: We are talking with a mother in the hospital. Her toddler is still sleeping after surgical repair of a perineal tear that extended from vagina to anus. No, explains the mother, nothing happened to her. No, no further care is needed. On awakening, the toddler would echo her mother and the narrative would vanish. Everything was fine. Except the little ripped body and the silenced self inside it.

Videotapes document the eloquence of the bodies of abused children (Lichtenberg 1978; Novick and Novick 1996). One would have to be blind to miss the frozen watchfulness, the avoidance of eye contact with the hurtful parent, the muscles stiffening as the body pulls away. Yet we miss these signs every day, and in adult forums, such as courts, they have very little standing (see Chapter 1).

One of the pleasing things about Bruce Perry's work (Chapter 1) is that he does keep his eye steadily on the child's body, even while all the other adults are immersed in their usual concerns—status or blame or rights or saving face. During the standoff in 1993 between federal agents and the Branch-Davidian cult in Waco, Texas, Dr. Perry had his steady eye on the pulses of the twenty-one children who had been evacuated from the compound. It was eight days before any child's pulse went below 120, even during sleep. Whatever lessons history finally draws from this moment in the American experience, one hopes that some part of it will encompass the pulse rates of those terrorized children.

By the 1980s, both of us were immersed in clinical practices in which adults who remembered chaotic childhoods were teaching us about the subsequent vicissitudes of childhood trauma. The confusions about the body were terrible. Am I pregnant? Am I not? The most fundamental questions about their bodies were completely insoluble, caught up in the same cloud of not-quite-knowing that had obscured the realities of the children's hurt bodies. A patient calls in tears, feeling badgered and caught between the specialist who says immediate surgery is required and the one who tells her it's all in her mind. What is so painful and difficult for her to explain is how confused she is about every aspect of her own bodily experience, which they assume she is so expert on. One patient devised the creative solution of moving to the site of a world-famous diagnostic clinic. She reasoned that there, at least, the diagnostic warfare could proceed in a more efficient manner.

In the most extreme instances, this loss of the grounding function of the body leads to simulated or bizarre bodily complaints and disastrous disconnection from the truth of one's own personal story. Some of these patients are diagnosed as having factitious disorder (Munchausen's syndrome). They tell us many different stories about their bodies and many different stories about their lives, but what they never tell us is the story of their childhood abuse. This we must learn from collateral sources, and the patients are adept at making certain we are too preoccupied with their diversionary actions ever to have time to discuss it (Goodwin 1988).

Richard Loewenstein's chapter (Chapter 3) summarizes the available literature on this confusing interface between past trauma and somatic disturbances, connects the confusion to the basic psychobiology of trauma (summarized in Chapters 1 and 2) and offers guidelines for therapists working with patients.

In the last chapter in this section (Nijenhuis and van der Hart), we follow the somatic symptoms in a particular case over time, classifying each symptom within Pierre Janet's careful and intricate nineteenth-century system as informed by contemporary trauma theory (Chapter 2). Readers may want to underline Janet's ideas about organic anesthesia and the potential here for losing the very consciousness of one's living existence as well as for rejecting the body as ego alien and not part of the self. (Each of these conditions will be discussed further in Chapter 13.) One of the appealing aspects of Janet's vision is that he sees the system as a whole without attempting to segregate bodily sensations from body image from body-ego functioning. The patient, Lisa, is experiencing problems in all these areas: She feels the touch of imaginary hands on her body, then looks down and realizes that those parts of her body have vanished and been replaced by "holes"; then she realizes that there are holes as well in her memory for those body parts and in her capacity to use them for her own ends (see Case 1 in Chapter 7 for a similar description).

We were particularly interested in the vignettes in these chapters that described eating disorders. Ten years ago, it was the effort to review and understand the eating disorders of our patients that convinced us finally of the pervasive and systematized nature of these bodily symptoms (Goodwin and Attias 1993, 1994). We were dealing not with random or occasional somatic problems or unique and interesting anecdotes, but with something that operated much more like a language, a language whose lawful syntax most of our patients seemed to be speaking in one dialect or another, if only we could understand. Any aspect of the eating symptom might contain clues that harkened back to the trauma: the time of day it occurred, the type of food that could or could not be eaten, the place where problems occurred, the imagined result of eating or not eating. There was a confusion of tongues with our colleagues, who imagined we were positing child abuse as a "cause" of eating disorders in the same way pneumococcus causes pneumonia; but for us it seemed more as if the symptom represented the patient's narrative picture of the trauma, but it was told in a language that not even its author could translate.

This section describes several cases quite similar to ours. In his third case (Chapter 1) Bruce Perry tells us about an eight-year-old boy in a group home who ends up in restraints after refusing to eat his hot dog. Perry traces the oropharyngeal stimulation of the hot dog to similar stimuli during forced fellatio, which were associated at that time with a state of fight-or-flight preparedness; that state has now become reactivated by the no longer neutral stimulation produced by the hot dog. When Nijenhuis and van der Hart describe in Chapter 4 the patient Lisa's idea that the penis of the abuser and his sperm are somehow still in her mouth, they classify this in nineteenth-century terms as a fixed idea, a positive hysterical symptom that is mobile or changeable. In Chapter 6 we describe yet another patient who accesses through art therapy a phallic structure that has accreted itself to her esophagus; here psychoanalytic ideas about body-image distortion are applied to understanding and categorizing the phenomenon. In Chapter 2 we learn that under threat we lose our appetite, but at moments when the predator relaxes, we may binge on excess calories to keep up our strength. When threat becomes chronic, corticosteroid elevation may produce physiologic changes that favor obesity. Both Chapters 1 and 2 remind us that brain changes associated with trauma make it extremely difficult for the subject to decode symptoms as trauma-related. All our protective mechanisms block access to aspects of those overwhelming moments; even when amnesia is not present for the story, alexithymia may block the making of emotional connections.

There are so many echoes across continents and centuries. Janet (Chapter 4) described patients who experience the body as "a collection of unrelated elements," as "thing-like" or "puppet-like"; they must look directly at a body part in order to move it coherently. We have perhaps heard similar experiences from our own patients, but not explored them as fully. One hears also the voice of D. W. Winnicott, working from an entirely different theoretical perspective than Janet (Chapter 10), describing a similar patient: "Her personality was not felt to be localised in her body, which was like a complex engine that she had to drive with conscious care and skill" (Winnicott, 1945, p.138).

REFERENCES

Damasio, A. R. (1994). *Descartes' error: Emotion, reason and the human brain.* New York: Putnam.

Goodwin, J. (1982). *Sexual abuse: Incest victims and their families.* Littleton, Mass.: Wright/PSG.

_____. (1988). Munchausen's syndrome as a dissociative disorder. *Dissociation* 1 (1): 54–60.

_____. (1989). *Sexual abuse: Incest victims and their families,* 2d ed. Chicago: Mosby/Yearbook.

_____. (1993). Childhood sexual abuse and nonepileptic seizures. In J. Rowan and J. R. Gages, eds., *Nonepileptic seizures* (pp. 181–192). New York: Butterworth.

Goodwin, J., and Attias, R. (1993). Eating disorders in survivors of multimodal childhood abuse. In R. Kluft and C. Fine, eds., *Clinical perspectives on multiple personality disorders* (pp. 327–341). Washington, D.C.: American Psychiatric Press.

Kafka, F. (1976). *The diaries: 1910–1923.* Ed. M. Brod. New York: Schocken.

Lichtenberg, J. (1978). The testing of reality from the standpoint of the body self. *Journal of the American Psychoanalytic Association* 26: 357–385.

Novick, J., and Novick, K. K. (1996). *Fearful symmetry: The development and treatment of sadomasochism.* Northvale, N.J.: Aronson.

Pessoa, F. (1991). *The book of disquiet.* Translated by Maria Jose de Lancastre. New York: The Serpent's Tail.

Scarry, E. (1985). *The body in pain: The making and unmaking of the world.* New York: Oxford University Press.

Winnicott, D. W. (1945). Primitive emotional development. *International Journal of Psychoanalysis* 26: 137–143.

CHAPTER 1

The Memories of States

How the Brain Stores and Retrieves Traumatic Experience

Bruce D. Perry

All organ systems in the human body have, to some degree, the property of memory: the capacity, unique to life forms, to bring elements of an experience from one moment in time to another. Memory is the foundation of every biological process—from reproduction to gene expression to cell division, from receptor-mediated communication to the development of more complex physiological systems (including neurodevelopment)—and it forms the basis of the immune, neuromuscular and neuroendocrine systems. Through complex physiological processes, elements of experience can even be carried across generations. Elements of the collective experience of the species are reflected in the genome, while the experience of the individual is reflected in the expression of that genome.

No biological system has a more sophisticated capacity to make and store internal representations of the external world—and the internal world— than the human central nervous system, the human brain. All nerve cells store information, and this storage is time-bound, contingent upon previous patterns of activity (Singer 1995; Thoenen 1995). Neurons are specifically designed to respond and modify themselves in response to external cues (e.g., neurohormones, neurotransmitters, neurotrophic factors); (Lauder 1998). These neurophysiological and molecular neurobiological properties have allowed the development of all of the complex functions mediated by the brain (thinking, feeling and acting). The cognitive, motor, emotional and state-regulating areas of the developed brain have organized in response to the experiences of the developing brain (Perry 1988, 1997; Brown 1997). And in *each* of the diverse brain systems that mediate specific functions, some element of previous experience is stored.

This storage involves complex neuromolecular processes: use-dependent changes in synaptic microarchitecture and intracellular alterations in various important chemicals involved in cellular communication and gene expression (Kandel 1989). The details—those that are known—are outside the scope of this chapter. Yet to understand that the physical properties of neurons change with experience is crucial to understanding the concept of memory. Simply stated, the brain changes with experience—*all* experience, good and bad. The focus of this chapter is how the brain changes by storing elements of a traumatic experience.

The human brain has evolved specialized capabilities that are the reflections and the "selections" of millions of years of evolutionary pressures—Nature's greatest hits. The brain allows the human to sense the external and internal environment, process this information, perceive and store elements of these sensations and act to promote individual survival and optimize the chances for successful mating—the key to the survival of the species.

In order to do this, the brain creates internal representations of the external world—it takes information once external to the organism, transforms it into patterned neuronal activity and, in a use-dependent fashion, creates and stores these representations (Kandel and Schwartz 1982; Maunsell 1995). A further remarkable characteristic of this internal representation is that the brain makes and stores associations between the bits of sensory information (e.g., sights, sounds, smells, positions and emotions) from a specific event (e.g., the pairing of the growl of the saber-toothed tiger and danger), allowing the individual to generalize to sensory information present in current or future events.

This chapter will discuss (1) the process of making internal representations during traumatic events; (2) the development of associations specific to the traumatic event; (3) the generalization of these associations from trauma-specific cues to nonspecific cues; and (4) the clinical implications of the storage and recall of trauma-related memories during childhood.

THE BRAIN: DEVELOPMENT AND PLASTICITY

The human brain is an amazing organ that acts to sense, process, perceive, store (create memories) and *act* on information from the internal and external environments to promote survival—survival of the clan. In order to carry out these functions, the human brain has evolved a hierarchical organization that ranges from the regulatory brain-stem areas to the complex, analytical cortical regions (Figure 1.1). All of the diverse functions of the brain are mediated by various combinations of widely distributed neurophysiological and neurochemical systems involving various brain areas— with more simple, regulatory functions (e.g., regulation of respiration, heart rate, blood pressure, body temperature) mediated by the "lower" parts of the brain (brain stem and midbrain) and the most complex functions (e.g., language and abstract thinking) by its most complex cortical structures.

The structural organization and functional capabilities of the mature brain develop throughout life, with the vast majority of the critical structural organization taking place in childhood. Brain development is characterized by (1) sequential development and "sensitivity" (growing from the brain stem to the cortex) and (2) use-dependent organization of these various brain areas. The neurophysiological and neuromolecular mechanisms underlying this use-dependent or activity-dependent neurodevelopment are the same that underlie the use-dependent development of memories. Indeed, use-dependent development and the resulting organization of the brain *are* memories—stored reflections of the collective experiences of the developing child.

For each of the hundreds of neurophysiological systems and areas of the brain, their mature organization and functional capabilities reflect some aspect of the quantity, quality and pattern of somatosensory experience present during the critical organizational periods of development (Bennett et al. 1964; Gunnar 1986; Lauder 1988; Perry 1988, 1997; Brown 1994; Singer 1995; Perry et al. 1995). This use-dependent property of brain development results in an amazingly adaptive malleability such that the brain develops capabilities suited for the type of environment it is growing in (Perry et al. 1995). Children reflect the world in which they are raised.

These various brain areas develop, organize and become fully functional at different stages during childhood. At birth, for example, the brain stem areas responsible for regulating cardiovascular and respiratory function must be intact, while the cortical areas responsible for abstract cognition have years before they are required to be fully functional. Once organized, any

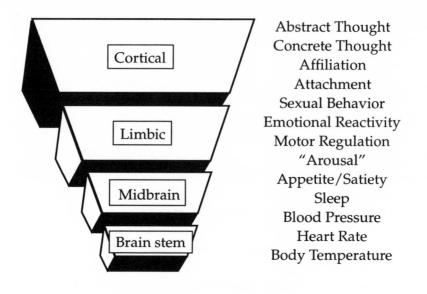

Figure 1.1   Hierarchy of Brain Function
The human brain is organized from the most simple (e.g., fewest cells: brain stem) to most complex (e.g., most cells and most synapses: frontal cortex). The various functions of the brain, from most simple and reflexive (e.g., regulation of body temperature) to most complex (e.g., abstract thought), are mediated in parallel with these levels. These areas organize during development and change in the mature brain in a use-dependent fashion. The more a certain neural system is activated, the more built-in this state becomes, creating an internal representation of the experience corresponding to this neural activation. This use-dependent capacity to make internal representations of the external or internal world is the basis for learning and memory.

brain area or system is less sensitive to experience—less likely to change in response to experience, less plastic. It is of critical importance, then, that by age three, when the brain is 90 percent and the body only 15 percent of adult size, the vast majority of the brain has been organized.

The degree of brain plasticity is related to two main factors—the stage of development and the area or system of the brain. Once an area of the brain is organized, it is much less responsive to the environment—it is less plastic. For example, after age three, experience-dependent modifications of the regulatory system are much less likely than experience-dependent modifications of cortically mediated functions such as language development (Figure 1.2). For the cortex, significant plasticity remains throughout life, such that

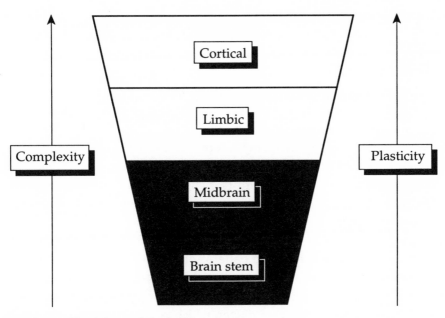

Figure 1.2   Plasticity and Brain Organization
Once the human brain has organized in childhood, it remains capable of changing in response to experience. Yet not all parts of the brain are equally changeable. With relatively brief cognitive experiences we can learn a new phone number but it is much more difficult to make a new motor memory. To make a new state memory—to modify the brain stem, however—is even more difficult. Prolonged or repeated activation of the neurophysiology of stress or alarm must occur to make state memories (see text). This is the reason therapeutic activities require prolonged and repetitive experience. The parts of the brain in which the dysfunctional symptoms arise are often midbrain and brain stem, which are relatively more difficult to modify than the cortex.

experiences can continue to alter, easily, neurophysiological organization and functioning.

THE BRAIN'S RESPONSE TO THREAT

The prime directive of the human brain is to promote survival and procreation. Therefore, the brain is "overdetermined" to sense, process, store, perceive and mobilize in response to threatening information from the external and internal environments (Goldstein 1995). All areas of the brain and body are recruited and orchestrated for optimal survival tasks during the threat. This total neurobiological participation in the threat response is important in understanding how a traumatic experience can impact and alter functioning in such a *pervasive* fashion. Cognitive, emotional, social, behavioral and physiological residues of a trauma may impact an individual for years— even a lifetime.

In order for any experience, traumatic or not, to become part of memory, it must be experienced by the individual. The first step in experiencing is sensation. The five senses of the human body have the amazing capacity to transform forms of energy from the external world (e.g., light, sound, pressure) into patterned activity of sensory neurons. The first stop for sensory input from the outside environment (e.g., light, sound, taste, touch, smell) and from inside the body (e.g., glucose levels, temperature) is the lower, more regulatory parts of the brain—the brain stem and midbrain.

As the sensory input comes into the brain stem and midbrain, it is matched against previously stored patterns of activation, and if unknown or if associated with previous threat, an initial alarm response begins (Aston-Jones et al. 1986). The alarm response begins a wave of neuronal activation in key brain-stem and midbrain nuclei, which contain neurons utilizing a variety of neurotransmitters (e.g., norepinephrine, dopamine, serotonin), neuromodulators and neuropeptides (e.g., ACTH, corticotrophin-releasing factor, vasopressin). At this point, the complex pattern of sensory neuronal activity associated with a specific visual image—or, in different areas of the midbrain, with a specific smell or sound—make connections with neurons in these parts of the brain.

A cascade of patterned neuronal activity is initiated in these primitive areas of the brain that moves up to more complex parts of the brain. In addition to sending these signals to higher parts of the brain, this cascade of activity also initiates a set of brain-stem and midbrain responses to the new information from the environment, allowing the individual to react in a near-reflexive fashion. In many instances, the brain's response to incoming sensory information will take place well before the signals can get to the higher, cortical parts of the brain, where they are "interpreted."

Activation of these key systems results in patterns of neuronal activation that move from brain stem through midbrain to thalamic, limbic and cortical areas. At the level of the brain stem and midbrain, there is very little subjective perception. It is at the level of the thalamic and limbic areas that the actual sensation of anxiety arises. Although the wave of neuronal activity that reaches the limbic area allows the individual to feel the sensation of anxiety, it is only after communication with cortical areas that the individual is able to make more complex, cognitive associations that allow interpretation of that internal state as anxiety (Singer 1995).

Simply stated, then, the fear response involves a tremendous mobilization and activation of systems distributed throughout the brain: Terror involves cortical-, limbic-, midbrain- and brain-stem–based neurophysiology (Gorman et al. 1989). Because the neuronal systems alter themselves in a use-dependent way in response to patterned, repetitive neuronal activation, a state of terror will result in patterned, repetitive neuronal activation in this distributed and diverse set of brain systems—resulting in a set of memories. In each of these areas—mediating cognitive, motor, emotional and state-regulating functions—elements of the traumatic event will be stored and memories of trauma will have been created (Terr 1983; Pynoos and Nader 1989; Schwarz and Kowalski 1991; Schwarz and Perry 1994).

This overview describes the sensing, storing and perceiving elements of the response to threat. At each level of the brain, as the incoming data are "interpreted" and matched against previous similar patterns of activation, a response is initiated. The brain responds to the potential threat. This immediate response capability is very important for rapid response to potentially threatening sensory signals—the classic examples being the immediate motor action of withdrawal of a finger after being burned or the jump that takes place following an unexpected loud noise (startle response). Clearly, in order for the brain to react in this immediate, "uninterpreted" fashion, the more primitive portions of the brain (i.e., brain stem and midbrain) must store patterns of previous sensory neuronal input associated with threat— there must be "state" memories, memories of previous patterns of sensory input that were connected with a bad experience (see below).

The classic response to the threatening cues involves activation of the autonomic nervous system. Originally described by Cannon (1929, 1914), who coined the term *fight or flight* reaction, the physiological manifestations of alarm and arousal frequently co-occur with the emotion of anxiety (e.g., profuse sweating, tachycardia, rapid respiration). These physical symptoms are manifestations of activation of the autonomic nervous system and the hypothalamic-pituitary axis (HPA); (Giller, Southwick and Perry, 1994); again, an adaptive response to the impending threat.

The physiological hyperreactivity of posttraumatic stress disorder (PTSD) is a cue-evoked state memory (see Figure 1.3). The brain has taken a pattern of neuronal activation previously associated with fear and will now act in response to this false signal. The recall of traumatic state memories underlies

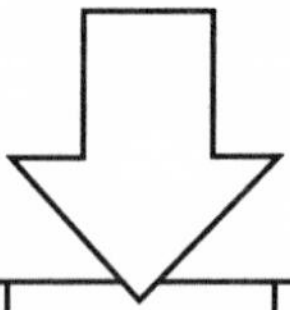

Adaptive Response	Rest *(Adult Male)*	Vigilance	Freeze	Flight	Fight
Hyperarousal Continuum	Rest *(Male Child)*	Vigilance	Resistance	Defiance	Aggression
Dissociative Continuum	Rest *(Female Child)*	Avoidance	Compliance	Dissociation	Fainting
Mental State	**CALM**	**AROUSAL**	**ALARM**	**FEAR**	**TERROR**

Figure 1.3   State-dependent Adaptations to Threat
Different children have different styles of adaptation to threat. Some children use a primary hyperarousal response, some a primary dissociative response. Most use some combination of these two adaptive styles. In the fearful child, a defiant stance is often seen. This is typically interpreted as a willful and controlling child. Rather than understanding the behavior as related to fear, adults often respond to the oppositional behavior by becoming more angry, more demanding. The child, overreading the nonverbal cues of the frustrated and angry adult, feels more threatened and moves from alarm to fear to terror. These children may end up in a very primitive minipsychotic regression or in a very combative state. The behaviors of the child reflect his attempt to adapt and respond to a perceived (or misperceived) threat.

many of the abnormally persistent characteristics of the once adaptive response to threat (Perry 1993, 1994, 1998). This persistence of the fear state and the ability of nonthreatening cues to become paired to a full-blown threat response is related to the remarkable capacity of the human brain to make associations.

THE BRAIN AND CATEGORIZING INFORMATION: ASSOCIATION AND GENERALIZATION

Neuronal systems are remarkably capable of making strong associations between paired cues (e.g., the growl of a tiger and threat). Associations between patterns of neuronal activity and specific sensory stimuli take place in all brain areas, yet complex associations involving the integration of multiple-sensory modalities require more complex brain areas (e.g., amygdala), and the most complex associations take place in cortical areas. Under ideal conditions, this threat-response capacity for association allows the brain to rapidly identify sensory information in the environment associated with threat, allowing the organism to act *rapidly* to promote long-term survival. Yet the remarkable capacity of the brain to take a specific event and generalize, particularly with regard to threatening stimuli, makes humans vulnerable to the development of false associations and false generalizations from a specific traumatic event to other nonthreatening situations. These processes are crucial to understanding memory and trauma.

As patterned neuronal signals come to the first synaptic connections in the regulatory areas of the brain, a cascade of response is started. The patterns of neuronal activity spread to other portions of the brain—up to the midbrain (thalamic, geniculate), creating patterns of activity responsible for different elements of perception. Other synaptic connections to limbic areas (hippocampus, amygdala) allow affective/emotional perception and interpretation of the incoming information. Still other synaptic connections to cortical primary sensory areas (to allow localization) and then to cortical association areas (to pair the elements of input—sight with sound and smell) create a complex perception. At each level of processing, more complex interpretation of the information is taking place, and more differentiated and specific interpretation of the experience is being made.

This increasingly complex and differentiated interpretation allows two things. The first is that the patterns of neuronal activity at each level can be matched with previous patterns and passed on to all other areas of the brain involved in perception and action. The second is the ability to form and act on these local associations being created. Associations between neuronal patterns of activity derived from specific sensory cues are matched against a catalogue of previous experiences. For an individual with a history of traumatic experience, a simple rise in heart rate induced by a nonthreatening experience (e.g., exercise; see Case 5, below) can trigger a whole cascade of brain-stem–mediated alarm response. In this person's past, the neuronal patterns of activation associated with increased heart rate were those associated with severe threat. The brain had stored this state memory and generalized this pattern to indicate threat.

Overgeneralization is an adaptive process. It was far preferable for the vulnerable human to be too cautious, remain too vigilant and overread nonverbal cues of threat. Learning the association between the growl of the saber-toothed tiger and danger should take only *one* experience. Not many individuals who required more than one trial to learn this had a chance to

Sense of Time	Extended Future	Days Hours	Hours Minutes	Minutes Seconds	Loss of Sense of Time
Primary Secondary Brain Areas	**NEOCORTEX** *Subcortex*	**SUBCORTEX** *Limbic*	**LIMBIC** *Midbrain*	**MIDBRAIN** *Brain stem*	**BRAIN STEM** *Autonomic*
Cognition	Abstract	Concrete	"Emotional"	Reactive	Reflexive
Mental State	**CALM**	**AROUSAL**	**ALARM**	**FEAR**	**TERROR**

Figure 1.4   State-dependent Cognition and the Response to Threat
One of the most important elements in understanding the child living in the vortex of violence is to recognize that all humans process, store, retrieve and respond to the world in a state-dependent fashion. When a child is in a persisting state of arousal due to persisting exposure to threat, the primary areas of the brain that are processing information are different from those in a child who can be calm.

pass on their genes. Indeed, it is likely that certain sensory cues are genetically coded to induce an alarm state; examples may include the pervasive nature of phobias to snakes or the stereotyped fashion in which infants exhibit distress at certain sudden loud auditory cues.

Because paired associations have been created in the regulatory, more primitive parts of the brain, a pattern of incoming sensory information may be interpreted as danger and acted upon in the brain stem, midbrain and thalamus milliseconds before it gets to the cortex to be interpreted as harmless. For a combat soldier from Vietnam, the sound of a firecracker will still elicit a fear response (e.g., increased heart rate, startle response), even though he knows it is a firecracker. This man's brain stem has interpreted and acted on the information before it has had a chance to get to the cortex to be interpreted in a more complex fashion. Brain-stem, midbrain and limbic associative capabilities are at the heart of trauma-related memories: emotional, motor and state memories.

At each level of increasing complexity, the local associations become more complex. The associations in the brain stem are simple and categorical. Associations in the amygdala are more complex and allow interpretation of emotional signals and cues, including facial expressions and the intentionality they convey (threat, affiliation). Associations in the cortex are the most complex and may involve a variety of abstract elements; associations can be made between previously unpaired cues and various levels of meaning, allowing abstract cognition (see Figure 1.4).

In PTSD, associations between specific complex cues (e.g., helicopters) may become linked to the limbic-mediated emotion (anxiety). Limbic activation may result from cortically mediated images (e.g., interpretation of a specific event as potentially threatening or imagining a specific traumatic event). Once these limbic areas are activated, there may or may not be activation of lower midbrain and brain-stem areas involved in the response to threat; the efferent wing of the alarm response may or may not be activated. The degree of activation of the rest of the threat-response neurobiology residing in the midbrain and brain stem depends, to some degree, upon the sensitivity of these systems. Indeed, it is likely that PTSD involves a sensitization of these systems to threat-related cues, internal or external (see below).

A sensitizing pattern resulting from a traumatic experience can dramatically change the sensitivity of the brain's alarm system (Kalivas et al. 1990). The result is a state of anxiety, even in the presence of what were originally nonthreatening cues. A sensitized stress-response apparatus is a likely etiology of trauma-related symptoms in children (Perry et al. 1995), where it has been demonstrated that exposure to chronic and repeated stressors alters a variety of brain-stem–related functions, including emotional and behavioral functioning (Perry 1994; Perry, Southwick and Giller 1990).

USE-DEPENDENT STORAGE OF EXPERIENCE: TYPES OF MEMORY

The brain changes in response to patterned neuronal activity (Perry 1988; Courchesne, Chisum and Townsend 1994; Perry et al. 1995). All parts of the brain are capable of changing in response to changes in neuronal activity; hence, all parts of the brain store information and have, in some sense, memory. Although the majority of research on memory has been in cognitive memory and, more recently, implicit and procedural memory, other brain areas, responsible for other functions, change in response to activation and, thereby, make memories. Simplistic categorization of these memories reflects major brain-mediated functions. Cognitive memories arise from use-dependent changes in neuronal patterns of activity present during cognition (e.g., learning names, phone numbers, language). Motor-vestibular memories arise from use-dependent activation of motor-vestibular parts of the brain (e.g., riding a bicycle, typing, dancing, playing the piano). Emotional, or affect, memories result from use-dependent changes in neuronal patterns of activity present during specific emotional experiences (e.g., grief, fear, mirth). Emotional memories may manifest as first impression or transference (LeDoux et al. 1990). State memories occur when a pattern of activation in state-regulating parts of the brain occurs with a sensitizing pattern or in a chronic, prolonged fashion (e.g., chronic domestic violence, traumatic stress). The specific nature of the memory, or storage, and the kind of information that is stored and recalled in each of these major areas (cognitive, emotional, motor, state) *differs*, depending upon the specific function of that given area or system (Selden et al. 1991; Shors et al. 1990).

As described above, there is an interactive and interconnected set of neuronal activities throughout various brain areas during a traumatic experience. Because the equilibrium activity of each major area of the brain is significantly altered during a traumatic event, each of these key areas is likely to store some new pattern of neuronal activation associated with the traumatic event. Since the brain stores information in a use-dependent fashion and the total-body response to a traumatic event activates so many key areas of the brain, trauma is more likely to result in strong emotional, motor and state memories in comparison with the typical experiences of everyday life. During familiar routines, the patterns of neuronal activity in the brain (especially in the regulatory systems) are familiar and similar to previously stored templates of activation. These systems, then, are in equilibrium during routine daily activities. Traumatic events disrupt these patterns of equilibrium. Patterns of neuronal activity present during the traumatic experience are unlike those present during routine daily activities and therefore will influence and alter functioning from the cortex (cognition) to the brain stem (core physiological state regulation).

Over time, a thought recalling the trauma may activate limbic, basal ganglia and brain stem areas, resulting in emotional, motor and arousal/state changes that are the functional residuals associated with the stored patterns of neuronal activation present in the original event (Greenwald, Draine and Abrams 1996). Conversely, a state—arousal—may result in activation of paired neuronal activity in the amygdala, resulting in an emotional change (LeDoux et al. 1988). This may or may not be sufficient to activate associated cognitive memories. Indeed in many cases, the individual is completely unaware of why he or she feels so fearful or depressed. The external or internal triggers may not be something the person is aware of. It is the nature of the human brain to store experience—all experience—and to generalize from

the specific to the general. As a rule children exposed to chronic abuse or neglect early in childhood will have little cognitive understanding of (insight
into) how the anxiety, impulsivity and social and emotional distress they
suffer are related to the brain's creation of memories during previous traumatic experience.

COGNITIVE AND AFFECTIVE (EMOTIONAL) MEMORY

The word *memory*, for most laypersons and mental-health professionals, has
come to signify some aspect of cognitive memory. In the recent past, the concept of emotional memory has received considerable attention, due in large
part to the excellent research on the function of the amygdala conducted by
such investigators as LeDoux et al. (1988, 1989, 1990) and Davis (1992). The
neurobiology and psychology of cognitive and affective memory have been
reviewed extensively elsewhere (Mesulam 1990; Davis 1992; LeDoux, Romanski and Xagoraris 1989; Schacter 1992; Squire 1992; Siegel 1996). The focus of the following discussion will be motor and state memory in relation
to these other forms of memory. (For more traditional discussions of motor
and state memory, see Knowlton, Maungels and Squire 1996; Greenwald,
Draine and Abrams 1996.)

MOTOR-VESTIBULAR AND STATE MEMORIES

In the same way that patterned neuronal activity (use) builds in cognitive
memories, so does certain motor activity such as playing piano or riding a
bicycle. The motor-vestibular movements of a roller coaster may elicit an internal state associated with the playful experiences of a small child being
tossed in the air by a parent. The fetal position clearly elicits a sense of soothing and calm. During the calmest, safest, warmest, least threatening time in
the history of the brain stem, the neuronal patterns of proprioception associated with the fetal position were associated with the neuronal patterns of
this calm, warm, safe, most soothing state. Therefore, as a motor memory,
when the child or adult rolls into the fetal position, the neuronal patterns
this evokes can evoke some elements of that original soothed state. Very few
people, feeling overwhelmed or sick, will lay on their backs in the spread-
eagle position.

Similarly, a major organizing sensory pattern of the developing brain stem
is the somatosensory pattern associated with maternal heart rate. During the

crucial final trimester, the neuronal apparatus of the brain stem is undergoing critical processes related to building the organizational capacity to regulate heart rate, blood pressure, body temperature and respiration; by birth, the primary environmental sensation is the repetitive, relentless and rhythmic sound and feel of mother's heart beating. The fetus's vibratory and auditory senses translate these maternal patterns into patterns of neuronal activation in the developing brain. And, as the brain is organizing in utero, these maternal patterns play a role as organizing templates for the brain. It is no surprise, then, that studies demonstrate that mothers, in all cultures, rock children at the same frequency (Hatfield and Rapson 1993). This frequency is between 70 and 80 beats per minute—the same as the resting mother's heart rate. This frequency of soothing may be related to the use of similar patterns of sound and movement in a host of healing or soothing rituals—again, practices observed through history and across cultures.

One of the most powerful examples of the connections between a motor memory and an emotional and state memory relates to oropharyngeal motor activity—eating. For individuals fortunate enough to have an attentive, nurturing caregiver, eating as an infant (the time when the patterns of oropharyngeal motor patterns related to eating are being built into the brain) becomes associated with eye contact, social intimacy, safety, calm, touch and cooing (Hatfield and Rapson 1993). This wonderful, soothing and interactive somatosensory bath that the nurturing caregiver provides literally organizes and grows the brain areas associated with attachment and emotional regulation (Perry et al. 1995; Perry 1997). Disruptions of this bath by neglect, depression, trauma or other chaotic, inconsistent experiences can result in abnormal development of the neurobiological systems and patterns of activity required for normal eating or relationship formation. The relationship between rumination and failure to thrive is a clear example of a disrupted maternal-infant somatosensory "dance." (For another example of a disturbed motor memory related to eating, see Case 3, below.)

USE-DEPENDENT LEARNING:
STATE-DEPENDENT STORAGE AND RECALL

As described above, the brain changes in a use-dependent fashion. All parts of the brain can modify their functioning in response to specific, repetitive patterns of activation. These use-dependent changes in the brain result in changes in cognition (this, of course, is the basis for cognitive learning),

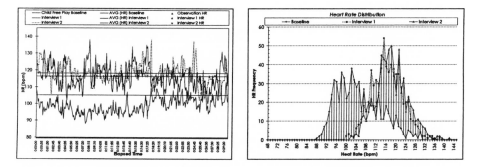

Figure 1.5   Physiological State Memory in a Child with PTSD

(*Left*) Continuous tracing of a free-play session (with the same adult therapist as during the structured interview: mean HR = 105) and two separate structured PTSD interviews (mean HR = 119) with a young male (age = 9). This boy met DSM-IV criterion for PTSD and exhibited prominent symptoms of physiological hyperreactivity (e.g., motor hyperactivity, anxiety, impulsivity, hypervigilance, sleep disturbance). (*Right*) HR distribution under the free-play and interview conditions. Note (1) the reproducibility of the increased baseline heart rate during interviews and (2) the separation of the free-play (baseline) distribution from the interviews.

emotional functioning (social learning), motor-vestibular functioning (e.g., the ability to write, type, ride a bike) and state-regulation capacity (e.g., resting heart rate). No part of the brain can change easily without being activated—you can't teach French to someone who is asleep or teach a child to ride a bike simply by giving verbal instructions.

Mismatches between modality of teaching and the receptive portions of a specific child's brain occur frequently. This is particularly true when considering the learning experiences of the traumatized child, who may be sitting in a classroom in a persistent state of arousal and anxiety, or dissociated. In either case, the child is essentially unavailable to process efficiently the complex cognitive information being conveyed by the teacher. This principle, of course, extends to other kinds of learning, social and emotional. The traumatized child frequently has significant impairment in social and emotional functioning. Social and emotional capabilities are learned; they develop in response to experiences, experiences these children often lack—or fail at. Indeed, hypervigilant children frequently develop remarkable nonverbal skills in proportion to their verbal skills ("street smarts"). It is common for them to overread (misinterpret) nonverbal cues: Eye contact means threat, a friendly touch is interpreted as an antecedent to seduction and rape—accurate in the world they came from, but now, one hopes, out of context. During development, these children spent so much time in a low-level state of fear (mediated by brain-stem and midbrain areas) that they were focusing consistently on nonverbal cues. In our clinic population, children raised in chronically traumatic environments demonstrate a prominent verbal-performance split on IQ testing (n = 108; WISC [Average Weighted Scores] Verbal = 8.2; WISC Performance = 10.4; Perry, in press).

This is consistent with the clinical observations of teachers that these children are bright, but can't learn easily. Often these children are labeled as learning disabled. These difficulties with cognitive organization contribute to a more primitive, less mature style of problem solving, with aggression often being employed as a tool.

This principle is critically important in understanding why a traumatized child—in a persistent state of arousal—can sit in a classroom and not learn. Even at rest, different areas of this child's brain are activated; different parts of the brain are controlling his or her functioning. The capacity to internalize new verbal cognitive information depends upon having portions of the frontal and related cortical areas activated, which, in turn, requires a state of attentive calm (Castro-Alamancos and Comori 1996), a state the traumatized child rarely achieves (Perry et al. 1995).

Children in a state of fear retrieve information from the world differently than children who feel calm (see Figures 1.3 and 1.4; Eich 1995; Kim and Fanslow 1992; McNally et al. 1990). We all are familiar with test anxiety. Imagine what life would be like if all experiences evoked the persisting emotion of anxiety. If a child in the specific moment is very fearful, whatever information is stored in cortical areas is inaccessible. In this regard, cognitively stored information does little good in the life-threatening moment. Simple didactic conflict-resolution models are doomed to fail unless they involve elements of role playing. Imagine how much you would trust an army that went through combat training by sitting in a classroom or the ER physician about to run her first code after only reading about it in a book. In the midst of most threatening experiences, situations where violence often takes place, the problem-solving information in the cortex is not easily accessed. It is of interest to note that information learned in song, rhyme or rap is more easily recalled when in a state of high arousal, due, of course, to the fact that this information is stored in a different fashion than traditional verbal cognitive information.

TRAUMATIC MEMORIES: CASE EXAMPLES

CASE 1: STATE AND AFFECT MEMORIES ELICITED IN A NONCONSCIOUS STATE

D. is a nine-year-old boy who was a victim of chronic and pervasive physical threat and abuse from his biological father. Between the ages of two and six he was physically and sexually abused by his father. At age six he was removed from the family. His mother acknowledged pervasive abuse.

At age eight, he was seriously injured in a fall. He suffered from serious brain injury that left him in a coma for eight months. He continues to be difficult to arouse and is nonverbal; no form of meaningful communication is noted. In the presence of his biological father, he began to scream and moan and his heart rate increased dramatically. Audiotapes of his biological father elicit a similar response.

Clearly, the sensory information associated with the father (sounds, smells) reaching this child's brain was capable of eliciting a state memory. This child's brain did not have the capacity to have conscious perception of the presence of his father. The auditory and olfactory sensory neuronal patterns that entered this boy's brain were associated, even at the level of his brain stem and midbrain, with past states of fear. Therefore, with exposure to this unique pattern, the boy's brain sensed, processed and acted on the information despite the fact that higher areas of his brain were damaged and incapable of full function. Exposure to his father elicited no cognitive, narrative memory; his agitation and increased heart rate were manifestations of affective and state memories that were the products of many years of traumatic terror associated with his father and all of his father's attributes.

CASE 2: STATE AND AFFECT MEMORY WITH NO ASSOCIATED COGNITIVE MEMORY

F. is a fifteen-year-old male. From birth to age eight, he was continually exposed to severe physical abuse from his biological father. He witnessed many episodes of his mother being severely beaten by this father. As he grew older, he attempted to intervene and was seriously injured on several occasions.

At age eight, his mother left his father. From that time on, he was noted to be quiet and withdrawn; in school he "tuned out" and was noted to be daydreaming. At age ten, he began having syncopal episodes of unknown origin. He received multiple evaluations by neurologists and cardiologists, who ruled out psychogenic causes of his fainting. During initial evaluation, the mother related the long history of domestic violence, abuse and a series of medical workups for a host of nonspecific symptoms including headaches, fainting, seizures, chest pains and chronic emotional and behavioral problems.

The boy's resting heart rate was 82. When asked about his biological father, his heart rate fell to 62 and he became very withdrawn. On a walk in the hall, when asked about his abuse, his heart rate fell below 60 and he fainted. He was placed on Trexan, an opioid receptor antagonist, with a marked decrease in his syncope. He has persisting problems.

This child exhibited a clear sensitization of the neurobiological systems involved in the dissociative response to threat. Sensitization of the brainstem catecholamine systems are involved in the hyperarousal, hypervigilance, startle response and sympathetic nervous system hyperreactivity in PTSD (Perry, Southwick and Giller 1990). Similar sensitization of the opioid systems involved in dissociation is likely to account for the symptoms of cue-specific bradycardia, syncope, daydreaming and a host of other dissociation-related signs and symptoms (Perry et al., submitted).

CASE 3: STATE AND AFFECT MEMORIES
EVOKED BY MOTOR MEMORIES

I first saw T. in the basement cafeteria-style lunchroom at the Residential Treatment Facility (excerpted from Perry, in press a). He—small, wiry, herky-jerky, runny nose, dirty shirt sleeves, always out of his chair, run-on speech—sat with six other young boys at a round table covered with an institutional plastic, red-checkerboard tablecloth. It was lunchtime and all of the children were eating hot dogs, beans and potato chips. All except T.

I was a new consultant to this center. Sixty children, the majority "in the system" after being removed from their abusive families and failing in an escalating series of least-restrictive placements—foster family to another foster family to a psychiatric hospital to a therapeutic foster home, back to the hospital to a residential treatment center for six months to a different foster family to this residential treatment facility. Failed placements, failing system.

T. stood out because he was loudly demanding that someone "cut my hot dog, cut my hot dog, cut my hot dog." It was a chant, a pressured, almost psychotic chant. A staff member came up to him and chided him for being a "baby" about not eating the hot dog without it being cut. The staff member, with some good intentions, felt that this was the time to take a stand and make T. "grow up."

"T., it's time you act your age. See, all the other kids are eating without my cutting this up. I won't cut it up." T. escalated, shouting louder, frantic. The staff member stood his ground. T. rose from his chair. The staff member commanded him to stay at the table. The confrontation ended with T. sobbing, hysterical, out of control, being physically restrained by two staff. He was led off to a quiet place to regroup, reorganize and, in some sense, to redevelop, emerging from his primitive, terrified disorganized state through various levels of psychological, cognitive and emotional organization back to his most mature level of functioning.

"You can't indulge this kind of demanding behavior," the staff member said to me as they carried T. from the cafeteria. The other children seemed familiar with these confrontations and with the resulting physical restraint. They kept eating. One of the children at his table looked at me and said, "This always happens when we have hot dogs."

Over the years I worked there, I came to see that T. would cut his bananas and take popsicles off of the stick and eat them with a spoon. He had a number of other unusual or bizarre eating habits. He had a host of swallowing difficulties. He needed to eat soft food, rarely eating foods that were solid. He chewed forever and frequently gagged. Although T. could tell anyone what these habits were, he had no idea why he had to do things that way.

"I just have to," he said.

"And if you don't?" I asked.

"I just get angry."

"Angry?"

"Well, I guess. Maybe scared. Mixed up. . . . I don't know."

T. was an eight-year-old boy who had been forced to fellate his father from birth. And later, other men, many other men. At age six he was finally taken from this life of pervasive, socialized abuse.

Normal oropharyngeal patterns of stimulation during development (primarily from eating) are associated with the development of normal eating and swallowing capabilities. Furthermore, these patterns of oropharyngeal stimulation take place in association with a caregiver's soothing touch, gaze, smell and warmth and the satiety of being fed. This should be one of the most soothing, comforting, positive sets of experiences an individual will ever have—and it follows us through life. Eating involves trainable neuromuscular events—motor memories, if you will—and these motor memories are linked to positive emotional, olfactory, gustatory and cognitive memories.

But for T., the development of oropharyngeal stimulation was associated with other things: fear, pain, gagging, suffocating in the flesh of a pedophile. No satiety, no calm, no comfort. Rather than the soothing warmth of the maternal breast, his brain internalized the confused, inconsistent, painful states associated with his abuse. Solid food in his mouth or his throat evoked the state memories ingrained during the critical formative stages of his first six years. Eating, for T., evokes fear and confusion. He has to eat to survive and there is some positive effect of eating, but often enough the evocative nature of the meal can erase these positive effects.

With each meal, some small part of T. relives the abuse of his early childhood, some set of deeply burned-in state memories are accessed. These rarely, if ever, come to his awareness as a cognitive memory. He will likely never be able to have the insight to make the association between his eating habits and his early abuse.

Each meal scratches at the slowly healing scars of his childhood.

He remains small for his age.

Case 4: Affect, Motor and State Memory Evoked by Cognitive Narrative Memory

C., a five-year-old girl, witnessed her father shoot and kill her mother and then himself. She started attending our clinic within days after the event, coming on a regular basis. Five weeks later, during a one-hour free-play therapy session, a semistructured PTSD interview was conducted (see Figure 1.6). When asked about the worst thing that ever happened to her, there was a marked alteration in her facial expression, she stopped playing, moved her face and head away from the interviewer and stared into space. After a long moment, she stated, "I wanted to stay up late last weekend and have pizza, but I had to go to bed." The rest of the interview was characterized by single-word responses, which minimized her distress over the traumatic nature of her parent's death.

This child exhibited a classic dissociative response when evocative cognitive cues of the murder/suicide were brought up. This dissociative state was protective and was evoked—a state memory—by merely thinking about the events. Her mood, motor movements and state of physiological regulation all were altered by this narrative memory. Narrative recall memory was

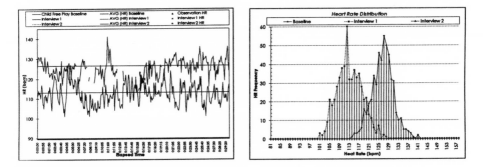

**Figure 1.6   Physiological State Memory in a Child
with Primary Dissociative Symptoms**

(*Left*) Continuous tracing of a similar free-play session as described above. This tracing is of a young girl (age = 8) who met criterion for PTSD. She exhibited primarily
dissociative and avoidant symptoms. During the structured interview, she exhibited
profound symptoms of dissociation, gave invalid and inaccurate responses to the
questions and had a marked decrease in her HR (mean = 112 compared to the free-
play mean of 128). (*Right*) HR distribution demonstrating almost complete separation of the two conditions, both with the same therapist/interviewer during the
same session.

strongly linked to affect, motor and state memories in this child, a common
finding in individuals following trauma (Burke, Heuer and Reisberg 1992).

CASE 5: COGNITIVE AND AFFECT MEMORIES
EVOKED BY STATE MEMORIES

T. is an eighteen-year-old female. She was brutally raped at age seventeen. She
had no previous history of psychiatric symptoms or treatment. She was seen
within a month after her rape for symptoms related to an acute trauma response (e.g., anxiety, sleep problems, guilt, dysphoria). A prominent memory
of the event was, "I felt my heart was going to burst it was beating so hard. I
felt it pounding against my chest." Prior to the event, she had exercised on a
regular basis, deriving significant pleasure from the activities. Since the time of
the rape, she had been unable to exercise. At multiple points during the treatment, she was free of anxiety, felt energetic and returned to exercising. She
would immediately find herself having intrusive ideations of the rape, dysphoria and anxiety. Ultimately the connection between her increased heart rate
and the affective and cognitive memories of the rape was identified. Once the

recognition was made that increased heart rate would trigger a cascade of emotions and recollections, she was able to guide herself through a form of progressive desensitization. Over time she was able to disconnect increased heart rate from the distressing affect and the cognitive recollections of the rape.

This example of a state memory eliciting intense affect and cognitive memory illustrates powerful associations that can exist between various neuronal systems and functions that are coactivated during a trauma. In many cases, the state-elicited distress is not associated with a clear cognitive recollection, nor is the manifestation of the symptom proximal in time to the trauma. In these situations, it is often very difficult to make the connections that allow for effective therapeutic intervention. Indeed, it is likely that many states of distress are activated by accessing state or affect memories without any clear cognitive or narrative associations to a specific trauma or experience. This is very common in young children who are preverbal or cognitively immature. Often their behaviors or symptoms are judged to be disconnected from past experiences, and traumatized children may get labeled as having attention-deficit hyperactivity disorder or conduct disorder based merely upon the current presentation of symptoms. These diagnostic labels, although often accurate, do not give the clinician any clues to etiology, prognosis or a treatment approach that would be suggested by knowing the relationships between past trauma and current functioning.

CASE 6: STATE MEMORY IN A PREVERBAL CHILD

K. is a three-year-old boy referred to our clinic following the murder of his eighteen-month-old sister by a caregiver. Over a series of nonintrusive clinical contacts, K. developed a sense of familiarity and comfort at our clinic. Approximately two months after the event, a semistructured interview was conducted. During the nonintrusive part of the interview, K. was spontaneous, interactive, smiling and age-appropriate in his play. When the direct questioning began, his heart rate increased, but his behaviors remained constant. Within five seconds of being asked about his sister, his heart rate dramatically increased and his play stopped. He broke eye contact, physically slowed and became essentially nonresponsive. This dissociative response was accompanied by a decrease in his heart rate to the previous baseline level of the free-play portion of the interview. Similar alterations in heart rate and induction of a protective dissociative response could be elicited by exposure to cues associated with the murder.

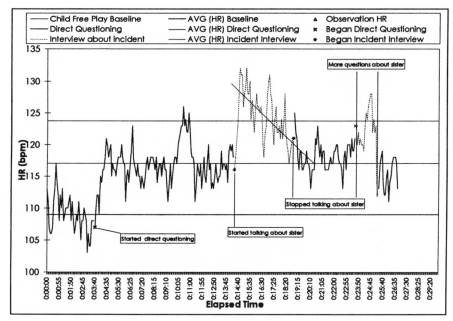

Figure 1.7   State Memory of a Witnessed Murder in a Three-Year-Old Child
A 3-year-old child witnessed the murder of his 13-month-old sister. During a therapeutic session, a free-play baseline heart rate was established. When direct, but nonthreatening, questioning began, his heart rate increased. Within 5 seconds of being
asked about his sister, a dramatic increase in heart rate was seen with an immediate
behavioral inhibition and dissociative response. His heart rate fell and nonintrusive
questioning resumed. When the issue was briefly mentioned again, an initial increase in heart rate, change in behavior, and dissociation-related decrease in heart
rate was observed (see test).

In this situation, this child, upon direct questioning, gave no verbal or narrative information about the event. This lack of a narrative memory, however,
did not mean that the child had not stored the experience. Clearly, he demonstrated clear and unambiguous evidence of emotional and state memories
when verbal or nonverbal cues were used to evoke the event (Figure 1.7).

TRAUMATIC MEMORY AND THE LAW:
VULNERABLE CHILDREN

Specific problems are posed by the child narrative when it is part of a forensic
proceeding. The focal conflict is that the law is a primarily verbal domain,

whereas communication in children, particularly about traumatic events, is primarily nonverbal. In the law words are essentially the only important element of a narrative; in traumatized children, the narrative words are mere shadows of what is being communicated as they recall the event. A child's recall of a traumatic event involves not just the shards of the event as recalled using cognitive memory, but also the intense fear of the emotional memory, the motor agitation of the motor memories and the physiological arousal (or dissociative response) of the state memory. Yet the syntax, semantics and grammar of these noncognitive narrations do not yet have the standing in court that the syntax, semantics and grammar of verbal language do.

Learning the language of trauma and translating its verbal and nonverbal elements will require many more years of investigation. Nonetheless, in this early stage of the investigation, it is the obligation of those of us working with maltreated children to bring to the attention of our peers and the rest of society four essential points: (1) this language does exist; (2) traumatic events, like other experiences, change the brain; (3) the brain stores elements of traumatic events as cognitive, motor, emotional and state memory, altering the functional capacity of the traumatized individual; and (4) by robbing millions of children each year of their individual potential, childhood trauma and neglect diminish the potential of families, communities and society.

TRAUMA, MEMORY AND HISTORY: TRANSGENERATIONAL MEMORY OF CULTURE AND SOCIETY

Traumatic events impact millions of children and adults worldwide each year. War, floods, earthquakes, rape, physical abuse, neglect—all create memories for individuals, families, communities and society. The memory of trauma is carried not only throughout the lives of individuals by their neurobiology, but also in the lives of families by family myths, childrearing practices and belief systems. Major traumatic events in the history of a people or culture are memorialized as well and carried forward across generations in literature, laws and social structures.

It is the unique property of living systems to carry forward elements of past experience; indeed, for all living systems the present is contingent upon and a reflection of that past experience. In a very true sense, a body collective—a group—is a living, dynamic system. And, in the same way that individuals carry their own history forward using the neurobiological mechanisms related to memory, each living group carries its memories forward in time. Yet living groups—families, clans, societies—carry this information forward using different mechanisms of recording and storage.

The methods for recording and storing the experiences of the group have evolved over the history of humankind. In our distant past, humans living in groups passed experience from generation to generation using oral tradition and sociocultural practices—language, arts, belief systems, rules, law—all were reflections of the past. And with each generation, past memory was modified, altered and amended by present experience. With the development of written language, a more efficient mechanism for passing information across generations became available. An increased rate of sociocultural advancement occurred, made possible by more efficient "remembering" of the lessons (good and bad) from the past. The "brain" of humankind—the libraries of the world—kept civilization alive through its darkest moments. Even if generation after generation during a given period in history did not take advantage of this memory, the information was not lost to humankind.

Later in history, again, with the introduction of the printing press, the past was more efficiently stored and passed on. Books became available to everyone. More people became literate. Information of all sorts—in the arts, sciences, social studies—was stored in books. Again, a tremendous advancement in human sociocultural evolution can be traced to this process, to literacy and widespread education. Information from the past, primarily cognitive information, enriched the present. The rate of creativity accelerated; invention and innovation—new ideas, machines, products, processes—were facilitated by the more efficient sociocultural memory allowed by books and literacy. Now, in the span of a lifetime, the accumulated and distilled experience of thousands of generations could be absorbed and acted upon to make sociocultural advancement.

Today we are in the early generations of a new era of recording, storing and transmitting information. Electronic media, photographs, films, tapes, videos—all immortalize the experiences of humankind. These media allow the memory of an individual, family, community or society to be passed from generation to generation in a unique and different way.

There is great hope for humankind in these advances. In the past, the inefficient methods of recording, storing and passing on the horrors of war, rape, neglect, abuse, starvation, misogyny and slavery allowed these lessons of living to be edited, modified, distorted and, with tragic consequences, forgotten. Only certain elements of the experience of war were passed across generations—the heroism of an individual, the success of the nation—and the emotional memory of war—the hate, rage, death and loss—forgotten.

Creative artists have always been the recorders and preservers of their cultures' emotional memory. In ways that standard recording of simple facts and figures cannot convey, a painting, poem, novel or film can capture the emotional memory of an experience. But in a society where artistic literacy and access to it are low, the emotional lessons of the past are easily lost. And when the last veteran of that distant war died, an element of the emotional memory of that horror died as well. In societies unable to carry the emotional memory of war to the next generation, history can much more easily repeat itself—or rather *we* can much more easily repeat history. But with documentary and creative film and video, which can convey both the fact and the emotion, perhaps it will be harder for us to forget the past—and, therefore, harder to repeat it.

How can we heal the scars of trauma to individuals and groups that haunt us today ? Can we ever make racism, misogyny and maltreatment of children distant memories? There are solutions. These conditions are not the inevitable legacy of our past. When an individual becomes self-aware, there is the potential for insight. With insight comes the potential for altered behavior. With altered behavior comes the potential to diminish the transgenerational passage of dysfunctional or destructive ideas and practices.

The challenge for our generation is to understand the dynamics and realities of our human living groups in a way that can result in group insight, which, inevitably, will lead to the understanding that we must change our institutionalized ignorance and maltreatment of children.

ACKNOWLEDGMENTS

This work was supported, in part, by grants from CIVITAS Initiative, the Hogg Foundation, the Children's Crisis Care Center of Harris County, Maconda O'Connor and an anonymous benefactor.

REFERENCES

Aston-Jones, G., Ennis, M., Pieribone, J., Nickel, W. T., and Shipley, M. T. (1986). The brain nucleus locus coeruleus: Restricted afferent control over a broad efferent network. *Science* 234: 734–737.

Bennett, E. L., Diamond, M. L., Krech, D., and Rosenzweig, M. R. (1964). Chemical and anatomical plasticity of the brain. *Science* 146: 610–619.

Briere, J., and Conte, J. (1993). Self-reported amnesia for abuse in adults molested as children. *Journal of Traumatic Stress* 6: 21–31.

Brown, J. W. (1994). Morphogenesis and mental process. *Development and Psychopathology* 6: 551–563.

Burke, A., Heuer, F., and Reisberg, D. (1992). Remembering emotional events. *Memory and Cognition* 20: 277–290.

Cannon, W. B. (1914). The emergency function of the adrenal medulla in pain and the major emotions. *American Journal of Physiology* 33: 356–372.

_____. (1929). *Bodily changes in pain, hunger, fear and rage.* New York: Appleton.

Castro-Alamancos, M. A., and Connors, B. W. (1996). Short-term plasticity of a thalamocortical pathway dynamically modulated by behavioral state. *Science* 272: 274–276.

Ceci, S. J., and Bruck, M. (1993). Suggestibility of the child witness: A historical review and synthesis. *Psychological Bulletin* 113: 403–439.

Clugnet, M. C., and LeDoux, J. E. (1990). Synaptic plasticity in fear conditioning circuits: Induction of LTP in the lateral nucleus of the amygdala by stimulation of the medial geniculate body. *Journal of Neuroscience* 10: 2818–2824.

Courchesne, E., Chisum, H., and Townsend, J. (1994). Neural activity-dependent brain changes in development: Implications for psychopathology. *Development and Psychopathology* 6 (4): 697–722.

Davis, M. (1992). The role of the amygdala in fear and anxiety. *Annual Review of Neuroscience* 15: 353–375.

Eich, E. (1995). Searching for mood-dependent memory. *Psychological Science* 6: 67–75.

Frankel, M. (1993). Adult reconstruction of childhood events in the multiple personality literature. *American Journal of Psychiatry* 150: 954–958.

Giller, E. L., Perry, B. D., Southwick, S., and Mason, J. W. (1990). Psychoneuroendocrinology of posttraumatic stress disorder. In M. E. Wolf and A. D. Mosnaim, eds., *Posttraumatic stress disorder: Etiology, phenomenology and treatment* (pp. 158–170). Washington, D.C.: American Psychiatric Press.

Goldstein, D. S. (1995). *Stress, catecholamines and cardiovascular disease.* New York: Oxford University Press.

Gorman, J. M., Liebowitz, M. R., Fyer, A. J., and Stein, J. (1989). A neuroanatomical hypothesis for panic disorder. *American Journal of Psychiatry* 146: 148–162.

Greenwald, A. G., Draine, S. C., and Abrams, R. L. (1996). Three cognitive markers of unconscious semantic activation. *Science* 273: 1699–1702.

Gunnar, M. R. (1986). Human developmental psychoneuroendocrinology: A review of research on neuroendocrine responses to challenge and threat in infancy and childhood. In M. E. Lamb, L. A. Brown and B. Rogoff, eds., *Advances in developmental psychology* (pp. 51–103). Hillsdale, N.J.: Erlbaum.

Hatfield, E., and Rapson, R. (1993). Love and attachment processes. In M. Lewis and J. M. Haviland, eds., *Handbook of Emotions* (pp. 595–605). New York: Guilford.

Kalivas, P. W., Duffy, P., Abhold, R. et al. (1990). Sensitization of mesolimbic dopamine neurons by neuropeptides and stress. In P. W. Kalivas and C. D. Carnes, eds., *Sensitization of the nervous system* (pp. 119–124). Caldwell, N.J.: Telford.

Kandel, E. R. (1989). Genes, nerve cells and remembrance of things past. *Journal of Neuropsychiatry and Clinical Neurosciences* 1: 103–125.

Kandel, E. R., and Schwartz, J. H. (1982). Molecular biology of an elementary form of learning: Modulation of transmitter release by cyclic AMP. *Science* 218: 433–443.

Kim, J., and Fanslow, M. (1992). Modality-specific retrograde amnesia of fear. *Science* 256: 675–677.

Knowlton, B. J., Mangels, J. A., and Squire, L. R. (1996). A neostriatal habit learning system in humans. *Science* 273: 1399–1401.

Lauder, J. M. (1988). Neurotransmitters as morphogens. *Progress in Brain Research* 73: 365–388.

LeDoux, J. E., Cicchetti, P., Xagoraris, A., and Romanski, L. R. (1990). The lateral amygdaloid nucleus: Sensory interface of the amygdala in fear conditioning. *Journal of Neuroscience* 10: 1062–1069.

LeDoux, J. E., Iwata, P., Cicchetti, D., and Reis, D. J. (1988). Different projections of the central amygdaloid nucleus mediate autonomic and behavioral correlates of conditioned fear. *Journal of Neuroscience* 8: 2517–2529.

LeDoux, J. E., Romanski, L., and Xagoraris, A. (1989). Indelibility of subcortical emotional memories. *Journal of Cognitive Neuroscience* 1: 238–243.

Loewy, A., and Spyer, K. 1990. *Central regulation of autonomic functions.* New York: Oxford University Press.

Madison, D. V., Malenka, R. C., and Nicoll, R. A. (1991). Mechanisms underlying long-term potentiation of synaptic transmission. *Annual Review of Neuroscience* 14: 379–397.

Maunsell, J. H. R. (1995). The brain's visual world: Representation of visual targets in cerebral cortex. *Science* 270:764–769.

McNally, R. J., Kaspi, S. P., Riemann, B. C., and Zeitlin, S. B. (1990). Selective processing of threat cues in posttraumatic stress disorder. *Journal of Abnormal Psychology* 99: 398–402.

Mesulam, M. (1990). Large-scale neurocognitive networks and distributed processing for attention, language and memory. *Annals of Neurology* 28: 597–613.

Perry, B. D. (1988). Placental and blood element neurotransmitter receptor regulation in humans: Potential models for studying neurochemical mechanisms underlying behavioral teratology. *Progress in Brain Research* 73: 189–206.

_____. (1993). Neurodevelopment and the neurophysiology of trauma: (I) Conceptual considerations for clinical work with maltreated children. *The APSAC Advisor* 6: 1–12.

_____. (1994). Neurobiological sequelae of childhood trauma: Posttraumatic stress disorders in children. In M. Murberg, ed., *Catecholamines in posttraumatic stress disorder: Emerging concepts* (pp. 253–276). Washington, D.C.: American Psychiatric Press.

_____. (1997). Incubated in terror: Neurodevelopmental factors in the "cycle of violence." In J. Osofsky, ed., *Children, youth and violence: The search for solutions* (pp. 124–148). New York: Guilford.

———. (1998). Anxiety disorders: Neurodevelopmental aspects of childhood responses to threat. In C. E. Coffey and R. A. Brumback, eds., *Textbook of pediatric neuropsychiatry* (pp. 580–594). Washington, D.C.: American Psychiatric Press.

———. (in press). *Maltreated children: Experience, brain development and the next generation.* New York and London: Norton.

Perry, B., Arvinte, A. Marcellus, J., and Pollard, R. (submitted). Syncope, bradycardia, cataplexy and paralysis: Sensitization of an opioid-mediated dissociative response following childhood trauma.

Perry, B. D., Pollard, R. A., Baker, W. L., Sturges, C., Vigilante, D., and Blakely, T. L. (1995). Continuous heart rate monitoring in maltreated children [Abstract]. *Annual Meeting of the American Academy of Child and Adolescent Psychiatry, New Research.*

Perry, B. D., Pollard, R., Blakely, T. W., Baker, W., and Vigilante, D. (1995). Childhood trauma, the neurobiology of adaptation and "use-dependent" development of the brain: How "states" become "traits." *Infant Mental Health Journal* 16 (4):271–291.

Perry, B., Southwick, S., and Giller, E. (1990). Adrenergic receptor regulation in posttraumatic stress disorders. In E. Giller, ed., *Advances in psychiatry: Biological assessment and treatment of posttraumatic stress disorder* (pp. 87–115). Washington, D.C.: American Psychiatric Press.

Phillips, R. G., and LeDoux, J. E. (1992). Differential contribution of amygdala and hippocampus to cued and contextual fear conditioning. *Behavioral Neuroscience* 106: 274–285.

Pynoos, R., and Nader, K. (1989). Children's memory and proximity to violence. *Journal of the American Academy of Child and Adolescent Psychiatry* 28: 236–241.

Schacter, D. L. (1992). Understanding implicit memory: A cognitive neuroscience approach. *American Psychologist* 47: 559–569.

Schwarz, E., and Kowalski, J. (1991). Malignant memories: Posttraumatic stress disorder in children and adults following a school shooting. *Journal of the American Academy of Child and Adolescent Psychiatry* 30: 937–944.

Schwarz, E., Kowalski, J., and McNally, R. (1993). Malignant memories: Posttraumatic changes in memory in adults after a school shooting. *Journal of Traumatic Stress* 6:95–103.

Schwarz, E. D., and Perry, B. D. (1994). The posttraumatic response in children and adolescents. *Psychiatric Clinics of North America* 17 (2): 311–326.

Selden, N. R. W., Everitt, B. J., Jarrard, L. E., and Robbins, T. W. (1991). Complementary roles for the amygdala and hippocampus in aversive conditioning to explicit and contextual cues. *Neuroscience* 42: 335–350.

Shors, T. J., Foy, M. R., Levine, S., and Thompson, R. F. (1990). Unpredictable and uncontrollable stress impairs neuronal plasticity in the rat hippocampus. *Brain Research Bulletin* 24: 663–667.

Siegel, D. J. (1996). Cognition, memory and dissociation. *Child and Adolescent Psychiatric Clinics of North America* 5: 509–536.

Singer, W. (1995). Development and plasticity of cortical processing architectures. *Science* 270: 758–764.

Squire, L. (1992). Declarative and non-declarative memory: Multiple brain systems supporting learning and memory. *Journal of Cognitive Neuroscience* 4: 232–243.

Terr, L. (1983). Chowchilla revisited: The effects of psychic trauma four years after a school-bus kidnapping. *American Journal of Psychiatry* 140: 1543–1550.

_____. (1991). Childhood traumas: An outline and overview. *American Journal of Psychiatry* 148: 10–20.

Thoenen, H. (1995). Neurotrophins and neuronal plasticity. *Science* 270: 593–598.

CHAPTER 2

Forgetting and Reexperiencing Trauma

From Anesthesia to Pain

Ellert R. S. Nijenhuis and Onno van der Hart

Traumatized individuals alternate, in varying degrees of mutual exclusiveness, between states of consciousness in which they experience their trauma over and over again, as if it were happening here and now, and episodes in which they are relatively unaware of trauma, on the surface undisturbed. This basic pattern of posttraumatic stress has been noted for the past hundred years by students of psychotraumatology (Brett and Ostroff 1985; Freud 1919; Horowitz 1986; Janet 1889, 1898, 1904; Kardiner 1946; Krystal 1969; Lindemann 1944; Myers 1940; Spiegel, Hunt and Dondershine 1988; van der Kolk and Ducey 1989).

In a little-known but important work, Myers (1940, 67) aptly referred to these alternating states as the "emotional personality" and the "apparently normal personality," metaphorical expressions we will use throughout this chapter. Studying severely traumatized combat soldiers with posttraumatic stress disorder (PTSD), Myers observed that the "emotional personality" suffers vivid, painful memories and images associated with overwhelming and threatening experience. As van der Kolk, van der Hart and Marmar put it: "'Memories' of the trauma are initially reexperienced as fragments of the sensory components of the event—as visual images; olfactory, auditory, or kinesthetic sensations; or intense waves of feelings that patients usually

39

claim to be representations of elements of the original traumatic event"(1996, 312). These reexperiences may intrude on the apparently normal personality, which tries to get away from the internally reproduced traumatic stress in all sorts of ways. It may become disconnected from the body, disconnected from positive and negative emotions as well as from memories, interests and social relationships, leaving the person in a state of somatic and psychological numbing.

This alternating pattern of intrusion and detachment can be traced back to psychic mechanisms during trauma that allowed the creation of one or more separate states or streams of consciousness. The human mind thus finds ways of registering the information presented and of responding to it, while at the same time keeping the event as well as traumatic reactions fully or partially out of normal consciousness. This may be adaptive under extremely threatening conditions, but this lack of integration of traumatic memories is also at the root of the complex biobehavioral changes that characterize PTSD and dissociative disorders, which can be understood as complex cases of PTSD (Spiegel 1984).

In this chapter we attempt to show that this duality in the response to traumatic experiences comprises a particular form of information processing, characterized subjectively by restriction of the field of consciousness and dissociation, which can partly be understood in terms of alternate-consciousness paradigms described by Pierre Janet nearly a century ago (Janet 1907; Crabtree 1992, 1993). As we will discuss, Janet's ideas are compatible with more recent behavioral descriptions of conditioned learning during extreme threat; together, these theories comprise an even more powerful explanatory paradigm for understanding the development of posttraumatic symptoms.

Although the distinction between intrusive reexperiencing of trauma and avoidance/numbing is basic, it does not capture the full range of complexity that may characterize posttraumatic responses. First, the alternations of state not only involve consciousness, but encompass complex psychological, behavioral, physiological and neurobiological responses. Second, severe threat may evoke more than two separate states. Patients with dissociative disorders, especially those with dissociative identity disorder (DID; American Psychiatric Association [APA] 1994) or dissociative disorder not otherwise specified (DDNOS; APA 1994; Ross, Anderson et al. 1992), show repetitive, far-reaching and sudden alterations of behavior, affect, sensation, perception and knowledge. According to Putnam, these patients have developed a range of "highly discrete states of consciousness organized around a prevailing affect, sense of self (including body image), with a limited repertoire of behaviors and a set of state-dependent memories" (1988, 103). We hypothesize that some of these dissociative states may relate to various defensive and recuperative reaction patterns similar to the automatic defensive reactions well described in animals under attack. Predatory attack involves various stages, each of which demands its own defensive reactions, and the defensive systems of prey include many different subsystems adapted to meet this variable threat.

Uncontrollable and repetitive intrusion of traumatic memories and related traumatic states—including dissociative (identity) states, fragments and other ego states—and the expenditure of continuous effort to avoid internal and external reminders of trauma, with consequent detachment from the body, emotions, self and social world, lead to exhaustion and, eventually, to chronic states of misery (Janet 1889, 1909). On the other hand, successful processing of traumatic memories implies integration of these states.

TRAUMATIC PERSONALITIES, RETRACTION
OF THE FIELD OF CONSCIOUSNESS AND DISSOCIATION

THE "EMOTIONAL PERSONALITY":
TRAUMATIC MEMORIES AS REENACTMENTS

The "emotional personality" (Myers 1940) stores traumatic experiences and reactions. Its traumatic memories are very different from processed narratives of trauma (Janet 1889, 1904, 1919/1925, 1928; van der Hart, Nijenhuis and van der Kolk, submitted; van der Kolk and van der Hart 1991). Normally processed memories strike the listener as narratives, stories told and retold that change over time and are adapted to an audience. Such memories are verbal, time-condensed, social and reconstructive in nature, while traumatic memories are often experienced as if the once overwhelming event were happening here and now. These hallucinatory, solitary and involuntary experiences consist of visual images, sensations and motor acts that engross the entire perceptual field. They are characterized by a sense of timelessness and immutability (Modell 1990; Spiegel, Frischholz, and Spira 1993) and have no social function (Janet 1928). Upon the reactivation of traumatic memories, access to other memories is obstructed or even inhibited.

When in the latent or dormant state, traumatic memories are usually not a hindrance (van der Hart, Steele et al. 1993). When reactivated, they, like harmful "parasites of the mind," overgrow consciousness (Charcot 1887; Janet 1894). Their reactivation may consume a considerable amount of time, partly reproducing the time line of the traumatic event (van der Hart, Nijenhuis and van der Kolk, submitted). The reexperiencing usually follows a fixed course of events and responses and cannot be interrupted, or can be interrupted only with excessive effort.

Research and clinical observation suggest that traumatic memories strongly involve the body. For example, van der Kolk and Fisler (1995) found that traumatic memories of subjects with PTSD were retrieved, at least initially, in the form of dissociated mental imprints of sensory and affective elements of the traumatic experience with little or no linguistic component. Sexually abused children also "remembered" their traumas in the form of sensory perceptions and behavioral responses (Burgess, Hartman and Baker 1995).

A traumatic memory is often associated with a different image of the body and sense of self. In some cases, it even involves a separate identity (McDougall 1926). For example, in dissociative child states, the DID patient usually looks upon him- or herself as a child, experiences and perceives the body as that of a child, displays childlike behaviors and skills and is strongly oriented to the traumatic past, which to the patient is the present. Hence, Myers's metaphorical expression "emotional personality" overlaps with current concepts of dissociative (identity) states.

Although nontraumatic sensory events usually are automatically and preconsciously synthesized into symbolic form, traumatic experiences in patients with PTSD and dissociative disorders seem to be encoded as sensorimotor and affective states that remain relatively unintegrated by the normal information processing that leads to autobiographical memory (van der Kolk and van der Hart 1991).

The "Apparently Normal Personality": Avoidance and Numbing

The "apparently normal personality" (Myers 1940) appears undisturbed, but may have partial or total amnesia for trauma and experience other losses, such as anesthesia. Also it may be inactivated to a greater or lesser extent when traumatic memories are triggered. Some patients may fail to recognize the traumatic nature of these intrusions and may experience them as mysterious nightmares or inexplicable somatoform symptoms (see Chapter 4). Leakage of traumatic information from one state to another is experienced as reexposure to trauma. The apparently normal personality may develop a phobia for these highly aversive, involuntary memory experiences (Janet 1919/1925, 661) and learn to avoid such mental events in various ways.

The simplest *passive-avoidance* strategy is not talking about the trauma or not exposing oneself to situations reminiscent of the trauma; for example, sexually abused individuals often avoid looking at or touching their bodies. *Intentional active avoidance* includes cognitive means such as thought suppression and diverting attention to other feelings, thoughts, activities and events, as well as behavioral means such as using increased doses of alcohol, cigarettes, drugs or medication (Putnam, Guroff et al. 1986; Solomon, Mikulincer and Avitzur 1988; Joseph et al. 1993). These avoidances may begin as intentional maneuvers, but in the long run they become quite automatic. Apparent normality can evolve into a detached lifestyle that relies on avoidance of intimacy and emotion and intense concentration on professional or occupational activities.

Although partial or complete traumatic reexperiencing constitutes *positive dissociative* symptoms, this posttraumatic pseudonormality is characterized by a range of losses or *negative dissociative* symptoms. Examples include loss of sensation and affect (bodily and emotional anesthesia), loss of knowledge (amnesia) and loss of familiarity with and attachment to one's body and identity (depersonalization). Some patients even fail to be aware of particular symptomatic losses (see Chapter 4), a condition that has become known as *"la belle indifférence d'une hystérique."*

RETRACTION OF THE FIELD OF CONSCIOUSNESS

Janet defined hysteria as "a form of mental depression characterized by the retraction of the field of personal consciousness and a tendency to the dissociation and emancipation of the systems of ideas and functions that constitute personality" (1907, 332). As he observed, these characteristics are most dominant during traumatic experiences that overwhelm the individual with intense fear or other vehement emotions, painful or offensive sensations and an intense feeling of helplessness. One result is that traumatized individuals remember best those aspects of the traumatic event toward which their attention was narrowly focused—the central details of the threatening event, the essential threat cues (Christianson 1992; Easterbrook 1959). Another result may be that certain sensory information is not perceived, experienced and stored at all by the "normal personality," but instead enters the memory of one or more dissociated states of consciousness (van der Hart and Nijenhuis 1995).

Janet was the first to analyze the dissociative nature of traumatic memories, and his discussion of the case of his patient Irene is still illuminating. Due to trying family circumstances, Irene was exhausted when her mother died and witnessing the death was an overwhelming experience for which she developed amnesia (Janet 1904; van der Kolk and van der Hart 1991). As a result, Irene in her normal state denied that her mother had died, but she continued to reexperience episodically the traumatic death.

Irene's dissociated ideas did not pertain only to her mother's death; they also involved her own body. Her reexperiencing included a wide range of movements, sensory perceptions and other somatoform reactions. During reactivations of that dramatic night, her image of her body mirrored her age and state at the time of mother's death.

SIMPLE AND COMPLEX DISSOCIATION

Irene's reenactments were far more complex than a simple flashback. In even more complex cases, dissociated memories emancipate themselves, in Janet's terms, and become even more elaborate and independent from the rest of the personality, seeming to embark on a life of their own.

Primary Dissociation.   The basic dividedness into an apparently normal state and a traumatic state, with its fixed ideas and disturbances of functions, has been labeled *primary dissociation* (van der Hart 1994). This condition characterizes simple PTSD, where major symptoms involve mentally and bodily reexperiencing the event through intrusive recollections, nightmares and flashbacks, sensitivity to and avoidance of associated stimuli and concomitant emotional numbing with feelings of detachment or isolation (Spiegel, Hunt and Dondershine 1988).

Secondary Dissociation.   Once a person is in a dissociated traumatic state, further dissociation in varying degrees of complexity may occur. A partial form of *secondary dissociation* (van der Hart 1994; van der Kolk, van der Hart and Marmar 1996) is reported frequently by incest survivors, victims of traffic accidents and combat-traumatized soldiers. "Dissociation between observing ego and experiencing ego" (Fromm 1965) involves the experience of mentally leaving the body and being able to observe what happens to it or what it is doing from a distance (Noyes, Hoenck and Kupperman 1977; Gelinas 1983). At the same time another part of the personality is emotionally and physically enduring the experience.

Although primary dissociation allows people to ignore or deny the reality of their traumatic experience and go on, apparently, as if nothing happened (Christianson and Nilsson 1984, 1989; Spiegel 1988), secondary dissociation implies a division between cognitive awareness and emotional experiencing of the painful affects, sensations and motor responses associated with the trauma. These acute peritraumatic dissociative responses include depersonalization, out-of-body experiences and altered body image (Bremner et al. 1993; Holen 1993; Koopman, Classen and Spiegel 1994; Marmar et al. 1994; Shalev et al. 1996).

Tertiary Dissociation.   Some authors define as traumatic dissociation only those mental distancing maneuvers described above (Terr 1994). However, the clinical literature on PTSD also reports more complex forms, including the development of "killer identities" in traumatized combat veterans (Brende and Benedict 1980; Bradshaw, Ohlde and Horne 1991). This *tertiary dissociation* involves the formation of separate ego states and can be found in patients with extreme dissociative disorders such as DID. Here some identities experience pain, but others are anesthetic; some are intensely fearful, while others experience aggression; still others know about, but escape experiencing, the trauma. Various trauma-ignorant identities continue to perform tasks in daily life, becoming aspects of the "apparently normal" personality, now also fragmented into various substates.

Although the label "emotional personality" conveys that in a sense all traumatic states involve a separate sense of self, that sense of self may not extend beyond dissociative or flashback episodes. However, if as a result of chronic trauma dissociation becomes a habitual way of coping, used even for minor stressors, this rudimentary separate identity may emancipate. Repeated trauma will extend its autobiographical memories and will reinforce previously stored experiences, reactions and images. Moreover, reactivations of traumatic memories may include perceptions of the actual present that are distorted under the influence of the restricted field of consciousness. For example, while engaging in sexual acts, a husband may suddenly become a former sexual abuser in the eye of the dissociative patient. When this misperception is not corrected, the dissociative identity involved may store this event as another rape. Misperceptions also occur when thoughts, fantasies or dreams the patient had at the time of trauma, or in a later stage are misfiled as actual events; Irene's reenactments of the tragic night included suicidal behavior, which she did not actually perform at the time of trauma. However, committing suicide may have crossed her mind. Thus, traumatic memories may include reconstructive as well as reproductive aspects (Janet 1928; van der Hart, Nijenhuis and van der Kolk, submitted).

PSYCHOLOGICAL AND SOMATOFORM DISSOCIATION

According to the *Diagnostic and Statistical Manual of Mental Disorders*, fourth edition (*DSM-IV*; APA 1994), the essential feature of dissociative disorders is a disruption in the usually integrated functions of consciousness, memory, identity or perception of the environment (APA 1994). However, many different strands of clinical observation and research (Janet 1889, 1901, 1907; Nemiah 1991; Nijenhuis 1990; van der Hart and Op den Velde 1995; Kihlstrom 1992, 1994; Nijenhuis et al. 1996, 1997, 1997b, 1998b) suggest that pathological dissociation also manifests itself in bodily symptoms, reactions and functions. We have labeled the phenomenon *somatoform dissociation* (Nijenhuis et al. 1996). Like psychological dissociation, it involves negative symptoms such as analgesia, anesthesia and motor inhibitions as well as positive symptoms such as site-specific pain and changing preferences of taste and smell (see Chapter 4).

High levels of psychological dissociation are found in patients with DID (Bernstein and Putnam 1986; Boon and Draijer 1993), patients with DDNOS (Ross et al. 1992; Coons 1992) and combat veterans with PTSD (Bremner et al. 1992, 1993; Spiegel, Hunt and Dondershine 1988). Vanderlinden et al. (1993b) reported that patients with DID attained significantly higher dissociation scores than patients with DDNOS, borderline personality disorder and PTSD. Recent evidence shows that somatoform disorders, DDNOS and DID are associated with increased levels of somatoform dissociation (Nijenhuis et al. 1997), as measured by the Somatoform Dissociation Questionnaire (SDQ-20; Nijenhuis et al. 1996, 1998b). Compared with psychiatric comparison patients, patients with *DSM-IV* somatoform disorders averaged significantly elevated scores, those with DDNOS had even higher scores and DID patients had the highest scores. All pairwise comparisons were significant and remained significant after statistical correction for general psychopathology.

DISSOCIATION OF IMPLICIT MEMORY

Clinical observation and some experimental evidence (Peters et al., in press) suggest that dissociation of implicit nonverbal memory can include state-dependent, dissociative bodily reactions, such as site-specific allergic reactions (e.g., in response to reexperiencing having sperm smeared on a specific part of the body) or other physical stigmata (such as notching and reddening of the skin near both wrists upon recalling being tied up). The patient we describe in Chapter 4 even displayed spontaneous bleeding of a facial scar upon recalling how it had originated. We were as amazed as she was when the scar totally disappeared after the new wound healed. A victim of a road accident who developed peritraumatic analgesia and PTSD also displayed spontaneous scar bleeding when, with great physical pain, he relived this trauma in therapy (Briggs 1993).

DOES TRAUMA INDUCE DISSOCIATION? EMPIRICAL DATA

As Janet observed, "[Traumas] produce their disintegrating effects in proportion to their intensity, duration and repetition" (1909, 1558). Indeed, high correlations between dissociation and self-reported intensity of trauma have been found. These studies involved children, adolescents and adults with dissociative disorders (e.g., Boon and Draijer 1993; Coons, Bowman and Milstein 1988; Hornstein and Putnam 1992; Loewenstein and Putnam 1990; Ross et al. 1991), PTSD, (e.g., Bremner et al. 1993), eating disorder (Vanderlinden et al. 1993a) and borderline personality disorder (e.g., Herman, Perry, and van der Kolk 1989).

A higher prevalence of traumatic incidents (Coons et al. 1988; Kemp, Gilbertson and Torem 1988), more severe reported childhood physical and sexual abuse and a younger age of onset of trauma have been found in dissociative disorder patients in comparison to patients with other psychiatric diagnoses (Boon and Draijer 1993; Fink and Golinkhoff 1990; Nijenhuis et al., in press d; Schultz, Braun and Kluft 1989). The degree of reported childhood and adult trauma predicted the level of psychological dissociation in borderline personality disorder (Shearer 1994). Studying dissociative disorder patients and psychiatric comparison patients, Nijenhuis et al. (in press d) found that somatoform dissociation was best predicted by the severity and duration of self-reported childhood sexual and physical abuse, even after statistically controlling for self-reported emotional neglect and abuse.

Sexual abuse seems particularly potent as a correlate of dissociation. In a study of consecutive rape victims at a French forensic center, Darves-Bornoz (1997) found that after six months 71 percent met criteria for PTSD, 69 percent for dissociative disorders and 66 percent for somatoform disorders. Of those who met criteria for PTSD, 85 percent also had dissociative disorder (85 percent) and 75 percent met criteria for somatoform disorder.

The validity of self-reported abuse, especially when it involves early memories, recovered memories and memories of sexual abuse, has been questioned (e.g., Frankel 1993; Loftus 1993). Are they constructions created by therapists in suggestible patients (Loftus 1993; Ofshe and Watters 1994)? To date, this claim has not been tested among dissociative disorder patients, and memories of abuse among general psychiatric patients have been found to be equally accurate whether recovered or continuously remembered (Dalenberg 1996).

Although retrospective assessment of trauma may yield false positives (reporting trauma that in fact did not occur), it may also yield false negatives (not reporting trauma that actually did occur). Dissociative symptomatology may involve memory distortion, compromising the validity of reports of trauma in either direction (Brown 1995; Loftus 1993) due to underreporting, overreporting and reporting mixtures of historically valid and invalid components (Kluft 1996). Another complexity is that corroboration or disproving of a part of a traumatic memory does not verify or falsify other recollections (Kluft 1996). In spite of these and related obstacles, independent corroboration of dissociative patients' traumatic memories, including formerly dissociated memories, has been found (Coons 1994; Hornstein and Putnam 1992; Kluft 1995; Martínez-Taboas 1996; Swica, Lewis and Lewis 1996).

The consistent finding that traumatic events evoke peritraumatic dissociation supports the hypothesized association between dissociation and trauma, as do findings that more intense traumatic exposure is associated with greater use of dissociation both at the time of trauma and later (Zatzick et al. 1994). The degree of peritraumatic dissociation was also influenced by subject characteristics, which included coping by means of escape-avoidance, and lower scores on the adjustment, identity, ambition and prudence scales of a personality inventory (Marmar et al. 1996). Future research should assess the degree to which such characteristics are associated with previous traumatization.

STRUCTURE AND CONTENTS OF TRAUMATIC MEMORIES: RELATIONSHIP TO ANIMAL MODELS

TRAUMATIC MEMORIES AND STIMULUS INFORMATION

By the beginning of the nineteenth century, it had been noted that the anniversary of a traumatic event, such as the unexpected death of a loved one, may reevoke the traumatic memory of this event, even though the person in an apparently normal state may be unable to recognize this reactivation or any connection with the date of the original traumatic event (van der Kolk 1989; Vijselaar and van der Hart 1992). Janet (1904, 1928) observed that traumatic memory can be evoked under other conditions as well, in situations reminiscent, either literally or symbolically, of some aspect of the original traumatic situation. These reminders range from sensory and emotional events, such as sounds, smells and situations (such as those requiring blind trust), to symbolic representations, such as having a child arrive at the age at which the parent was molested (APA 1994; Blank 1985; Foa, Steketel and Rothbaum 1989; Gelinas 1983; Jones and Barlow 1990; Spiegel, Frischholz and Spira 1993; Steele and Colrain 1990; van der Hart and Friedman 1992; van der Kolk 1994). These events are generally referred to as triggers, reactivating stimuli or conditioned stimuli.

Classical Conditioning of Trauma.   Upon exposure to extreme stress, previously neutral stimuli may become, through salient association with trauma, *conditioned* stimuli (Davey 1992; Eelen, Van den Bergh and Bayens 1990; Hearst 1989). These classically conditioned stimuli will thereafter tend to reactivate the traumatic memory. All kinds of phobias may result. For example, victims of chronic abuse may become phobic of trust, attachment, dependency or even human contact in general. Since any emotional arousal may become a conditioned stimulus, even positive emotions may pose a threat. Hence, a *phobia of normal human contact and normal life* may result.

Conditioned stimuli do not reactivate a single isolated response, but complex psychophysiological states. The reactivation comes as a unit, consistent with evidence in cognitive psychology for state-dependent memory (Bower 1981). Therefore, conditioned stimuli have the capacity to reactivate dissociated states.

For practical purposes, the following types of reactivating stimuli can be distinguished: (1) sensory data, (2) time-related stimuli, (3) daily life events,

(4) events during therapeutic sessions, (5) emotional states, (6) physiological states, and (7) current trauma (van der Hart and Friedman 1992).

Behavioral Avoidance. Exposure to traumatic memories is aversive and instigates avoidance and escape reactions. Chronic traumatization, which begins at an early age, yields far more conditioning than later and restricted traumatization, rendering impossible total behavioral avoidance of all conditioned stimuli. Also, behavioral avoidance will fail when conditioned stimuli appear in unpredictable and uncontrollable ways or when, due to dissociation of the relevant knowledge, patients are not aware that certain stimuli will reactivate the painful past.

TRAUMATIC MEMORIES AND RESPONSE INFORMATION

Threat calls for defense of psychological and physical integrity. Defense, or *coping*, consists of the cognitions and behaviors used to assess and reduce stress and to moderate the tension that accompanies it. Thus coping includes two functions: (1) a problem-focused function (channeling resources to solve the stress-creating problem) and (2) an emotion-focused function, also described as mental escapism (easing the tension aroused by the threat by intrapsychic activity, such as denying or changing one's attitude toward the threatening circumstances) (Lazarus 1993; Solomon, Mikulincer and Avitzur 1988; Wolfe et al. 1993).

For severe threat, the kind of coping that will be available or wise depends on the nature of the stressor, the stage of imminence and characteristics of the threatened organism. Sometimes flight, assertive behavior or fight may be instrumental in avoiding further danger, but, as Solomon, Mikulincer and Avitzur (1988) point out, there are traumatic situations in which trauma survivors could have done little to change things. For example, applying problem-solving coping (attempted flight, fight or assertiveness) would be inevitably frustrating and nonproductive for a child being physically or sexually abused or witnessing violence. In some situations, active motor defense may actually increase danger and therefore be less adaptive than passive, mental ways of coping. As victims of child abuse recount, active resistance is likely to evoke anger in a perpetrator and related prolongation or aggravation of abusive behavior. Further, futile actions reinforce a sense of sadistic domination in the perpetrator and a sense of utter helplessness in the victim.

ANIMAL DEFENSIVE STATES

Animals do not respond to aversive, threatening stimuli idiosyncratically, but with well-defined behavioral and physiological states tuned to optimize survival chances in successive stages of predator imminence (Bolles 1970; Bolles and Fanselow 1980; Fanselow and Lester 1988). These states are mutually inhibitory, and there is evidence suggesting that the various defensive subsystems (e.g., affiliative behaviors, freezing, aggression) are mediated by different neurochemical systems (Kalin and Shelton 1989). Imminence varies in terms of space (physical distance between prey and predator) and time (frequency of previous predatory exposure in a particular location). Different stages of imminence evoke abrupt and specific shifts from one behavioral and physiological state to another and include *preencounter*, *postencounter* and *circa-strike defensive subsystems* and *recuperation*.

In the absence of threat, animals engage in normal, functional activities (food seeking, eating, procreation and nurturing). Upon meeting a potentially dangerous situation, preencounter defense is evoked, with normal activities immediately inhibited. For example, food abstinence for prolonged periods facilitates alert attention to potential predatory threat, and intermittent bingeing (rapid consumption of meals of increased size) prevents loss of body mass. Postencounter defense consists of short-lived flight, followed by freezing and silencing. These inhibitory responses serve survival in that predators are less capable of detecting nonmoving objects, and predatory attack is evoked by movement of prey (Suarez and Gallop 1981). Freezing becomes the dominant defensive response at the stage of attack characterized by low survival value of flight or counterattack (Fanselow and Lester 1988). Circa-strike defense includes analgesia and emotional anesthesia. These responses inhibit pain-directed behavior and panic, which might interfere with remaining immobile and silent and continued watchfulness for attack. Circa-strike defense also includes the startle response, short-lived flight and fight and subsequent return to freezing. Recuperative responses (return of pain perception, wound care, rest) are evoked upon the survival of attack.

SIMILARITIES BETWEEN ANIMAL DEFENSE
AND RECUPERATION AND HUMAN DISSOCIATION

Rivers (1920) and Nijenhuis et al. (1998c) observed striking similarities between the animal threat response and human dissociation. Some research findings are consistent with the proposed parallel (for a review, see Nijenhuis et al., in press e). DID and DDNOS patients often report freezing, analgesia and anesthesia, as well as disturbed eating (Boon and Draijer 1993). Symptoms in these three categories were among the five symptoms that best discriminated dissociative from general psychiatric patients (Nijenhuis et al., in press a; see also Chapter 4, this volume). Analgesia and anesthesia have been documented in survivors of many different kinds of trauma. Albach (1993) and Draijer (1990) reported that the majority of the sexually abused women they studied experienced analgesia; retrospectively assessed freezing, dissociation and anxiety during incestuous abuse were the best predictors for the development of PTSD (Albach and Everaerd 1992). Survivors of an earthquake (Cardeña and Spiegel 1993) as well as of a disaster at sea (Cardeña et al., in press) experienced transient analgesic effects, and reminders of traumatic events were found to reactivate analgesia (van der Kolk et al. 1989).

Traumatic Memories and Meaning Information

People are meaning-making creatures. As we develop, we organize our world according to a personal theory of reality, some of which may be conscious, but much of which is an unconscious integration of accumulated experience (Harber and Pennebaker 1992; Janet 1889; van der Kolk and Ducey 1989). As Horowitz (1986), Mandler (1988) and Epstein (1991) have pointed out, conceptions of oneself and the world are organized according to relatively stable cognitive *schemas* about competence and dependence, power and helplessness, trust and distrust and so on. These schemas, or basic assumptions (Janoff-Bulman 1985, 1992), contain certain notions about the degree to which one sees oneself as an active or passive agent, as a lovable or hateful person, about the world as a benevolent or dangerous place, and other people as sources of pleasure or danger (Epstein 1991; Janoff-Bulman 1985, 1992). Schemas generally reflect and follow life experiences and will be extremely disrupted by trauma.

Trauma and Cognitive Interference.   Extreme arousal may add to disturbed cognitive functioning, probably due to massive release of stress hormones (van der Kolk 1994). As Janet already believed, severe threat may evoke vehement emotions that interfere with cognition (Janet 1889, 1904, 1909, 1919/1925). He also thought that if an event is too upsetting for people to be able to make sense of, it cannot be properly stored in memory, that is, put into cognitive schemas that allow for integration of the experience. Trauma may leave the person in a state of "unspeakable terror." Janet described how traumatized individuals become attached to the trauma and have difficulty integrating new personality-significant experiences as long as the traumatic memories remain unassimilated. These individuals "are attached to an unsurmountable obstacle. The patient is unable to tell the story of the events as they occurred and yet, he remains confronted with the situation in which he was unable to play a satisfactory role" (Janet 1919/1925, 660). It is "as if their personality development has stopped at a certain point and cannot be expanded anymore by the addition or assimilation of new elements" (Janet 1898, 135). Eventually, Janet suggested, patients just want to get away from it all and forget the situation: "Complete avoidance is characterized by complete absence of allusion to sensitive objects or the anxiety associated with them. It is as if the event, or even the function, never existed" (Janet 1935, 325).

Trauma as Schema-Discrepant Information.   Many students of trauma have noted that tragic experiences challenge people's notions about themselves and may profoundly reorganize existing mental schemas (Epstein 1991; Bowlby 1969, 1973; Horowitz 1986; Janet 1935). Overwhelming and unbearable experiences that do not fit into people's personal schemas may be assimilated into existing schemas ("Maybe it wasn't really rape"; "I must have done something bad, since good people don't get raped"). Further, people may accommodate their schemas to the experience by altering their conceptions of the world, other people and themselves. Especially in absence of social support, such accommodations may be maladaptive ("There is no safe place in the world"; "They hurt me because I am bad and deserve punishment") (Hollon and Garber 1988; Resick and Schnicke 1992). As Epstein put it, a traumatic resolution involves an accommodation that "embraces the trauma"; with adoption of a belief system and lifestyle fashioned around the trauma. However, those most successful at coping with a distressing experience do not generalize from that experience to the totality of existence, but rather view it merely as one terrible event that occurred at a particular place at a particular time (Epstein 1991). They may view the world as an unpredictable, dangerous and uncontrollable place—but *within limits*.

Dissociative State-Dependent Schemas.   Because they rely on diverging life experiences, dissociative memory structures will, as a rule, contain schemas that differ from each other and from the apparently normal state. A dissociative state that encompasses conditioned freezing is likely to look upon itself and the body as weak, powerless and guilty. It may misinterpret its defensive freezing ("I did not resist"), and it may adopt a name that fits this lack of behavioral resistance as well as the body's rape-induced sexual responses ("Slut"). Its image of the body will relate to the one that prevailed at the time of the trauma ("It is dirty"; "I have small breasts"; "I am thirteen years of age"). To the extent that coconsciousness between states exists, other dissociative identities may reinforce these accusations in order to protect their own self-images ("Slut is to blame"). Meanwhile, other states may give quite different self-descriptions ("I am a strong and aggressive man"). In case of simultaneous activation of states, conflicting senses of the self, the body and the world may clash, resulting in "inner fights and battles" that further strengthen separateness.

As a result of chronic traumatization, such dissociative states may develop elaborate schemas of self, body and world. Some profess a deeply engrained sense of helplessness ("I am a thing"), shame ("I am dirty") or aggression and hate directed toward self or others ("My body is evil"; "Every man is a monster"). Such cognitive schemas may promote further abuse as adults, either as victims (Kluft 1990) or as perpetrators. Secondary shaping of dissociative states by sociocultural influences may also be involved (Gleaves 1996).

CHRONIC DISSOCIATION AND POSTTRAUMATIC DECLINE

Continued Dissociation

Since traumatic memory states are highly emotionally charged and tied to restricted levels of mental functioning, spontaneous posttraumatic integrative tendencies are not likely. If external or personal pressure for integration of trauma and relearning are absent, trauma will continue to haunt the mind and the body.

Posttraumatic integrative tendencies are enhanced by social support and social interference with dissociative avoidance. For example, realization of the death of a loved one is supported by the burial, sadness of others, consolation, conversations, legal consequences and the need to dispose of possessions. In their review of the literature, Jones and Barlow (1990) conclude that social support moderates the expression of PTSD, much as it does for other emotional disorders, and that its absence is detrimental. Dissociation is probably reinforced by social denial, pressure for secrecy, induction of guilt, lack of support and continued traumatization and betrayal (Freyd 1996).

Reactivated traumatic memories may themselves retraumatize the survivor who "forgets" the intrusive memory through dissociative mechanisms (van der Hart et al. 1993; van der Kolk 1994). In this case, remembering has led not to successful reprocessing, but to a new dissociative episode.

Continued dissociation not only interferes with emotional processing, but also inhibits the development of other ways of coping and, consequently, general adaptation. As summarized by Solomon, Mikulincer and Avitzur (1988), several researchers proposed that the optimal coping style consists of the largest possible repertoire of coping responses (Billings and Moss 1981; Folkman and Lazarus 1980; Pearlin and Schooler 1978). Even if intrapsychic coping aids in maintaining emotional balance, the nonuse of problem-solving strategies will in the end have negative psychological outcomes (Solomon, Mikulincer and Avitzur 1988). Solomon, Mikulincer and Avitzur on this basis hypothesized that among combat stress-reaction casualties, a style that emphasizes problem-solving coping will be associated with less PTSD, whereas intrapsychic coping and extensive behavioral avoidance will be associated with more severe PTSD, which was confirmed in their study. Wolfe et al. (1993) in their study of readjustment patterns in Vietnam combat veterans found that active, nonavoidant (or problem-focused) coping characterized the functioning of well-adjusted Vietnam veterans. In contrast, the high-symptom groups reported using significantly higher levels of mental escapism and externalization and extensive behavioral avoidance.

Posttraumatic Decline.   Janet noticed that many traumatized patients experience a slow decline in their ability to deal with both old and new stressors unless they become involved in actions that allow them to gain mastery over failures to act appropriately during the traumatic events (Janet 1919/1925, 663). Several factors seem to contribute to this state of exhaustion, fatigue and loss of control.

Stimulus-controlled Reactivation of Traumatic Memories: Keane et al. (1985) argue that two principles—higher-order conditioning and stimulus generalization—account for the observation that the number of cues capable of evoking the traumatic memory may greatly increase over time. Avoidance behavior will become ever more extended, while it also becomes progressively more difficult to avoid all cues that elicit traumatic memories. More frequent intrusions of traumatic memories and related alarm responses reflect more loss of control, reinforce a sense of helplessness and cause further elevation of the general level of arousal. Increased use of dissociation as a defense is called for. However, it may be assumed that dissociation consumes energy, as was demonstrated in hypnotic experiments (Stevenson 1976). Hence, the patient's resources may become exhausted, and increasing misery ensues.

Chronic Hyperarousal: The posttraumatic individual will react to these events with chronic hyperarousal and concomitant cognitive symptoms of hypervigilance to trauma-related cues, the conditioned stimuli (Chemtob et al. 1988; McFarlane 1994; van der Kolk and Ducey 1989). It also has been shown that hyperarousal in general increases the frequency of intrusive thoughts (Rainey et al. 1987; Southwick et al. 1993). Thus, a response that is supposed to prepare for ongoing threat paradoxically ensures that the individual will experience a steady stream of trauma-related intrusive thoughts and images, together with their emotional and sensory concomitants (Jones and Barlow 1990).

Chronic Narrowing of Attention: Threat-related arousal is accompanied by narrowing of attention to other, potentially gratifying experiences and increases the likelihood of interpreting ambiguous information as threatening. It inhibits new learning, leaving the patient fixated on the past (Spiegel, Frischholz and Spira 1993).

Neurobiological Aspects of Chronic Decline: The burgeoning literature on this subject, which cannot be discussed here, suggests that trauma, PTSD and dissociation are associated with demonstrable neurophysiologic and neuroanatomic changes (Krystal et al. 1995; van der Kolk 1994). Learning how these changes interconnect with the clinical features of traumatic decline and recovery maps the agenda for the next generation of research in this area.

SUMMARY

Exposure to traumatic events interferes globally with the normal integrative processing of experience. Traumatic memories come to reside in mental compartments that are not fully connected with the larger systems of explicit and implicit memory. As a result, the victim alternates between states in which trauma is painfully reexperienced and apparently normal states that nonetheless involve significant losses of self-attributes. Dissociation apparently facilitates adaptation in the short term, but is also the source of long-term pathology. Social support in the aftermath of trauma stimulates integration. When this is lacking or when trauma persists, dissociation may become a permanent adaptation. However, sooner or later, dissociative systems start to fail. More and more stimuli become triggers, reactivating intrusive traumatic memories. The trauma sufferer becomes phobic of inner realities and exhausted in the downward spiral of dissociative decline.

It is at this stage that such individuals come to therapists for treatment. Resolution of this state of misery ultimately implies the successful processing of traumatic memories and thus the integration of the "emotional" and "apparently normal" personality states. Controlled stepwise therapeutic exposure to and reinterpretation of feared external and internal worlds may be necessary in order to heal these divided minds.

REFERENCES

Albach F. (1993). Freud's veerrleidingstheorie. *Incest, trauma en hysterie.* Middelburg: Stichting Petra.

Albach, F., and Everaerd, W. (1992). Posttraumatic stress symptoms in victims of childhood incest. *Psychotherapy and Psychosomatics* 57 (4): 143–151.

American Psychiatric Association (1994). *Diagnostic and statistical manual of mental disorders,* 4th ed. *(DSM-IV).* Washington, D.C.: American Psychiatric Association.

Bernstein, E. M., and Putnam, F. W. (1986). Development, reliability, and validity of a dissociation scale. *Journal of Nervous and Mental Disease* 174: 727–735.

Billings, A. G., and Moss, R. H. (1981). The role of coping responses and social resources in attenuating the stress of life events. *Journal of Behavioral Medicine* 4: 139–157.

Blank, A. A. (1985). The unconscious flashback to the war in Viet Nam veterans: Clinical mystery, legal defense, and community problem. In S. M. Sonnenberg, and J. A. Talbot, eds., *The trauma of war: Stress and recovery in Viet Nam veterans* (pp. 293–308). Washington, D.C.: American Psychiatric Press.

Bolles, R. C. (1970). Species-specific defense reactions and avoidance learning. *Psychological Review* 77: 32–48.

Bolles, R. C., and Fanselow, M. S. (1980). A perceptual-defensive-recuperation model of fear and pain. *The Behavioral and Brain Sciences* 3: 291–301.

Boon, S., and Draijer, N. (1993). *Multiple personality disorder in the Netherlands: A study on reliability and validity of the diagnosis.* Amsterdam: Swets and Zeitlinger.

Bower, G. H. (1981). Mood and memory. *American Psychologist* 36: 129–148.

Bowlby, J. (1969). *Attachment and loss.* Vol. 1. New York: Basic Books.

———. (1973). *Attachment and loss.* Vol. 2. New York: Basic Books.

Bradshaw, S. L., Jr., Ohlde, C., and Horne, J. B. (1991). The love of war: Vietnam and the traumatized veteran. *Bulletin of the Menninger Clinic* 55: 96–103.

Bremner, J. D., Southwick, S. M., Brett, E., Fontana, A., Rosenheck, R., and Charney, D. S. (1992). Dissociation and posttraumatic stress disorder in Vietnam combat veterans. *American Journal of Psychiatry* 149: 328–332.

Bremner, J. D., Steinberg, M., Southwick, S. M., Johnson, D. R., and Charney, D. S. (1993). Use of the Structured Clinical Interview for *DSM-IV* dissociative disorders for systematic assessment of dissociative symptoms in posttraumatic stress disorder. *American Journal of Psychiatry* 150: 1011–1014.

Brende, J. O., and Benedict, B. D. (1980). The Vietnam combat delayed stress syndrome: Hypnotherapy of "dissociative symptoms." *American Journal of Clinical Hypnosis* 23: 34–40.

Brett, E. E., and Ostroff, R. (1985). Imagery and post-traumatic stress disorder. *American Journal of Psychiatry* 142: 417–424.

Briggs, A. C. (1993). A case of delayed post-traumatic stress disorder with "organic memories" accompanying therapy. *British Journal of Psychiatry* 163: 828–830.

Brown, D. (1995). Pseudomemories: The standard of science and standard of care in trauma treatment. *American Journal of Clinical Hypnosis* 37: 1–24.

Burgess, A. W., Hartman, C. R., and Baker, T. (1995). Memory presentations of childhood sexual abuse. *Journal of Psychosocial Nursing* 33: 9–16.

Cardeña, E., and Spiegel, D. (1993). Dissociative reactions to the San Francisco Bay Area earthquake of 1989. *American Journal of Psychiatry* 150: 474–478.

Cardeña, E., Holen, A., McFarlane, A., Solomon, Z., Wilkinson, C., and Spiegel, D. (in press). A multisite study of acute-stress reaction to a disaster. In *Sourcebook for the DSM-IV*. Vol. 4. Washington, D.C.: American Psychiatric Press.

Charcot, J. M. (1887). *Leçons sur les maladies du système nerveux faites à la Salpêtrière.* Vol. 3. Paris: Progrès Médical en A. Delahaye and E. Lecrosnie.

Chemtob, R., Roitblat, H. L., and Hamada, R. S. (1988). A cognitive action theory of post-traumatic stress disorder. *Journal of Anxiety Psychology* 2: 253–275.

Christianson, S. A. (1992). Emotional stress and eyewitness memory: A critical review. *Psychological Bulletin* 112: 284–309.

Christianson, S. A., and Nilsson, L. G. (1984). Functional amnesia as induced by psychological trauma. *Memory and Cognition* 12: 142–155.

———. (1989). Hysterical amnesia: A case of aversively motivated isolation of memory. In T. Archer and L. G. Nilsson, eds., *Aversion, avoidance, and anxiety: Perspectives on aversively motivated behavior* (pp. 289–310). Hillsdale, N.Y.: Erlbaum.

Coons, P. M. (1992). Dissociative disorder not otherwise specified: A clinical investigation of 50 cases with suggestions for typology. *Dissociation* 5: 187–196.

———. (1994). Confirmation of childhood abuse in child and adolescent cases of multiple personality disorder and dissociative disorder not otherwise specified. *Journal of Nervous and Mental Disease* 182: 461–464.

Coons, P. M., Bowman, E. S., and Milstein, V. (1988). Multiple personality disorder: A clinical investigation of 50 cases. *Journal of Nervous and Mental Disease* 176: 519–527.

Crabtree, A. (1992). Dissociation and memory: A two-hundred year perspective. *Dissociation* 5: 150–154.

———. (1993). *From Mesmer to Freud: Magnetic sleep and the roots of psychological healing.* New Haven: Yale University Press.

Dalenberg, C. J. (1996). Accuracy, timing and circumstances of disclosure in therapy of recovered and continuous memories of abuse. *Journal of Psychiatry and Law* 24: 229–275.

Darves-Bornoz, J. M. (1997). Rape-related psychotraumatic syndromes. *European Journal of Obstetrics and Gynecology* 71: 59–65.

Davey, G. C. L. (1992). Classical conditioning and the acquisition of human fears phobias: A review and synthesis of the literature. *Advances in Behavior Research and Therapy* 14: 29–66.

Draijer, N. (1990). *Seksuele traumatisering in de jeugd: Gevolgen op lange termijn van seksueel misbruik door verwanten.* Amsterdam: SUA.

Easterbrook, J. A. (1959). The effect of emotion on cue utilization and the organization of behavior. *Psychological Review* 66: 183–201.

Eelen, P., Van den Bergh, O., and Bayens, F. (1990). Fobieën: leertheorieën. In J. W .G. Orlemans, W. Brinkman, W. P. Haayman and E. J. Zwaan, eds., *Handboek voor Gedragstherapie* (C.15.4 1–29). Deventer: Van Loghum Slaterus.

Epstein, S. (1991). The self-concept, the traumatic neurosis, and the structure of personality. In D. Ozer, J. M. Healy, Jr., and A. J. Stewart, eds., *Perspectives in personality.* Vol. 3, Part A (pp. 63–98). London: Jessica Kingsley.

Fanselow, M. S., and Lester, L. S. (1988). A functional behavioristic approach to aversively motivated behavior: Predatory imminence as a determinant of the topography of defensive behavior. In R. C. Bolles, and M. D. Beecher, eds., *Evolution and learning* (pp. 185–212). Hillsdale, N.J.: Erlbaum.

Fink, D., and Golinkhoff, M. (1990). Multiple personality disorder, borderline personality disorder, and schizophrenia: A comparative study of clinical features. *Dissociation* 3: 127–134.

Foa, E. B., Steketee, G., and Rothbaum, B. O. (1989). Behavioral/cognitive conceptualizations of post-traumatic stress disorder. *Behavior Therapy* 20: 155–176.

Folkman, S., and Lazarus, R. S. (1980). An analysis of coping in a middle-aged community sample. *Journal of Health and Social Behavior* 21: 219–239.

Frankel, F. H. (1993). Adult reconstruction of childhood events in the multiple personality literature. *American Journal of Psychiatry* 150: 954–958.

Freud, S. (1919). Einleitung zur Psychoanalyse der Kriegsneurosen. G.W. Band 12.

Freyd, J. J. (1996). Betrayal trauma: the logic of forgetting childhood abuse. Cambridge, Mass.: Harvard University Press.

Fromm, E. (1965). Hypnoanalysis: Theory and two case excerpts. *Psychotherapy: Theory, Research, and Practice* 2: 127–133.

Gelinas, D. (1983). The persisting negative effects of incest. *Psychiatry* 46: 312–332.

Gleaves, D. H. (1996). The sociocognitive model of dissociative identity disorder: A reexamination of the evidence. *Psychological Bulletin* 120: 42–59.

Harber, K. D., and Pennebaker, J. W. (1992). Overcoming traumatic memories. In S. A. Christianson, ed., *The handbook of emotion and memory: Research and theory* (pp. 359–386). Hillsdale, N.J.: Erlbaum.

Hearst, E. (1989). Fundamentals of learning and conditioning. In R. C. Atkinson, R. J. Herrnstein, G. Lindzey and R. D. Luce, eds., *Stevens' handbook of experimental psychology.* Vol. 2, *Learning and conditioning,* 2d ed. (pp. 3–109). New York: Wiley.

Herman, J. L., Perry, J. C., and van der Kolk, B. A. (1989). Childhood trauma in borderline personality disorder. *American Journal of Psychiatry* 146: 390–395.

Holen, A. (1993). The North Sea oil rig disaster. In J. P. Wilson and B. Raphael, eds., *International handbook of traumatic stress syndromes* (pp. 471–478). New York: Plenum.

Hollon, S. D., and Garber, J. (1988). Cognitive therapy. In L. Y. Abrahamson, ed., *Social cognition and clinical psychology: A synthesis* (pp. 204–253). New York: Guilford.

Hornstein, N. L., and Putnam, F. W. (1992). Clinical phenomenology of child and adolescent dissociative disorders. *Journal of the American Academy of Child and Adolescent Psychiatry* 31: 1077–1085.

Horowitz, M. J. (1986). *Stress response syndromes*, 2d ed. New York: Jason Aronson.

Janet, P. (1889). *L'automatisme psychologique*. Paris: Félix Alcan. Reprint: Société Pierre Janet, Paris, 1973.

_____. (1894). Histoire d'une idée fixe. *Revue Philosophique* 37: 121–163. Also in P. Janet (1898), *Névroses et idées fixes*. Vol. 1 (pp. 156–212). Paris: Félix Alcan. Reprint: Société Pierre Janet, Paris, 1990.

_____. (1898). *Névroses et idées fixes*. Vol. 1. Paris: Félix Alcan. Reprint: Société Pierre Janet, Paris, 1990.

_____. (1901). *The mental state of hystericals*. New York: Putnam. Reprint: University Publications of America, Washington D.C., 1977.

_____. (1904). L'amnésie et la dissociation des souvenirs par l'émotion. *Journal de Psychologie* 1: 417-453. Also in P. Janet (1911), *L'Etat mental des hystériques*, 2d ed. (pp. 506–544). Paris: Félix Alcan. Reprint: Lafitte Reprints, Marseille, 1983.

_____. (1907). *The major symptoms of hysteria*. London/New York: Macmillan. Reprint of second edition: Hafner, New York, 1965.

_____. (1909). Problèmes psychologiques de l'émotion. *Revue de Neurologie* 1551-1687.

_____. (1911). *L'Etat mental des hystériques*. Paris: Félix Alcan, 2d extended ed. Reprint: Lafitte Reprints, Marseille, 1983.

_____. (1919). *Les médications psychologiques*. 3 vols. Paris: Félix Alcan, Reprint: Société Pierre Janet, Paris, 1986. English edition: *Psychological healing*. 2 vols. New York: Macmillan, 1925. Reprint: Arno Press, New York, 1976.

_____. (1928). *L'évolution de la mémoire et la notion du temps*. Paris: A. Chahine.

_____. (1929). *L'Evolution de la personalité*. Paris: A. Chahine. Reprint: Société Pierre Janet, Paris, 1984.

_____. (1935). Réalisation et interprétation. *Annales Médico-Psychologiques* 93 (2): 329–366.

Janoff-Bulman, R. (1985). The aftermath of victimization: Rebuilding shattered assumptions. In R. Figley, ed., *Trauma and its wake*. Vol. 1 (pp. 15–35). New York: Brunner/Mazel.

_____. (1992). *Shattered assumptions: Towards a new psychology of trauma*. New York: Free Press.

Jones, J., and Barlow, D. H. (1990). The etiology of posttraumatic stress disorder. *Clinical Psychology Review* 10: 299–328.

Joseph, S., Yule, W., Williams, R., and Andrews, B. (1993). Crisis support in the aftermath of a disaster: A longitudinal perspective. *British Journal of Clinical Psychology* 32: 177–185.

Kalin, N. H., and Shelton, S. E. (1989). Defensive behaviors in infant rhesus monkeys: Environmental cues and neurochemical regulation. *Science* 243: 1718–1721.

Kardiner, A. (1941). *The traumatic neuroses of war.* New York: Paul Hoeber.

Keane, T. M., Fairbank, J. A., Caddell, J. M., Zimering, R. T., and Bender, M. E. (1985). A behavioral approach to assessing and treating post-traumatic stress disorder in Vietnam veterans. In C. Figley, ed., *Trauma and its wake* (pp. 257–294). New York: Brunner/Mazel.

Kemp, K., Gilbertson, A. D., and Torem, M. (1988). The differential diagnosis of multiple personality disorder from borderline personality disorder. *Dissociation* 1: 41–46.

Kihlstrom, J. F. (1992). Dissociative and conversion disorders, In D. J. Stein, and J. Young, eds., *Cognitive science and clinical disorder* (pp. 247–270). San Diego/New York: Academic Press.

_____. (1994). One hundred years of hysteria. In S. J. Lynn and J. W. Rhue, eds., *Dissociation: Clinical and theoretical perspectives* (pp. 365–395). New York: Guilford.

Kluft, R. P. (1990). Incest and subsequent revictimization: The case of therapist-patient sexual exploitation, with a description of the sitting duck syndrome. In R. P. Kluft, ed., *Incest-related syndromes of adult psychopathology* (pp. 263–289). Washington D.C.: American Psychiatric Press.

_____. (1995). The confirmation and disconfirmation of memories of abuse in DID patients: A naturalistic clinical study. *Dissociation* 8: 251–258.

_____. (1996). Treating the traumatic memories of patients with dissociative identity disorder. *American Journal of Psychiatry, Festschrift Supplement* 153: 103–110.

Koopman, C., Classen, C., and Spiegel, D. (1994). Predictors of posttraumatic stress symptoms among survivors of the Oakland/Berkeley, Calif., firestorm. *American Journal of Psychiatry* 151: 888–894.

Krystal, H. (1969). *Massive trauma.* New York: International Universities Press.

Krystal, J. H., Bennett, A., Bremner, J. D., Southwick, S. M., and Charney, D. S. (1995). Toward a cognitive neuroscience of dissociation and altered memory functions in posttraumatic stress disorder. In M. J. Friedman, D. S. Charney and A. Y. Deutch, eds., *Neurobiological and clinical consequences of stress: From normal adaptation to PTSD* (pp. 239–269). Washington D.C.: American Psychiatric Press.

Lazarus, R. S. (1993). Why should we think of stress as a subset of emotion. In L. Goldberger and S. Brezniz, eds., *Handbook of stress,* 2d ed. (pp. 21–39). New York: Free Press.

Lindemann, E. (1944). Symptomatology and management of acute grief. *American Journal of Psychiatry* 101: 141–148.

Loewenstein, R. J., and Putnam, F. W. (1990). The clinical phenomenology of males with multiple personality disorder: A report of 21 cases. *Dissociation* 3: 135–144.

Loftus, E. F. (1993). The reality of repressed memories. *American Psychologist* 48: 518–537.

Mandler, G. (1988). Memory: Conscious and unconscious. In P. R. Solomon, G. R. Goethals, C. M. Kelly and B. R. Stephens, eds., *Memory: Interdisciplinary approaches.* New York: Springer.

Marmar, C. R., Weiss, D. S., Metzler, T. J., and Delucchi, K. (1996). Characteristics of emergency personnel related to peritraumatic dissociation during critical incident exposure. *American Journal of Psychiatry, Festschrift Supplement* 153: 94–102.

Marmar, C. R., Weiss, D. S., Schlenger, W. E., Fairbank, J. A., Jordan, B. K., Kulka, R. A., Hough, R. L. (1994). Peritraumatic dissociation and posttraumatic stress in male Vietnam theater veterans. *American Journal of Psychiatry* 151: 902–907.

Martínez-Taboas, A. (1996). Repressed memories: Some clinical data contributing towards its elucidation. *American Journal of Psychotherapy* 50: 217–230.

McDougall, W. (1926). *An outline of abnormal psychology.* London: Methuen.

McFarlane, A. C. (1994). Individual psychotherapy for post-traumatic stress disorder. *Psychiatric Clinics of North America* 17: 393–408.

Modell, A. (1990). *Other times, other realities: Toward a theory of psychoanalytic treatment.* Cambridge, Mass.: Harvard University Press.

Myers, C. S. (1940). *Shell shock in France 1914–18.* Cambridge: Cambridge University Press.

Nemiah, J. C. (1991). Dissociation, conversion, and somatization. In A. Tasman and S. M. Goldfinger, eds., *American Psychiatric Press Annual Review of Psychiatry.* Vol. 10 (pp. 248–260). Washington, D.C.: American Psychiatric Press.

Nijenhuis, E. R. S. (1990). Somatische equivalenten bij dissociatieve stoornissen. *Hypnotherapie* 12: 10–21.

_____. (1994). *Dissociatieve stoornissen en psychotrauma.* Houten: Bohn Stafleu Van Loghum.

_____. (1995). Dissociatie en leertheorie: trauma-geïnduceerde dissociatie als klassiek geconditioneerde defensie. In K. Jonker, J. L. L. Derksen, and F. J. Donker, eds., *Dissociatie: een fenomeen opnieuw belicht* (pp. 35–61). Houten: Bohn Stafleu Van Loghum.

Nijenhuis, E. R. S., Spinhoven, Ph., Vanderlinden, J., van Dyck, R., and van der Hart, O. (in press a). Somatoform dissociative reactions as related to animal defensive to predatory threat and injury. *Journal of Abnormal Psychology.*

Nijenhuis, E. R. S., Spinhoven, Ph., van Dyck, R., van der Hart, O., and Vanderlinden, J. (1996). The development and the characteristics of the Somatoform Dissociation Questionnaire (SDQ–20). *Journal of Nervous and Mental Disease* 184: 688–694.

_____. (1997). Wezenlijke kenmerken van somatoforme en dissociative stoornissen. Presentation at the Conference on Somatic Complaints, Conversion and Dissociation, Utrecht, Society of Psychosomatic Medicine, April 11.

_____. (1997b). The development of the Somatoform Dissociation Questionnaire (SDQ–5) as a screening instrument for dissociative disorders. *Acta Psychiatrica Scandinavica* 96: 311–318.

_____. (1998a). Degree of somatoform and psychological dissociation in dissociative disorder is correlated with reported trauma. *Journal of Traumatic Stress 11:* 711–730.

_____. (1998b). The psychometric characteristics of the Somatoform Dissociation Questionnaire: A replication study. *Psychotherapy and Psychosomatics 67:* 17–23.

Nijenhuis, E. R. S., Vanderlinden, J., and Spinhoven, Ph. (1998c). Animal defensive reactions as a model for trauma-induced dissociative reactions. *Journal of Traumatic Stress 11:* 243–260.

Noyes, R., Hoenck, P. R., and Kupperman, B. A. (1977). Depersonalization in response to life-threatening danger. *Psychiatry* 164: 401–407.

Ofshe, R., and Watters, E. (1994). *Making monsters: False memories, psychotherapy, and sexual hysteria*. New York: Scribner.

Pearlin, L., and Schooler, C. (1978). The structure of coping. *Journal of Health and Social Behavior* 19: 2–21.

Peters, M. L., Consemulder, J., Uyterlinde, S., and van der Hart, O. (in press). Apparent amnesia on experimental memory tests in dissociative identity disorder: An exploratory study. *Consciousness and Cognition*.

Putnam, F. W. (1988). The switch process in multiple personality disorder. *Dissociation* 1: 24–33.

_____. (1989). *Diagnosis and treatment of multiple personality disorder*. New York: Guilford.

Putnam, F. W., Guroff, J. J., Silberman, E. K., Barban, L., and Post, R. M. (1986). The clinical phenomenology of multiple personality disorder. *Journal of Clinical Psychiatry 47*: 285–293.

Rainey, J. M., Aleem, A., Ortiz, A., Yeragani, V., Pohl, R., and Berehou, R. (1987). Laboratory procedure for the inducement of flashbacks. *American Journal of Psychiatry* 144: 1317–1319.

Resick, P. A., and Schnicke, M. K. (1992). Cognitive processing therapy for sexual assault victims. *Journal of Consulting and Clinical Psychology* 60: 748–756.

Rivers, W. H. R. (1920). *Instinct and the unconsciousness: A contribution to a biological theory of the psycho-neuroses*. London: Cambridge University Press.

Ross, C. A., Anderson, G., Fraser, G. A., Reagor, P., Bjornson, L. and Miller, S. D. (1992). Differentiating multiple personality disorder and dissociative disorder not otherwise specified. *Dissociation* 5: 87–91.

Ross, C. A., Miller, S. D., Bjornson, L., Reagor, P., Fraser, G. A., and Anderson, G. (1991). Abuse histories in 102 cases of multiple personality disorder. *Canadian Journal of Psychiatry* 36: 97–101.

Schultz, R., Braun, B. G., and Kluft, R. P. (1989). Multiple personality disorder: Phenomenology of selected variables in comparison to major depression. *Dissociation* 2: 45–51.

Shalev, A. Y., Peri, T., Canetti, M. A., and Schreiber, S. (1996). Predictors of PTSD in injured trauma survivors: A prospective study. *American Journal of Psychiatry* 153: 219–225.

Shearer, S. L. (1994). Dissociative phenomena in women with borderline personality disorder. *American Journal of Psychiatry* 151: 1324–1328.

Solomon, Z., Mikulincer, M., and Avitzur, E. (1988). Coping, locus of control, social support, and combat-related posttraumatic stress disorder: A prospective study. *Journal of Personality and Social Psychology* 55: 279–285.

Southwick, S. M., Krystal, J. H., Morgan, C. A., Johnson, D., Nagy, L. M., Nicolaou, A., Heninger, G. R., and Charney, D. S. (1993). Abnormal noradrenergic function in posttraumatic stress disorder. *Archives of General Psychiatry* 50: 266–274.

Spiegel, D. (1984). Multiple personality disorder as a post-traumatic stress disorder. *Psychiatric Clinics of North America* 7: 101–110.

_____. (1988). Dissociation and hypnosis in post-traumatic stress disorders. *Journal of Traumatic Stress* 1: 17–33.

Spiegel, D., Frischholz, E. J., and Spira, J. (1993). Functional disorders of memory. In A. Tasman and S. M. Goldfinger, eds., *American psychiatric press review of psychiatry.* Vol. 12 (pp. 747–782). Washington, D.C.: American Psychiatric Press.

Spiegel, D., Hunt, T., and Dondershine, H. E. (1988). Dissociation and hypnotizability in post traumatic stress disorder. *American Journal of Psychiatry* 145: 301–305.

Stevenson, J. A. (1976). Effect of posthypnotic dissociation on the performance of interfering tasks. *Journal of Abnormal Psychology* 85: 398–407.

Suarez, S. D., and Gallop, G. G. (1981). An ethological analysis of open-field behavior in rats and mice. *Learning and Motivation* 9: 153–163.

Swica, Y., Otnow Lewis, D., and Lewis, M. (1996). Child abuse and dissociative identity disorder/multiple personality disorder: The documentation of childhood maltreatment and the corroboration of symptoms. *Child and Adolescent Psychiatric Clinics of North America* 5: 431–447.

Terr, L. (1994). *Unchained memories: True stories of traumatic memories, lost and found.* New York: Basic Books.

van der Hart, O. (1994). Psychisch trauma, dissociatieve verschijnselen en meervoudige persoonlijkheidsstoornis: Complicaties in de gynaecologische en verloskundige praktijk. In A. A. W. Peters, I. M. M. Foeken, and Ph. Th. M. Weijenborg, eds., *Gevolgen van geweld voor de gynaecologische en verloskundige praktijk* (pp. 51–62). Leiden: Boerhave Commissie RU Leiden.

van der Hart, O., and Friedman, B. (1992). Trauma, dissociation and triggers: Their role in treatment and emergency psychiatry. In J. B. van Luyn et al., eds., *Emergency psychiatry today* (pp. 137–142). Amsterdam: Elsevier.

van der Hart, O., and Nijenhuis, E. R. S. (1995). Amnesia for traumatic experiences. *Hypnos* 22: 60–73.

van der Hart, O., and Op den Velde, W. (1995). Posttraumatische stoornissen. In O. van der Hart, ed., *Trauma, dissociatie en hypnose* (pp. 103–145). Lisse: Swets and Zeitlinger.

van der Hart, O., Steele, K., Boon, S., and Brown, P. (1993). The treatment of traumatic memories: Synthesis, realization, and integration. *Dissociation* 6: 162–180.

van der Hart, O., Nijenhuis, E. R. S., and van der Kolk, B. A. (submitted). Traumatic memories: Between reproductions and reconstructions.

van der Kolk, B. A. (1989). The compulsion to repeat the trauma. *Psychiatric Clinics of North America* 12: 389–411.

_____. (1994). The body keeps the score: Memory and the evolving psychobiology of posttraumatic stress. *Harvard Review of Psychiatry* 1: 253–265.

van der Kolk, B. A., and Ducey, C. P. (1989). The psychological processing of traumatic experience: Rorschach patterns in PTSD. *Journal of Traumatic Stress* 2: 259–274.

van der Kolk, B. A., and Fisler, R. (1995). Dissociation and the fragmentary nature of traumatic memories: Overview and exploratory study. *Journal of Traumatic Stress* 8: 505–525.

van der Kolk, B. A., Greenberg, M. S., Orr, S. P., and Pitman, R. K. (1989). Endogenous opioids, stress induced analgesia, and posttraumatic stress disorder. *Psychopharmacology Bulletin* 25: 417–422.

van der Kolk, B. A., and van der Hart, O. (1991). The intrusive past: The flexibility of memory and the engraving of trauma. *American Imago* 48: 425–454.

van der Kolk, B. A., van der Hart, O., and Marmar, C. R. (1996). Dissociation and information processing in posttraumatic stress disorder. In B. A. van der Kolk, A. C. McFarlane, and L. Weisaeth, eds., *Traumatic stress: The effects of overwhelming experience on mind, body, and society* (pp. 301–331). New York: Guilford.

Vanderlinden, J., Vandereycken, W., van Dyck, R., and Vertommen, H. (1993a). Dissociative experiences and trauma in eating disorders. *International Journal of Eating Disorders* 13: 187–193.

Vanderlinden, J., van Dyck, R., Vandereycken, W., Vertommen, H., and Verkes, R. J. (1993b). The dissociation questionnaire (DIS-Q): Development of a new self-report questionnaire. *Clinical Psychology and Psychotherapy* 1: 21–27.

Vijselaar, J., and van der Hart, O. (1992). The first report of hypnotic treatment of traumatic grief. *International Journal al Hypnosis* 40: 1–6.

Wolfe, J., Keane, T. M., Kaloupek, D. G., Mora, C. A., and Wine, P. (1993). Patterns of positive readjustment in Vietnam combat veterans. *Journal of Traumatic Stress* 6: 179–193.

Zatzick, D. F., Marmar, C. R., Weiss, D. S., and Metzler, T. (1994). Does trauma-linked dissociation vary across ethnic groups? *Journal of Nervous and Mental Disease* 182: 576–582.

CHAPTER 3

Assessment and Management of Somatoform Symptoms in Traumatized Patients

*Conceptual Overview
and Pragmatic Guide*

Richard J. Loewenstein
and Jean Goodwin

The association between traumatic life events and somatoform symptoms has been described repeatedly in the medical literature for over 150 years (Loewenstein 1990). Despite this historical finding and more sophisticated modern studies that support it, physicians and psychiatrists remain relatively unaware of the phenomenon. This professional blind spot has costs not only to the individual patients who receive inadequate assessment and treatment, but to society as a whole. It is well known that inappropriate medical interventions for somatoform symptoms lead to substantial unnecessary expenditure of health-care dollars (Cummings 1992; Smith, Monson and Ray 1986). There is a similar cost to society due to the medical sequelae of childhood maltreatment, a finding that is just beginning to be appreciated (Felitti et al. 1998).

The potential scope of these interrelated problems is considerable. Surveys report that during any week, 60 to 80 percent of the general population will suffer a somatic symptom (Cassem 1987; Kellner 1985). Other data show

67

that 60 percent of visits to physicians at a large California HMO studied over many years were for complaints without discoverable physical or biological difficulties (Cummings 1992). In these studies, another 20 to 30 percent of patients were seeking help for "stress-related" disorders such as irritable bowel syndrome (IBS).

To be sure, somatization is a complex problem with many determinants. These can include undiagnosed or misdiagnosed medical disorders; somatic symptoms due to *DSM-IV (Diagnostic and Statistical Manual of Mental Disorders)* disorders such as anxiety affective, psychotic and trauma disorders, as well as malingering and factitious disorders. Further, these conditions are not mutually exclusive; more than one can coexist in an individual patient (Ford 1983).

Conceptualization of somatoform disorders exists at the theoretical interface of the mind and the body; the person, the family and the culture; and the patient, the physician and the medical care system. Lazare (1981) suggests a "multidimensional approach" to somatization "in which there are both separate and simultaneous biologic, psychodynamic, sociocultural, and behavioral explanations" (p. 746).

In 1990, I published a review of the literature on the relationship of somatization and somatoform disorders to a history of childhood abuse, particularly, childhood sexual abuse (Loewenstein 1990). I reviewed the classical literature on hysteria, beginning with the works of Briquet (Briquet 1859) and Freud (Breuer and Freud 1893, 1895). Then I reviewed the more recent literature supporting the association between traumatic experiences and the development of somatoform disorders in adults and children. A large body of data from case reports as well as systematic studies supports the view that a substantial subset of patients with somatoform disorders have antecedent histories of abuse and trauma. In these studies, childhood trauma, particularly childhood sexual abuse, was thought to be a significant factor in the development of somatoform disorders in children, adolescents and adults.

In this chapter, I will extend the literature review to include studies published since 1990 that document the relationship between an antecedent history of childhood abuse and somatoform disorders. Further, data on the psychophysiologic and neurobiologic sequelae of abuse and trauma will be applied to understanding somatoform phenomena in this population. In addition, an overview will be given for the management of the trauma survivor with significant somatization.

MEDICAL SEQUELAE OF TRAUMA AND ABUSE

Trauma and abuse appear to be associated with significant direct negative consequences to health and subjective well-being, including "poor self-reported health, morbidity (as indicated by physical exam or laboratory tests), utilization of medical services, and mortality" (Schnurr 1996, 1). This observation has been reported across many populations, including combat veterans, survivors of childhood abuse, individuals subjected to interpersonal violence as adults and those subjected to natural disasters. Syndromal posttraumatic stress disorder (PTSD) itself is also associated with poorer health status.

Rosenberg and Krugman (1991) review the medical problems that commonly affect individuals subjected to childhood physical abuse, sexual abuse and/or neglect (see Table 3.1). These include scarring from beatings, burning or biting; limb and spine deformities due to fractures caused by abuse; and complications caused by failure to provide the child adequate medical attention after abuse-related injuries. Genital and anal mutilation may occur as part of specific sadistic acts by abusers or due to trauma occurring in the course of abuse. Urinary-tract pathology due to trauma and/or repeated infections may also be a consequence of childhood abuse.

Neurological damage can be caused by violent head trauma, shaking and similar acts. This can result in acquired mental retardation, seizure disorders, cerebral palsy, blindness, deafness and learning disabilities. Supervisional neglect can lead to accidental poisoning with alcohol and/or prescription, over-the-counter and/or street drugs as well as to abuse by extrafamilial caretakers. Medical neglect can lead to many threats to health, for example, never receiving childhood immunizations, lack of basic dental care, and permanent damage related to untreated common childhood disorders such as ear infections. Other forms of sensory impairment, speech disorders and developmental problems can also result from neglect of basic medical care. In some families, one might more accurately speak of medical abuse rather than medical neglect; one mother sewed up her daughter's cuts with string and a sewing needle, rather than take her to the emergency room.

Sexually transmitted diseases (STDs), including HIV infection, may result from abuse and can deprive the child of health, fertility or life. Incest pregnancy can occur with a variety of devastating effects, including induced abortions, some of which may be secret, illegal or even performed by the perpetrator or his or her associates.

TABLE 3.1

Physical Manifestations of Abuse in Children and Adults

Scars, deformities, mutilation from beatings, bites, fractures
Oral-facial trauma
Genital and anal injuries from abuse
Specific sadistic mutilation of breasts, genitals, and other organs
Traumatic accidents
Ingestion of poisons, medications, street drugs
Neurological and cerebral insults
Mental Retardation
Damage to special senses (hearing, vision, smell, taste)
Sexually transmitted diseases
Recurrent Urinary Tract Infections
Incest pregnancies, incest abortions
General medical neglect (lack of medical care, immunizations, etc.)

(Based on Rosenberg & Krugman, 1991)

Springs and Friedrich (1992) reported that a variety of health-risk behaviors and medical problems were more common in women with a history of childhood sexual abuse in a primary-care population (Table 3.2). Twenty-two percent of the 511 women in this clinic population reported childhood abuse. Health-risk behaviors predicted by abuse history included earlier age of onset and heavier smoking, greater likelihood of abuse of alcohol or drugs, earlier sexual experiences with more partners, earlier pregnancy and less frequent Pap smears. Medical problems more frequent in the abuse group included a higher incidence of pelvic inflammatory disease (PID), breast disease, yeast infections, overweight and frequent surgeries. The latter finding has been reported frequently in the literature with a subgroup of abused women categorized as "polysurgery" addicts (Engel 1959).

Subsequent studies in larger population groups have extended these findings. Felitti et al. (1988) studied 9,508 adults in a large HMO. Data were acquired on respondents' history of "adverse childhood experience" including psychological, physical or sexual abuse; domestic violence directed at the mother; or living with household members with a history of substance abuse, mental illness, suicidality or incarceration. Subjects with 4 or more categories of adverse experiences, compared to those with none, had a 4–12 fold increased risk for drug abuse, alcoholism, depression and suicide attempts. These subjects also showed a 2–4-fold increase in risk for smoking, poor subjective health status, sexually transmitted diseases and more sexual

TABLE 3.2

Health-Risk Behaviors and Medical Illnesses More Commonly Found Among Abused Individuals in a Primary Care Setting

Earlier age of onset and heavier smoking
Alcohol and drug abuse
Earlier sexual intercourse onset, more partners
Earlier pregnancy
Less frequent Pap smears
Sexually Transmitted Diseases and Pelvic Inflamatory Disease
Breast disease
Frequency of yeast infections
Overweight
More surgeries
Depression and suicide attempts
Poor subjective sense of health

(From Springs and Friedrich 1992; Felitti et al. 1988)

partners. They were also at greater risk for severe obesity. These was a "graded relationship" between adverse childhood experiences and adult disease including cancer, ischemic heart disease, chronic lung disease, liver disease and fractures. Multiple exposures to adverse life events in childhood predicted multiple health-risk factors in adulthood.

TRAUMATIC EXPERIENCES
AND SOMATOFORM DISORDERS

One can look at the relationship between traumatic experiences and somatization from different vantage points. A number of reports describe patients with somatoform disorders such as somatization disorder, pain disorder or conversion disorder and attempt to explore the relation between traumatic experiences and these conditions (Walker et al. 1992; Walker et al. 1993).

From another perspective, there is a growing literature that describes symptoms and behavioral problems in individuals reporting a history of traumatic experiences, particularly childhood physical and sexual abuse. Many of these studies describe high rates of multiple somatic symptoms in this population (Maynes and Feinauer 1994; McCauley et al. 1995; McCauley et al. 1997; Saxe et al. 1994). Typical symptom patterns include headaches, face and head pain, musculoskeletal complaints, gastrointestinal problems, genitourinary difficulties, breathing problems, menstrual problems, fatigue and pseudoneurological symptoms such as pseudoepilepsy, fainting and weakness. *DSM-IV* disorders commonly diagnosed in the trauma-survivor population include affective disorders, PTSD and other anxiety disorders, dissociative disorders, eating disorders and substance-abuse disorders. These may also contribute to the somatic symptoms commonly reported by this population.

Despite the robust findings across studies, methodological issues make some comparisons among studies problematic. Researchers may have different theoretical biases, basic paradigms and study populations, for example, primary versus tertiary care and psychiatric versus general medical populations. There may be differing study designs and assessment measures, for example, retrospective versus prospective, questionnaire versus patient interview, or different sample sizes, response rates and varying definitions of abuse and abuse severity. Unless carefully questioned, traumatized individuals commonly underreport their trauma experiences, particularly those of physical and sexual violence (Carlson et al. 1998; Williams 1994)). On the other hand, concern has been raised about possible overreporting of traumatic experiences in some populations (Chu 1998).

Several recent studies look at large populations of patients and assess the relationship between traumatic experiences, PTSD, and somatization. McCauley and her colleagues (1995, 1997) have reported on the health consequences of adult domestic violence and childhood abuse, respectively, in over 1900 women in an urban primary-care internal-medicine practice.

One hundred and eight of 1,952 respondents (5.5 percent) had experienced domestic violence in the previous year, assessed by stringent criteria on a self-report measure. Four hundred and eighteen (24 percent of those reporting) had experienced domestic violence sometime in their adult lives. Of those reporting abuse in the past year, 30 (39 percent) reported two to three episodes of abuse; 21 (27.3 percent) reported four or more abuse episodes. Forty-nine percent (of 103 responses) reported "high-severity abuse," including use of weapons, burning and choking and/or hitting, resulting in broken bones or head or internal injuries.

Women who had experienced recent domestic violence were significantly more likely to have more physical symptoms (mean = 7.3) and had higher scores on measures of depression, anxiety, somatization and interpersonal sensitivity, compared with nontraumatized women form the same cohort. Patients reporting six or more somatic symptoms were five times more likely to report abuse than subjects with between zero and two somatic symptoms.

Symptoms associated with current abuse included loss of appetite, eating binges or self-induced vomiting, abdominal or stomach pain, diarrhea, vaginal discharge, pelvic or genital pain, fainting or passing out, headaches, sleeping problems, nightmares, shortness of breath, chest pain and urinary problems. Other findings included higher rates of substance abuse, partner substance abuse, suicide attempts, and ER visits, but not psychiatric admissions in the domestic violence group.

In a subsequent report, McCauley et al. (1997) evaluated childhood physical and/or sexual abuse in the same population. Of 1,931 subjects, 424 (22 percent) reported a history of childhood sexual and/or physical abuse. The abuse subjects reported significantly more somatic symptoms, with a mean of 6.2 symptoms. Somatoform symptoms significantly associated with a history of childhood abuse included: back pain, frequent and severe headaches, pelvic and genital pain, tiredness, abdominal pain, vaginal discharge, breast pain, choking sensation, diarrhea, constipation, urinary problems, chest pain, face pain, shortness of breath and frequent bruising.

Abused women had significantly higher mean scores on measures of anxiety, depression, somatization and interpersonal sensitivity/low self-esteem. High scores on these measures predicted membership in the childhood-abuse group. Women reporting both adult victimization and childhood abuse had higher levels of physical and psychological symptoms than women reporting only childhood abuse. Abused women were more likely to have been psychiatrically hospitalized, to have been suicidal and to have had substance-abuse problems.

Van der Kolk et al. (1996) reported on dissociation, PTSD, affect dysregulation and somatization in a population of 395 traumatized individuals seeking treatment and 125 nontreatment-seeking traumatized subjects as part of the *DSM-IV* PTSD field trials. Subjects were studied using a variety of standardized measures. The authors found highly significant intercorrelations between PTSD, dissociation, somatization and affect dysregulation in subjects with a current or lifetime history of PTSD. Even subjects who did not meet criteria for current PTSD, but who had a lifetime history of PTSD, suffered from high levels of dissociation, somatization and affect dysregulation. Mental-health treatment was sought for dissociation and affect dysregulation, but not for somatization. It was thought that patients with a predominance of somatoform symptoms related to traumatization might be more likely to seek assistance in the medical care system, perhaps with costly and ineffective results.

Interestingly, studies of patients with dissociative identity disorder/multiple personality disorder (DID/MPD) have consistently reported high rates of dissociation, high rates of comorbid PTSD (90–100 percent in some samples) and very high rates of intercurrent somatization (Armstrong and Loewenstein 1990; Loewenstein 1990; Saxe et al. 1994). Many of these patients are described as also meeting diagnostic criteria for Briquet's syndrome/somatization disorder (BS/SD), conversion disorder and pain disorder (see Chapter 4, this volume). High rates of somatoform disorders have been described in other populations of dissociative patients, such as those with dissociative amnesia (DA; Coons and Millstein 1992).

In our own data from the Sheppard Pratt Health Systems Trauma Disorders Program, 98 percent of 148 dissociative disorder patients met *DSM-III-R/DSM-IV* criteria for a somatoform disorder based on structured interview data. Ninety-five percent of the patients reported physical and/or sexual abuse as a child, with 92 percent reporting childhood sexual abuse and 84 percent describing childhood physical abuse. This sample of patients reported a mean number of 15.72 somatoform symptoms. Patients meeting diagnostic criteria for somatization disorder had a mean of 22.4 somatic symptoms. One patient endorsed 34 somatoform symptoms! These patients also reported high rates of medical care utilization, with frequent emergency room visits, outpatient medical visits and hospitalization for both emergency and nonemergency medical and surgical care. Our estimate was that utilization rates were several times that for the general population (Smith et al. 1986).

Systematic studies looking at trauma, childhood abuse and dissociation in patients with specific somatoform disorders, such as Briquet's syndrome/somatization disorder, have found similar associations between somatization, dissociation and abuse (Morrison 1989; Pribor et al. 1993). Pribor et al. (1993) studied 100 women in the *DSM-IV* field trials for somatization disorder. More than 90 percent of women meeting criteria for Briquet's syndrome (BS) reported a history of sexual, physical or emotional abuse as a child or adult (in this study all patients meeting *DSM-III-R* and *DSM-IV* criteria for somatization disorder were analyzed together as patients with BS). Eighty percent of the BS women reported sexual abuse before the age of seventeen. Abused individuals had significantly higher rates of somatoform symptoms, compared with nonabused women. Dissociative Experiences Scale (DES; Bernstein and Putnam 1986) scores were also significantly elevated in abused individuals, but this correlated more strongly with the presence of a sexual abuse history than with somatization.

In a parallel development, a series of systematic studies from researchers in psychiatry, internal medicine, gastroenterology, neurology, orthopedics and gynecology have demonstrated much higher rates of childhood and adult sexual trauma and abuse, affective symptoms and/or dissociation, compared with controls in patients with unexplained chronic pelvic pain, irritable bowel syndrome (IBS), gastroesophageal reflux disorder (GERD), pseudoseizures, fibromyalgia, late luteal phase dysphoric disorder (LLPDD), morbid obesity, chronic low back pain and migraine headaches (Walker et al. 1992, 1993; Loewenstein 1990; Scarcini et al. 1994). A subgroup of eating-disorder patients with high rates of childhood abuse and high DES scores has also been described (Demitrack et al. 1990).

Scarcini et al. (1994) used standardized pain/nocioception paradigms to study patients with IBS, GERD and noncardiac chest pain (NCCP). A history of childhood sexual abuse was much more prevalent in GERD (92 percent) and IBS patients (82 percent), compared with NCCP patients, who reported a frequency of childhood sexual abuse similar to that of the general population (27 percent). Abused patients reported more psychiatric symptoms, pain symptoms, anxiety, tension, reactivity to everyday "hassles" and disability.

Abused patients had significantly lower pain-threshold levels and were much more likely to judge neutral stimuli as noxious. Thus, relatively normal or minor discomforts related to the body would be interpreted as noxious. Abuse subjects were thought to be "hypervigilant" for noxious internal and external stimuli.

Accordingly, a cognitive vicious circle was described in which the abused subjects' hypervigilance, hopelessness, negative self-perceptions and self-blame led to increased pain perception, pain complaints and disability. Repeated lack of medical explanation for the pain and repeated unsuccessful interactions with health care providers reinforced the self-blame, hopelessness, disability and futile search for magical relief.

ASSESSMENT, MANAGEMENT AND TREATMENT OF SOMATIZATION IN THE PATIENT WITH A HISTORY OF TRAUMA

Clinicians of every sort and level of experience face difficulties in providing effective care for patients with chronic somatoform disorders. This is particularly so where somatization and a history of maltreatment, victimization and abuse coincide. In this section, we will focus on the pitfalls that await the clinician in evaluating and managing the somatizing patient with a history of abuse. In addition, we will describe clinical strategies that may assist the clinician in work with this difficult patient population. It may be helpful to articulate some common areas of difficulty at the outset.

The clinical situation with the somatizing patient is inherently ambiguous. In many clinical situations, there is no definitive medical test to "prove" that a symptom or symptom cluster is caused by a somatoform condition as opposed to a medical illness. In fact, somatoform symptoms, medical symptoms and amplification of medical symptoms can all coexist in the same patient. At different times, any one (or more) of these may explain an upsurge in symptoms.

Accordingly, the clinician and the patient must both learn to tolerate ambiguity in assessment of symptoms. Repeated medical workup, multiple invasive procedures and extensive search for arcane medical explanations for symptoms should be carefully weighed against the possible risks. These include reinforcement of somatization, potential side effects and complications of procedures (requiring further medical evaluation and treatment), and failure to treat somatoform disorders psychotherapeutically while the seemingly endless search for medical pathology goes on.

The diagnosis of somatization should not imply a pejorative view of the patient. Chronic somatization is a serious, costly clinical problem. It does not imply that "nothing is wrong." All partners in the somatization situation need to understand that somatoform symptoms are just as "real," although etiologically different, from symptoms more usually understood as "medical" in origin. We tend to be dominated by Cartesian dualism about the mind and the body. In fact, epistemologically, conceptualization of medical and somatoform symptoms involve the same process of our organizing human phenomena into categories of health and illness (Sedgwick 1982). Clinically, it is helpful to remember that all disorders have both a somatic and psychic representation. *All* symptoms are "in the mind," since this is the center of awareness of all physical processes for human beings.

Further, it is well established that perception of symptoms, thresholds and styles for conveying physical distress, and expectations of helping persons may be influenced by sociocultural factors, personality variables, level of anxiety and perceived locus of control, among others. (Leigh 1983). Neurobiological factors may also account for some of the differences in pain perceptions in clinical populations. For example, Pitman and his colleagues (Pitman, van der Kolk, Orr & Greenburg, 1990) found that combat veterans with PTSD had a higher baseline threshold for perception of certain types of exogenous pain compared with combat veterans without PTSD. Data were developed linking this finding to alterations in endorphin function thought to be related to traumatization.

Many trauma patients show simultaneous or oscillating numbing and lack of concern over externally validated physical difficulties, alternating with hypersensitivity and preoccupation with somatic problems that defy physical explanation. These oscillations can be viewed as parallel to the basic process of numbing/intrusion seen in PTSD. Maladaptive cognitive patterns in trauma patients characterized by minimization of significant problems and "catastrophizing" minimal ones also parallel this process (Fine 1990).

The adult survivor of childhood abuse and trauma, especially repeated trauma, may be subject to a variety of psychological processes that complicate his/her participation in the process of assessment of symptoms. These include chronic depersonalization often combined with a sense of chronic alienation and rejection of the body. Some patients are relatively unconcerned about repeated self-injury and its medical sequelae. These patients also may ignore severe symptoms indicative of significant medical problems. At other times, the same patients will become doggedly, obsessively focused on somatoform symptoms that either are without clear medical explanation or are due to relatively minor or nonprogressive medical problems. They may repeatedly seek medical consultation and procedures to "prove" that a significant medical problem is present.

Many patients with a history of severe early trauma will have significant difficulty giving a clear medical history or participating in the medical workup. Studies suggest that individuals with histories of abuse are unlikely to report this unless specifically asked about abuse in the medical or psychiatric history (Briere 1993). In addition, the patient may be amnesic for important parts of his/her life history and unable to report accurately because of this. Patients may fail to report important information because of shame and embarrassment over abuse or maltreatment. Patients may be limited in the ability to undergo physical examinations because of posttraumatic reactivity to being touched, taking off clothing, and/or having specific parts of the exam such as pelvic or rectal examinations. Some patients will avoid medical care altogether, just as others compulsively seek medical workup.

Additionally, trauma patients may report adverse experiences with medical professionals in the past. These can include reported failure of the medical profession to realize that the patient was being abused when brought for medical care as a child, including for injuries or illnesses related to abuse and/or neglect. The patient may report psychological insensitivity, emotional abuse and even medical cruelty at the hands of medical professionals and allied personnel. Some patients report sexual exploitation by medical professionals in either childhood or adulthood. On the other hand, some patients report that encounters with medical professionals and/or hospitalization were among the only benign experiences during an early life characterized by extremes of cruelty, brutality, sadism and neglect. These patients may develop a "Munchausen"-like pattern of seeking medical care as an attempt to find solace in life.

It can be difficult to find the proper balance in assessing and providing treatment for these complex patients. There may be a pressure for the roles of medical and psychotherapeutic professionals to become blurred. The psychiatrist becomes the internist, the internist becomes the psychotherapist, and the nonmedical therapist may attempt to act as a physician. The classic case of Anna O exemplifies the story of the physician who becomes over-involved with a compelling somatizing patient, with problematic outcome for both parties (Loewenstein 1993). Increasingly aggressive and heroic diagnostic and treatment strategies frequently lead to the same result: continued severe symptoms and complaints. If additional complications arise from recommended interventions, this may amplify even further the patient's sense of futility, misunderstanding and desperation. Ultimately, the most common outcome is the angry rejection of the patient. The patient is bewildered and devastated that the promise of "cure" has now been replaced by another painful loss and reinforcement of the idea of blame and badness: "It's all in your mind! Go see the psychiatrist!"

The patient comes to the psychiatric assessment already hurt, confused, angry and oppositional: "They tell me it's all in my mind, but I know something is wrong with my body." Despite this, the psychiatrist's proper task is, with the patient, to help clarify the biopsychosocial components of the patient's symptoms. The psychiatrist also may serve as an intermediary for the patient vis-à-vis the medical care system. The psychiatrist (or other mental health clinician) can begin to form an alliance with the patient by educating the patient about the problems of evaluating somatization that have been outlined above.

An overview of the patient's history of childhood trauma can often clarify for the clinician traumatic antecedents of the patient's style of interaction with the medical care system. If there was medical neglect, the patient may unconsciously believe that only an "emergency" presentation will result in being cared for: "In my family, unless the bone was sticking out of my arm, they wouldn't take me to the doctor." The clinician can then clarify how this understandable stance can create many problems in getting adequate medical care and forming positive relationships with medical providers. The patient can be taught more adaptive ways to relate to the health care system based on the patient's actual current medical needs. Separating "past from present" may allow the traumatized patient more freedom in seeking health care and participating in the examination and workup.

It is often helpful to observe that it is a shame that the individuals who reportedly abused and/or neglected the patient are still experienced as such a forceful presence in the patient's life. They thus continue to interfere with the patient's right to basic health care. Trauma patients are often surprised at the idea that they have a "right" to health care. This formulation is often very helpful in assisting even those patients with profound phobic avoidance of medical assessment to participate in routine care and even to undergo procedures they perceive as markedly aversive.

Living in a kind of "emergency mode" is a common style of existence for many childhood trauma survivors. These patients commonly find it amazing that clinicians can listen *better* if routine complaints are not presented as emergencies. It may be helpful to remind the patient that when clinicians go into an emergency mode, they are focused on very broad clinical decisions: Does the patient need to be in the hospital? Can the patient be managed on an acute basis as an outpatient? If so, what other emergency interventions might be required? And so on. A helpful metaphor is to remind the patient that when the fireman is taking you out of the burning building, he is not in a frame of mind to listen to your life story: "Why don't you sit on the curb over there. When we have the fire put out, then maybe I can listen to your story."

There are several other broad principles of care that apply to medical complaints in trauma survivors. The patient needs to have confidence that the treater's first priority is to rule out life-threatening conditions—whether medical or psychosocial. This may make the patient more open to accepting the clinician's view of the ambiguity and uncertainty that is inherent in the clinical situation. Medical factors should not be minimized, however. At least some of the patient's problems may be due either to medical illnesses or to conditions like IBS that have both medical and stress-related aspects. Not infrequently, a new medical problem or exacerbation of an old one is missed since the patient is perceived as a "crock," and/or the patient's mal-adaptive style of communicating with caregivers interferes with adequate assessment.

Psychotherapy for patients with chronic trauma disorders is usually more successful if the patient is encouraged to be an active collaborator in the treatment. This does not mean, however, that the clinician relinquishes clin-ical judgement and responsibility for structuring treatment goals and mak-ing clinical decisions. Rather, this stance involves the recognition by both parties that clinical gains are unlikely unless the patient makes an active commitment to risk engagement in the therapeutic process. Byck (1978) points out that: "There is a convenient myth that doctors give treatment. Doctors rarely treat; they usually give advice . . . [T]he patient goes forth to treat himself" (p. 110).

Conversely, the traumatized patient frequently perceives the clinician as being in "control" of the therapeutic process. The patient often reacts as if his/her autonomy is threatened by the clinician's advice and interventions. Reflexively saying "no" or persisting in maladative solutions to problems are common reactions of patients in this situation. It is important to point out to the patient that the clinician, far from being in full control, is more likely to be reactive to the patient's style of communication and statement of problems. For example, if the patient insists that he/she is going to act in a life-threatening or severely self-destructive way, the clinician's reaction is predictable. Unless safety can be reestablished, some involuntary interven-tion to protect the patient can be anticipated.

Our cultural split between mind and body creates a climate in which it can be very difficult for patients or their loved ones to grasp the absolute ambiguity that characterizes these somatic symptoms. The patient, espe-cially if dissociative, may have no basis for understanding that discomfort is perceived, modified and expressed through the mind and is therefore de-pendent on psychological state, anxiety level, mood, sense of cognitive con-trol, as well as a host of other individual and cultural factors. Conversely, in highly hypnotizable dissociative patients, serious physical problems can be completely masked by dissociative disengagement with the body character-ized by profound numbing of physical perception and/or minimization of significant symptoms. Patients respond positively, however, if they are edu-cated about these issues. Frequently, they can readily find examples in their own history to confirm these observations. They then become more astute observers of their own internal psychological and physical states.

As sequential physical and psychological interventions prove successful in resolving symptoms, the patient may move from certainty that their cause is purely physical, then back to uncertainty to certainty in the other direction—"it's a post-traumatic symptom"—and finally back to the fundamental doubleness that characterizes these symptoms. As in the riddle, "What has four wings and flies?" the answer is easy once you allow yourself to envision two birds, rather than just a single rare and monstrous creature. Serious medical illness and childhood trauma often coexist. Once dissociation is cleared away, we often find that more problems than one have been concealed by it.

Several case examples illustrate this frequent pattern. A dissociative patient repeatedly underwent workup and physical therapy for chronic back pain out of proportion to the physical findings. Psychological explorations were repeatedly unrevealing about hidden dynamics relating to somatization. When, in exasperation, her psychotherapist suggested that the patient use her limited financial resources for a specialized pain rehabilitation program rather than psychotherapy, she revealed a group of alters who accounted for the persistence of the pain complaints: "We've been hiding Daddy in our back." Cognitive-behavioral therapy and working through of traumatic recollections with these self-aspects provided significant symptomatic relief and functional improvement with decreased hypervigilance, improved sleep and significantly reduced muscle tension. The patient no longer required physical and rehabilitation therapy.

However, several years later, the pain and disability returned. Unfortunately, this time, psychosocial interventions remained of relatively little assistance. The patient had progressed dramatically in psychotherapy, was mostly integrated and had begun to enjoy life for the first time. Now, she was diagnosed with spinal stenosis. As this condition progressed, producing significant disability, the patient experienced marked grief about the lost years of dysfunction related to PTSD and DID. She felt profoundly unfairly treated: Just when she might have been able to enjoy her life, she experienced a disabling physical condition. This in turn had to be worked through therapeutically to facilitate adjustment and rehabilitation.

A patient whose menstrual-related migraines had just been diagnosed announced, in an alter-identity state, "those are my father's headaches." She worked through memories of sexual abuse that she recalled frequently occurred during her menstrual periods. Ultimately, several types of interventions were necessary in order for her to gain better control of her migraine pain. Substance abuse treatment helped her give up reliance on opiates for pain control; cognitive-behavioral therapy focused on trauma-related issues; a systematic medical approach focused on diet and rational pharmacology; and hypnotherapy provided another symptom control measure for PTSD symptoms and migraine pain.

In another case, somatic symptoms were caused entirely by newly diagnosed diabetes mellitus. However, the meaning of this medical diagnosis for the patient triggered an exacerbation of her posttraumatic, depressive and dissociative symptoms. One of her reported intrafamilial abusers had also suffered from this illness. For the patient, the new diagnosis symbolized her fearful fantasy that the legacy of her unfortunate childhood was irreversible and inscribed in her genome. In addition, there was a related fear that her unconscious identifications with her abuser could never be undone: "I'll never be rid of her." She felt cursed from the grave by her relative.

Severely dissociative patients can so compartmentalize their lives that there are medical and psychiatric clinicians working with them who do not know of the existence of one another. For example, one young woman pursued a complex treatment plan in the psychiatry clinic for depression. The emergency room staff knew her because of multiple visits for unsubstantiated rape complaints. She visited the obstetric clinic almost monthly insistent that she was pregnant, but always registering a negative test. Until these complaints could all be heard together, there was no hope of understanding them as a traumatic sequence that reenacted in detail childhood sexual abuse. The latter history was documented in still a fourth medical record, again unknown to any of the other three treatment teams.

Our health care system does not systematically encourage coordination of care. However, some habits of practice can facilitate teamwork: Whenever possible, obtain old and concurrent records; share records or leave even the briefest of telephone messages with other members of the treatment team. Knowing that the door is open for communication is often what is most important. A few minutes of explanation or reassurance around a new development or a crisis may be all that is needed to allow treatment to progress.

As the treatment focus shifts from search for cure to coping and health promotion, many sessions will include a psychoeducational focus with attention to the trauma-related symptoms that interfere with prudent and wise self-care. Smoking and substance abuse may have developed as symptom management techniques. The idea of relinquishing them may lead to panic. If staying busy is what has held anxiety at bay, medical advice "to rest" may feel like a catastrophe. Where medication has been used to obliterate certain negative feeling states, the notion of judicious use of medication may be unintelligible. Exercise or physical therapy may suddenly put patients in touch with their bodies that they have previously tried to dismiss, discount, detach from and disown. Psychological paralysis may ensue with inability to utilize these treatments. Conversely, some patients may develop inappropriate erotized or frankly sexual involvement with physical therapists and "body workers" that complicate medical and psychotherapeutic interventions. These boundariless relationships around manipulation of the body also frequently appear to recapitulate traumatic scenarios, relationships and/or attempts to defend against recollection of these.

At times the situation can be clarified by pointing out conflicts between two coping tracks: "The old way and the new way." The idea of a new healthy way of living may be approached first in imagery using metaphors about healing, cleansing, renewal, growth, safety and serenity. It is important to remember that symptoms serve many functions: to substitute for missing memories, to communicate distress, to symbolize crucial relationships, to contain internal conflicts, to manage interpersonal issues. If gentle probing elicits a great deal of resistance around the idea of losing a particular symptom, the focus must shift from symptom relief to understanding the symptom's many meanings and functions.

The idea that the body is impervious, unaffected by what happens to it has often been a central defense in coping with abuse. This view must be amended in all of these patients, but especially those whose pathological stress-reduction "techniques"—eating disorders, substance abuse, smoking—are beginning to take a toll on their physical well-being. Osteoporosis, dental disease, morbid obesity and its complications, liver disease, pulmonary disease, HIV infection, carcinoma become the focus of medical attention, often complicated by the patient's difficulties in adaptive engagement with the medical care system. The clinician is now confronted with an even more demoralized, depleted, hopeless, self-destructive, grief-stricken patient with reduced motivation for meaningful therapeutic work. The patient's trauma-based coping methods of dissociation, acting out, and addictive and compulsive behaviors only compound adaptation to severe illness. Limited social supports and/or enmeshment in pathological family systems add to the difficulty in working with these patients. These cases are among the most difficult to manage and treat among the trauma-survivor population.

PSYCHOPHARMACOLOGICAL MANAGEMENT

As discussed above, the psychiatrist's main tasks are to manage psychiatric symptoms—in many cases, posttraumatic and dissociative symptoms—so that they do not further confuse the somatic problems and to assist the patient in interacting positively with the medical treatment team. Pharmacotherapy must often begin with an attempt to rationalize a regimen of more and less inappropriate medications and/or medication dosages. Often, these have accrued as overwhelmed treaters have tried to manage the patient's refractory plethora of symptoms, complaints and dysphoria. The patient may have become desperately over-reliant on medications that provide marginal relief often at the cost of problematic (often covert) side effects. The somatizing trauma patient may be fixed on having *something* to take, rather than risking dysphoria. Patients may resist nonpharmacological interventions, obdurately insisting that there must be a pill for every symptom. Inpatient staffs who treat these patients are frequently nonplussed by the patient's need to take a pill, often *any* pill if they are having difficulties with physical discomfort, anxiety or dysphoria.

Side effects may result in additional medications being prescribed. Opiates given for pain may lead to constipation causing more pain, requiring more medicines to treat these side effects. Sedation or disinhibition by anxiolytic or analgesic medications may also complicate the patient's ability to think, process and evaluate sensory information whether from somatic sensations or form the outside world. Insisting that the patient attempt to bear reduction or discontinuation of medicines that cause more problems than they solve is an essential task for the psychiatrist treating these patients.

On the other hand, while it is essential to help the patient discontinue truly inappropriate medications, in some cases it may be counterproductive to be a purist. A particular agent may not be optimal from a purely rational point of view. However, it may provide some helpful symptom control or containment. It may provide a needed placebo for a problem the patient finds intolerable. Consequently, the potential psychological disruption of an immediate medication change may outweigh the theoretical gains that are envisioned.

Countertransference exasperation in the caregivers may complicate this situation. A patient had to be hospitalized psychiatrically after her internist precipitously and angrily began discontinuing her long list of medications. Unfortunately, although the patient was on a number of medications of marginal efficacy, he elected initially to discontinue the patient's effective SSRI antidepressant. This resulted in a profound pseudopsychotic reaction in which the patient manifested recrudescence of depression, probable SSRI withdrawal symptoms, marked depersonalization and a posttraumatic panic that all helpful treatment would be "taken away." This paralleled the patient's recollections of childhood punishments in which objects she loved reportedly were destroyed or discarded.

This same patient precipitated many of her own difficulties, however. Like so many somatizing trauma patients, she obdurately clung to the idea that a pill should be found for every symptom. She was resistant to the idea that many PTSD, dissociative and somatic symptoms at best are only partially medication-responsive. She had been taught a variety of behavioral and self-hypnotic symptom management techniques. Although she found them helpful, she either refused or "forgot" to use them. She sought repeated medical evaluations and medication trials. She suffered from an unusual, stable endocrine disorder making it that much more difficult to resist additional medical tests for her manifold and shifting symptoms.

This case illustrates a major issue in the psychopharmacological management of the complex PTSD patient. Medications may be efficacious for depressive, PTSD, anxiety, OCD and some pseudopsychotic symptoms in this population. However, medication response is likely to be partial, and readily obscured by symptoms engendered by additional life stress. A helpful metaphor for these patients is to liken medications to a "shock absorber" for an automobile. Shock absorber efficacy may depend on the characteristics of the vehicle, the type of shock absorber used, and the overall characteristics of the terrain the vehicle must negotiate. Shock absorbers may need to be repaired or reinforced under particularly rough driving conditions. If the road is particularly rough, one may not appreciate what the shock absorbers are doing. Remove them, however, and one becomes much more appreciative of the job they have done all along.

Collaboration between clinician and patient in assessment of level of symptoms and efficacy of medication interventions becomes even more essential when medication response is partial in this way. Patients may become quite adept at wondering: "If I wasn't taking this, and all this was going on in my life, what level of symptoms would I have?"

The "trauma frame of reference" is often the most helpful organizing construct to assist the clinician in making real progress with these complex patients. Many of them really can make improvements in their physical well-being and in their relationship with the medical care system. In addition, data suggest that costs of care for somatoform disorders is considerable and may be reduced by more appropriate psychosocial interventions, particularly around trauma-based symptoms (Smith et al. 1986).

SUMMARY

The literature on somatization consistently supports a relationship with traumatic life events. Medical and somatoform symptoms described in studies of traumatized patients have an almost numbing consistency from study to study. Traumatic experiences, particularly domestic violence and child abuse, are the largest single preventable cause of psychiatric morbidity in our culture. In addition, it is now clear that they are related to significant adverse medical health consequences as well. In order to be successful, treatment must remain centered in the dual psychic and somatic nature of these clinical problems. Clinicians are more successful if they can be tolerant of ambiguity, humble in the face of their realistic limitation and accepting of the long-term nature of these patients' problems. The process of trying to live inside one's body in a positive and healthy way is a core aspect of trauma recovery.

REFERENCES

Armstrong, J. G., and Loewenstein, R. J. (1990). Characteristics of patients with multiple personality and dissociative disorders on psychological testing. *Journal of Nervous and Mental Disease* 178: 448–454.

Bernstein, E. M., and Putnam, F. W. (1986). Development, reliability, and validity of a dissociation scale. *Journal of Nervous and Mental Disease* 174: 727–735.

Breuer, J., and Freud, S. (1893–1895). Studies in hysteria. In J. Strachey, ed., vol. 2 of *The complete psychological works of Sigmund Freud.* London: Hogarth Press.

Briquet, P. (1859). *Traite de l'hysterie.* Paris: J. Bailliere.

Byck, R. (1978). Psychologic factors in drug administration. In K. L. Melmon and H. F. Morrelli, eds., *Clinical pharmacology: Basic principles in therapeutics,* 2nd ed. (pp. 110–126). New York: Macmillan.

Carlson, E. B., Armstrong, J., Loewenstein, R., and Roth, D. (1998). Relationships between traumatic experiences and symptoms of posttraumatic stress, dissociation, and amnesia. In J. D. Bremner and C. R. Marmar, eds., *Trauma, memory, and dissociation* (pp. 205–227). Washington, D.C.: American Psychiatric Press.

Cassem, N. H. (1987). Functional somatic symptoms and somatoform disorders. In T. P. Hackan and N. H. Cassem, eds., *Massachusetts general hospital handbook of general hospital psychiatry,* 2d ed. Boston: Littleton, PSG Publishers.

Chu, J. A. (1998). Dissociative symptomatology in adult patients with histories of childhood physical and sexual abuse. In J. D. Bremner and C. R. Marmar, eds., *Trauma, memory, and dissociation* (pp. 179–202). Washington, D.C.: American Psychiatric Press.

Coons, P. M., and Millstein, V. (1992). Psychogenic amnesia: A clinical investigation of 25 cases. *Dissociation* 5 (2): 73–79.

Cummings, N. (1992). Psychologists: An essential component to cost-effective, innovative care. *Psychotherapy in Private Practice* 10: 137–143.

Demitrack, M. A., Putnam, F. W., Brewerton, H A., Brandt, H. A., and Gold, P. W. (1990). Relation of clinical variables to dissociative phenomena in eating disorders. *American Journal of Psychiatry* 147: 1184–1188.

Engel, G. L. (1959). "Psychogenic" pain and the pain-prone patient. *American Journal of Medicine* 26: 899–918.

Felitti, V. J., Nordenburg, D., Williamson, D. F., Spitz, A. M., Edwards, V., Koss, M. P., and Marks, J. S. (1988). Relationship of childhood abuse and household dysfunction to many of the leading causes of death in adults. The adverse childhood experiences (ACE) study. *American Journal of Preventative Medicine* 14(4): 245–258.

Fine, C. G. (1990). The cognitive sequelae of incest. In R. P. Kluft, ed., *Incest-related disorders of adult psychopathology* (pp. 161–182). Washington D.C.: American Psychiatric Press.

Ford, C. V. (1983). *The somatizing disorders: Illness as a way of life.* New York: Elsevier Biomedical.

Kellner, R. (1985). Functional somatic symptoms and hypochondriasis: A survey of empirical studies. *Archives of General Psychiatry* 42: 821–833.

Lazare, A. (1981). Conversion symptoms. *New England Journal of Medicine* 305: 745–748.

Leigh, H., ed. (1983). *Psychiatry in the practice of medicine.* Menlo Park, Calif.: Addison-Wesley.

Loewenstein, R. J. (1990). Somatoform disorders in victims of incest and child abuse. In R. P. Kluft, ed., *Incest-related disorders of adult psychopathology* (pp. 75–113). Washington D.C.: American Psychiatric Press.

———. (1993). Anna O: Reformulation as a case of multiple personality disorder. In J. Goodwin, ed., *Rediscovering childhood trauma: Historical casebook and clinical applications* (pp. 139–167). Washington, D.C.: American Psychiatric Press.

Maynes, L. C., and Feinauer, L. L. (1994). Acute and chronic dissociation and somatized anxiety as related to childhood sexual abuse. *American Journal of Family Therapy* 22: 165–175.

McCauley, J., Kern, D. E., Kolodner, K., Schroeder, A. F., DeChant, H. K., Ryden, J., Derogatis, L. R., and Bass, E. B. (1995). The battering syndrome: Prevalence and clinical characteristics of domestic violence in primary care internal medicine practice. *Annals of Internal Medicine* 123 (17): 737–746.

_____. (1997). Clinical characteristics of women with a history of childhood abuse: Unhealed wounds. *Journal of the American Medical Association* 277 (17): 1362–1368.

Morrison, J. (1989). Childhood sexual abuse histories of women with somatization disorder. *American Journal of Psychiatry* 146: 239-241.

Pitman, R. K., van der Kolk, B. A., Orr, S. P., and Greenburg, M. S. (1990). Naloxone-reversible analgesic response to combat-related stimuli in posttraumatic stress disorder: A pilot study. *Archives of General Psychiatry* 47: 541–544.

Pribor, E. F., Yutzy, S. H., Dean, T., and Wetzel, R. D. (1993). Briquet's syndrome, dissociation, and abuse. *American Journal of Psychiatry* 150: 1507–1511.

Rosenberg, D. A., and Krugman, R. D. (1991). Epidemiology and outcome of child abuse. *Annual Review of Medicine* 42: 217–224.

Ross, C., Heber, S., Norton, G., and Anderson, G. (1989). The dissociative disorders interview schedule. *Dissociation* 9: 169–188.

Saxe, G. N., Chinman, G., Berkowitz, R., Hall, K., Lieberg, G., Schwartz, J., and van der Kolk, B. A. (1994). Somatization in patients with dissociative disorders. *American Journal of Psychiatry* 151: 1329–1334.

Scarcini, I. C., McDonald-Haile, J., Bradley, L. A., and Richter, J. E. (1994). Altered pain perception and psychophysical features among women with gastrointestinal disorders and history of abuse: A preliminary model. *American Journal of Medicine* 97: 108–118.

Schnurr, P. P. (1996). Trauma, PTSD, and physical health. *PTSD Research Quarterly* 2 (3): 1–6.

Sedgwick, P. (1982). *Psychopolitics.* New York: Harper and Row.

Smith, G. R., Monson, R. A., and Ray, D. C. (1986). Psychiatric consultation in somatization disorder. *New England Journal of Medicine* 314: 1407–1413.

Springs, F. E., and Friedrich, W. N. (1992). Health risk behaviors and medical sequelae of childhood sexual abuse. *Mayo Clinic Proceedings* 67: 527–532.

van der Kolk, B., Pelcovitz, D., Roth, S., Mandel, F. S., McFarlane, A., and Herman, J. L. (1996). Dissociation, somatization, and affect dysregulation: The complexity of adaptation to trauma. *American Journal of Psychiatry*, Festschrift Supplement 153: 83–93.

Walker, E. A., Katon, W. J., Neraas, K., Jemelka, R. P., and Massoth, D. (1992). Dissociation in women with chronic pelvic pain. *American Journal of Psychiatry* 149: 534–537.

Walker, E. A., Katon, W. J., Roy-Byrne, P. P., Jemelka, R. P., and Russo, J. (1993). Histories of sexual victimization in patients with irritable bowel syndrome or inflammatory bowel disease. *American Journal of Psychiatry* 150: 1502–1506.

Williams, L. M. (1994). Recall of childhood trauma: A prospective study of women's memories of child sexual abuse. *Journal of Consulting and Clinical Psychology* 6: 1167–1176.

CHAPTER 4

Somatoform Dissociative Phenomena
A Janetian Perspective

Ellert R. S. Nijenhuis
and Onno van der Hart

It is through the study of mental stigmata that the malady of hysteria must be diagnosed and understood. Each of them shows very well that the subject has sustained a loss in his personality and that he is no longer master of his own thought.

Pierre Janet (1893)

The observation that dissociation and the dissociative disorders resulting from it affect a wide range of mental and physical functions was basic to nineteenth-century views on hysteria. In that era hysteria encompassed symptom complexes that today would be diagnosed as dissociative disorders, somatoform disorders, sexual disorders, eating disorders and personality disorders.

Pierre Janet, the French pioneer in the field of trauma and dissociation, defined hysteria as "a form of mental depression characterized by the retraction of the field of personal consciousness and a tendency to the dissociation and emancipation of the systems of ideas and functions that constitute personality" (Janet 1907/1965, 332). Such "systems of ideas and functions" could belong to either psyche or soma. In the introduction to his medical thesis, *L'État mental des hystériques,* Janet quoted Briquet (1859), who stated: "Hysteria is a disease which modifies the whole organism" (Janet 1893/1901, xiii). And Janet immediately added: "If it disturbs nutrition and all the physiological functions, it disturbs also the psychological phenomena, which are one of the functions of the organism."

Contemporary North American views on dissociation tend to be more restrictive and completely or partially disregard the alterations in somatoform functions and reactions that so frequently accompany pathological dissociation. For example, the third edition of the *Diagnostic and Statistical Manual of Mental Disorders (DSM-III-R)* defined the essential feature of the dissociative disorders as "a disturbance or alteration in the normally integrative functions of identity, memory, or consciousness" (American Psychiatric Association [APA] 1987, 269). In the fourth edition, *DSM-IV* (APA 1994), it was hesitantly added that this disturbance could also affect perception of the environment. Consequently, in this diagnostic system, somatoform symptoms, which nineteenth-century French psychiatrists would have considered dissociative, are diagnosed instead as somatization disorder, pain disorder, conversion disorder, sexual disorder or body dysmorphic disorder—disorders not understood or classified as dissociative in nature. In contrast, the latest edition of the *International Classification of Diseases*, the *ICD-10* (World Health Organization [WHO] 1992), recognizes that dissociation may affect somatoform functions and reactions: "The common theme shared by dissociative disorders is a partial or complete loss of the normal integration between memories of the past, awareness of identity and immediate sensations, and control of bodily movements" (p. 151).

However, even this current international definition is more restrictive than what Janet had in mind. As defined in *ICD–10*, dissociative disorders of movement and sensation involve only *loss* of sensations and *loss* of or *interference* with movements. Disorders involving *additional* sensations such as pain are to be included in the somatoform disorders, and somatization disorder is not classified as a dissociative disorder.

Janet (1893, 1894, 1901, 1907) distinguished between two major categories of hysterical symptoms, the mental stigmata and the mental accidents. The *mental stigmata* reflect functional losses, such as losses of sensation (anesthesia), memory (amnesia), motor control, will (abulia) and character traits (modifications of character). The *mental accidents* involve intrusions, such as additional sensations, movements and perceptions, up to the extremes of complete interruptions of the habitual state of consciousness through reactivations of dissociative secondary existences. These dissociative states display psychological and somatoform features that diverge from those characteristic of the habitual state. Interestingly, Janet's dichotomy does not follow a mind-body distinction.

Both categories apply equally to psyche and soma, which, he insisted, should not be radically divided: "There is no reason why we should begin over again here the old quarrel about the physical and the moral, which, from a scientific standpoint, is altogether idle" (Janet 1893/1901, xiii). Rejecting philosophical (Cartesian) dualism, he held that the brain and the mind are indivisible, a position that anticipated modern views on the matter (Edelman 1992).

Janet may also have anticipated other advances in neurophysiology in regarding hysteria as a mental disturbance based on a "cerebral insufficiency" involving unidentified "(neuro)physiological modifications which accompany and provoke" it (Janet 1894/1901, 528). In present-day language, Janet was describing hysteria as a disorder of information processing. A century later, those neurophysiological modifications that Janet hinted at are beginning to be studied (Krystal et al. 1995; see also Chapter 1, this volume).

Although in principle psyche and soma are indivisible, *phenomenologically* the two types of dissociation can be categorized separately (Kihlstrom 1992, 1994). Further, the symptoms of both categories fall into two broad classes, negative and positive, paralleling the familiar division between positive and negative symptoms in schizophrenia. In our view, this distinction also parallels Janet's mental stigmata (negative symptoms) and mental accidents (positive symptoms).

To gain a clearer view on the matter, see Table 4.1, which categorizes dissociative symptoms according to the double dichotomy described above. The first dichotomy divides *psychological* and *somatoform* dissociation. *Somatoform dissociation* designates dissociative symptoms that phenomenologically involve the body. The adjective *somatoform* indicates that the physical symptoms suggest, but cannot be explained by, a medical condition or the direct effects of a substance. Hence, in this chapter we will use the adjective *somatoform* instead of *somatic* unless we describe symptoms that could perhaps be an expression of a somatic disease. *Dissociation* describes the existence of a disruption of the normal synthesis between "systems of ideas and functions that constitute the personality." This disruption relates to mental and neurophysiological processes still not completely understood. The second dichotomy divides *negative dissociative symptoms* (mental stigmata) from *positive dissociative symptoms* (mental accidents). Accordingly, somatoform dissociation includes negative and positive somatoform manifestations of disrupted mental synthesis.

In addition to the *ICD-10*'s recognition of somatoform dissociation, several clinicians have emphasized the need to return to Janet's pioneering

TABLE 4.1

A Phenomenological categorization of dissociative symptoms

	Psychological dissociation	*Somatoform dissociation*
Mental stigmata, or negative dissociative symptoms	Amnesia Abulia Modifications of character (loss of character traits predominantly affects) Suggestibility	Anesthesia (all sensory modalities) Analgesia Loss of motor control (movements, voice, swallowing, etc.)
Mental accidents, or positive dissociative symptoms	Subconscious acts, hysterical accidents Fixed ideas (flashbacks) Hysterical attacks (reexperiencing) Somnambulism (altered states) Deliriums (dissociative psychosis)	Subconscious acts, hysterical accidents Fixed ideas: single intrusive somatoform symptoms Hysterical attacks: complexes of somatoform symptoms influencing the habitual state Somnambulism: alterations of state including complex somatoform alterations Deliriums: alterations of state including grotesque somatoform alterations

studies in order to further understanding of the somatoform aspects of dissociation (Kihlstrom 1992, 1994; Nijenhuis 1990; van der Hart and Friedman 1989; van der Hart and Op den Velde 1991). Consistent with these clinically based opinions, several recent studies have shown that patients with *DSM-III-R* (or *DSM-IV*) dissociative disorders suffer from many somatoform symptoms (Pribor et al. 1993; Ross et al. 1989; Saxe et al. 1994). It has also been found that patients with particular somatoform disorders, for instance, pseudoseizures (Bowman and Markand 1996) and chronic pelvic pain (Walker et al. 1992), show elevations on measures of psychological dissociation (as on the Dissociative Experiences Scale [DES]) (Bernstein and Putnam 1986]). Although *ICD-10* recognizes pseudoseizures as a dissociative disorder, in North America these various somatoform phenomena have generally not been grouped with dissociative disorders (Bowman and Markand 1996).

To test the feasibility of our provisional classification of dissociative symptoms, we have applied it in several ways. We returned to Janet's original classification of hysterical symptoms to determine whether our categories adequately contained the symptoms described in Janet's historical cases. We have also applied this classification to a contemporary case involving a traumatized individual with dissociative identity disorder (DID), in which the symptoms of psychological and somatoform dissociation were intertwined.

The study of traumatized individuals is of interest; Janet was able to show in many cases of hysteria the traumatic origins of both psychological and somatoform dissociation (Janet 1889, 1898, 1911; van der Kolk and van der Hart 1989). This is currently an area of great clinical and scientific controversy. Some authors have suggested that memories of trauma may be a result of fantasy and suggestion, especially if the patient was not aware of some or all traumatic memories in advance of the start of therapy (Loftus 1993). By presenting a DID patient whose previously dissociated traumatic memories could be partially validated, we attempt to reaffirm the connection between actual trauma and psychological and somatoform dissociative phenomena that Janet postulated.

In this chapter we also report briefly on yet another application of these concepts—the development of a self-report instrument measuring somatoform dissociation, the Somatoform Dissociation Questionnaire (SDQ-20; Nijenhuis et al., 1996, in press b), and a brief dissociative disorders screening version derived from it (SDQ-5; Nijenhuis et al., 1997b, 1998b).

MENTAL STIGMATA AND MENTAL ACCIDENTS

Let us look more closely at Janet's distinction between mental stigmata and mental accidents (cf. van der Hart and Friedman 1989) as put forth in his original and careful clinical studies of hysteria (1889, 1893/1901, 1894/1901, 1907, 1909, 1911). *Mental stigmata* referred to general markers of hysteria and were regarded as permanent and persistent deficit symptoms that would beset patients until full recovery, reached only upon the reintegration of the personality. Janet estimated that mental stigmata appear in two-thirds of hysterical (dissociative disorder) patients. As these patients may be little aware of the exact nature of their mental stigmata or may be indifferent to them, their self-reports should be regarded as imprecise. Janet (1907) distinguished two classes of mental stigmata: (1) *proper stigmata*, which appear exclusively in hysteria, and (2) *common stigmata*, which are shared by hysteria and other mental disorders, notably psychasthenic neuroses. Janet understood common stigmata as related to a *lowering of the mental level*; these symptoms included feelings of incompleteness, lapses of all the mental functions, the lack of feeling and of will (abulia) and the inability to begin and end activities. Hysteria's proper stigmata relate to the *retraction of the field of consciousness* and include suggestibility and unconscious acts, absentmindedness carried to unconsciousness and alternations of symptoms. Somatoform mental stigmata include anesthesia, analgesia and movement disorders.

Mental accidents are hysteria's acute, transient features, which appear briefly or intermittently. Since patients are usually aware of them, they experience this category of symptoms as distressing or painful. Janet (1894/1901, 1907) distinguished the following types of mental accidents: subconscious acts, fixed ideas, hysterical attacks (in which traumatic events are reexperienced), somnambulistic states (altered states of consciousness, memory and identity) and deliriums (dissociative psychotic episodes). Here we will discuss hysterical stigmata and accidents as manifested both in Janet's historical cases and contemporary dissociative patients, primarily in relationship to somatoform phenomena.

Hysteria's mental stigmata and mental accidents can be described in terms of negative and positive symptoms, respectively. The mental stigmata, as negative symptoms, are directly based on the dissociation and emancipation of the "systems of ideas and functions that constitute personality." Normally, Janet (1909) added, these systems of ideas and functions are *synthesized* among each other to form coherent mental structures, which are then integrated into previously synthesized mental structures.

Examples of nonsynthesized systems range from a simple image, memory or thought (together with attendant feelings, bodily manifestations and a rudimentary but alternate sense of self) to a complex dissociative identity state such as is found in DID (APA 1994; Breuer and Freud 1893–1895/1955; Janet 1889; van der Hart and Friedman 1989). The phenomena belonging to dissociated systems are not perceived or processed by personal consciousness. This is what produces mental stigmata, the gaps in perception and function that we call negative symptoms.

When memory systems remain chronically dissociated they may become centers or identities that take on a life of their own and can uncontrollably intrude on personal consciousness. These intrusive parallel perceptions and parallel existences are what have been called the positive symptoms of hysteria.

Both the stigmata and accidents that hysterical (dissociative disorder) patients manifest are extremely changeable, because they are highly dependent on the mental state (ego center or identity) dominating consciousness at that particular point in time. Rapid changes of symptoms may occur because of rapid transitions from one state to another. These symptoms also are contradictory; it can be demonstrated, for instance, that a patient who displays visual, auditory or kinesthetic anesthesia (hysterical blindness, deafness or insensibility pertaining to touch) at the same time does in fact see, hear or feel. According to Janet (1889, 1893/1901, 1907), this peculiar characteristic (which has evoked the erroneous idea that hysterics are simulators) is based on the existence of dissociative states, which may alternate in consciousness or may be simultaneously active. For example, while in a particular psychophysiological state, a hysterical (dissociative disorder) patient may be analgesic, but when the same patient is in another state he or she may sense pain quite well. Janet (1889) demonstrated this in a series of experiments with his patient Lucie, who, as "Lucie," was anesthetic, but as "Adrienne" was not. When "Lucie" dominated consciousness and was insensitive to pain stimuli, the dissociative identity "Adrienne" could still describe and express her pain through "automatic writing" (cf. van der Hart and Horst 1989).

MENTAL STIGMATA:
NEGATIVE DISSOCIATIVE SYMPTOMS

As stated above, hysteria's stigmata include a wide range of functional losses. Here we present an overview of those stigmata we would categorize as involving negative symptoms, or retractions of the field of personal consciousness.

ANESTHESIA

Anesthesia refers to the absence or diminution of normal sensibility (more properly called hypoesthesia). All sensory modalities (propriocepsis, kinesthesia, nocicepsis [perception of pain], vision and audition, as well as the senses of smell and taste) may be disturbed by it, separately or simultaneously. Janet distinguished localized, systematized and generalized anesthesia.

Localized anesthesia presents at a particular, localized area of the body, for instance, the left side of the body (hemianesthesia), the face or sharply defined spots. Charcot (1887) observed that localized anesthesias may appear in geometrical segments, mappings that do not correspond to anatomically distinct enervations. *Systematized anesthesia* follows a single subconscious idea or a system of ideas that determines what will and will not be perceived. For example, the subject may see all the persons or objects in a room except one particular person or object. *Generalized anesthesia* affects a sense in general, as in cases of hysterical blindness, deafness or the inability to feel touch, temperature, texture and pain in all bodily regions.

In one or another of these forms, anesthesia occurs in the majority of hysterical (dissociative disorder) patients (Janet 1893/1901). However, in contrast to somatically determined anesthesias, hysterical anesthesias are often ignored and unreported. In most hysterical cases, anesthesia is modified or disappears more or less completely for variable periods of time. This *changeability*, or *mobility* (Janet, 1893/1901), of stigmata can occur during hysterical attacks, sleep, intoxications or somnambulistic states (i.e., dissociative identity states, discussed below). The mobility of anesthesia could also be provoked by "artificial somnambulism," that is, the induction of hypnosis, and in some cases by waking suggestions.

A current DID patient, Ms. L. occasionally described anesthesia on the left side of her body. While engaged in a friendly conversation with her therapist, Ms. L.'s left hand, apparently unnoticed by her, reached for her shoe, took it and brought it upward to a throwing position. The therapist watched these movements and brought his hands up into a defensive position. Ms. L. saw this and his look toward her left side; alarmed, she too looked abruptly to her left side and let the shoe fall. Subsequent exploration of this incident revealed that a dissociative identity state with an intense dislike of the therapist was angered by the friendly conversation and was able to take control of the patient's left arm and hand in an attempt to hurt the therapist. Here the identity without anesthesia tried to exploit Ms. L.'s symptom in order to express dissenting views about therapy. Once this state was activated, touch stimuli on the left side were perceived, even though the patient in the habitual state of consciousness remained anesthetic and unaware. In this case the subconscious parallel perceptions were accompanied by actions that also escaped personal consciousness. In other words, this patient demonstrated parallel information processing—each state was receiving its own perceptual input.

Thus, like the other mental stigmata, anesthesias are typically *state-dependent* (Janet 1889, 1898, 1907). For example, the famous nineteenth-century

DID patient Louis Vivet had at least six dissociative identities, which were, among other things, characterized by differences in sensation and motion (Bourru and Burot 1895; Janet 1907). In one state, Louis Vivet was insensible and paralyzed on his left side; in another state he was paralyzed on his right side; in a third state he was paraplegic, and so on.

Analgesia Another frequent hysterical symptom (Janet 1889, 1893/1901), analgesia is defined as insensibility to pain, with the sense of touch remaining unimpaired. While being pricked, cut or burned (by themselves or others), analgesic patients will neither experience nor show any conscious sign of pain. Even subconscious sensations of pain seem to play a very small role (Janet 1893). Witm., a patient with feet absolutely anesthetic, went to bed without testing the temperature of her hot-water bottle. The next day the soles of her feet showed large burns. When specifically asked, a secondary identity of hers reported having experienced pain, but it had not removed the feet from the bottle, leading Janet to conclude that this second state believed it had only imagined feeling the pain.

Janet further observed that analgesic and anesthetic patients may be unable to assess temperature, exemplified by the inability to distinguish hot from cold water. One of our DID patients remarked: "When I take a bath, I can estimate the temperature of the water only by looking at the color of my skin."

Organic Anesthesia Janet gave the name *organic anesthesia* to "the loss of those vague sensations that are informing us of the presence and life of our organs" (1893/1901, 56). He added that some patients not only cease feeling the touch of their limbs, but lose the consciousness of their existence as well. In extreme cases these phenomena resemble parietal lobe syndromes in which parts of the body are rejected as ego alien and/or experienced as foreign bodies not part of the self. Janet added that the sensations of hunger, thirst and fatigue and the desire to urinate may also be lost.

For example, an incestuously physically and emotionally abused woman with dissociative disorder not otherwise specified (DDNOS) (APA 1994) was almost chronically and generally anesthetic. Since she was never aware of any urge to urinate, she suffered both diurnal and nocturnal enuresis. These symptoms were resistant to behavior therapy and other kinds of treatment that did not take her dissociative condition into account. However, sensation did return when a dissociative child identity state reworked memories of being touched by the harsh hands of a sexually abusive brother. As this child alter, in tears, reexperienced the desire to be held and comforted, she reclaimed the capacity to sense touch, texture and warmth.

Genital Anesthesia   Janet noted that genital sensations may be completely or intermittently lacking in some cases. This was manifested in his patient Maria, who, upon the onset of her illness, lost all interest in her husband and children, whom she formerly dearly loved but whom she now abandoned (Janet 1893/1901). When her husband died, she could not have cared less: "I have forgotten him." With the loss of love, she also lost all shame. She was not obscene, but profoundly indifferent, and wholly anesthetic in the genital part. Maria claimed incomprehension of the possibility of genital pleasure, saying: "Why, I have children, and I do not know yet why people maintain that there is pleasure in it." However, for brief intervals Maria came out of her "psychological feebleness" (Janet 1893/1901, 206). During these periods she temporarily lost her stigmata, mourned the loss of her husband and her children, and regained genital sensibility. Maria also demonstrates another mental stigma that we will mention only in passing, the *modifications of character*. Maria's modifications of character seem to derive from her loss of affects and thus would be categorized in our system as negative psychological dissociative symptoms.

Kinesthetic Anesthesia   Janet distinguished between anesthesias for movements that are self-initiated (active) and those for movements that are caused by someone else manipulating the body (passive). Anesthesia often implies *ataxia*, the inability to direct one's movements with eyes closed. Lasègue's syndrome, a classic hysterical variant, involves difficulties in initiating voluntary movement and unawareness of movement without the help of sight. For example, Janet's patient Lucie was unable to make the slightest movement in the dark.

Usually, these characteristics do not seem to trouble the subjects, who, during daily life, perform all the movements without complaint, unaware of the crucial role that vision has assumed in movement capacity. Since hysterical patients tend to "forget" anesthetic members, visual input may act as a reminder.

Tactile Anesthesia   Apart from losing the sensibility of pain (analgesia), dissociative disorder patients may lack the sense of touch. They then are unable, with eyes closed, to identify objects placed in their hands, and they will not sense being touched. In these cases, awareness of being touched is mediated by visual perception.

Visual Anesthesia   Janet had a special interest in retractions of the visual field, a characteristic that many hysterical (dissociative disorder) patients display. The degree of constriction is state-dependent, but is also influenced by physiological variables such as rest, alcohol and menstrual periods and psychological variables such as emotions, stress and cognition. For example, in her habitual mental state, his patient Bertha had a very constricted visual field, but in a dissociative state this stigma completely disappeared. Phenomenologically, the symptom may appear as "tunnel vision."

Visual anesthesia may be localized. An example is provided by patients who seem to have totally lost vision in one eye. As with all the other mental stigmata, this *unilateral amaurosis*, a localized visual anesthesia, is of a contradictory nature in that it can be experimentally shown that visual stimuli projected to the affected eye are still processed, although subconsciously.

Visual anesthesia can also be of a systematized nature. As Janet (1893/1901) explained, while remaining in a dissociative state a patient may see only a certain category of objects that relate to ideas of special significance to that state.

Like the other anesthesias, visual anesthesias are mobile. Janet's patient Bertha usually was hemianesthetic on the left side, with extreme contractions of both sides of her visual field. However, after a hysterical attack she became totally anesthetic and at times completely blind (generalized visual anesthesia) for some hours.

Other Anesthesias   Much of what has already been said in this section is equally applicable to auditory, gustatory and olfactory anesthesia.

AMNESIA

Hysterical (dissociative) amnesia, a stigma that, according to Janet (1893/1901), is almost as frequent as anesthesia, pertains not to memory loss, but to state-dependent inaccessibility of memories for present and past events (Janet 1889, 1893/1901, 1898). Thus, in contrast to organic amnesia, hysterical amnesia implies the preservation of memories. In fact, seemingly lost memories are stored in particular dissociative states and may or may not be accessible to other states, and this (in)accessibility can be unilateral or bilateral (Janet 1907). Due to this state-dependent memory storage and retrieval, dissociative amnesia is a *mobile* phenomenon: Patients know or do not know, depending on their state of consciousness. And, as more than one state can be concomitantly reactivated, amnesia is also *contradictory* in its presentation: Patients can, although unwittingly, still be influenced by apparently lost memories. For example, while remaining in a dissociative child state and moving like a child, a patient may yet demonstrate adult intellectual capacities. Furthermore, "lost" knowledge and skills may be relearned much faster than would be the case if such mental contents were not in fact present. In short, dissociative barriers are far from absolute.

According to Janet (1889), dissociated knowledge predominantly, but not exclusively, involves autobiographical memory. Such knowledge of personal history is defined today as an aspect of explicit memory, that is, knowledge available to conscious awareness. Dissociative amnesia can also include state-dependent inaccessibility of motor and other skills. Such skills deficits are regarded today as manifestations of implicit memory, knowledge that is unavailable to consciousness, but that affects performance. Thus, even though hysterical amnesia is a mental dysfunction, Janet (1893/1901) maintained that alterations of memory also affect the body and its functions. Janet saw movements as the outward manifestation of certain images, holding that hysterical paralyses are the outward expression of the amnestic loss (inaccessibility) of these images about movement. Such paralyses usually are of a systematized type involving a particular group of movements and skills, for example, standing and walking (astasia-abasia), writing or sewing, while leaving many others unaffected. Janet observed that such losses of movement may be accompanied by (often systematized) intellectual amnesias, for instance, forgetting particular events or being unable to recognize familiar people.

MOTOR DISTURBANCES

Janet observed that voluntary movements of hysterical (dissociative disorder) patients tend to be slackened, undecided and ill-directed. These patients may have difficulty performing complex acts that necessitate several different simultaneous movements, resulting in a simplification of voluntary movement. In his view, such disturbances result from anesthesia and a retraction of the field of consciousness. According to Janet, the observed weakening of voluntary movement was more related to abulia, a common mental stigma pertaining to a defect of the will and of conscious attention. However, when Lasègue's syndrome or one of its abnormal varieties (cf. Janet, 1893/1901) is present, motor disturbances are usually more pronounced. These patients are unable to move their body parts voluntarily without looking at them, but can, given this visual input, perform complex motor acts without effort.

Catalepsy is another motor disturbance related to amnesia. The patient's limbs can be easily moved about by another person, but when a limb is put into some position, even the strangest, it will tend to stay in that position for a long time, as if the patient had completely forgotten the member.

Contractures may also relate to anesthesia and forgetting the body. For example, Maria had a tendency to hyperflexion on the anesthetic left side of her body, but not on the still sensitive right side. Upon the disappearance of the anesthesia, the motor contractures vanished with it. Although partial catalepsies often are undone by increasing attention to the "forgotten" limb, looking at a contracture does not arrest the symptom. In Janet's mind, both catalepsy and contracture are determined by a retraction of the field of personal consciousness with a concomitant dissociative loss of the relevant motor images.

A modern example concerns a DID patient with a chronic contracture (including anesthesia) of her right hand in the form of a *main d'accoucheur*—the hand contracted in the form of a cone with fingers conjoined (Babinski and Froment 1918). The contracture developed after a traffic accident, actually a suicide attempt, in which the hand was injured. In the course of psychotherapy, she asked the therapist if he could help her to regain control over her right hand. He contacted the part of her personality responsible for the contraction. This identity explained that she had seen the traffic accident as a means of killing herself, because she could no longer tolerate the emotional pain of her loneliness. When she eventually discovered that her hand and wrist had been injured, she decided to perpetuate the problem: That way at least a part of herself was dead, while the physical pain experienced by this identity distracted her from the unbearable emotional pain of loneliness. Through bringing both identities in contact with each other (until then, they had been ignorant of each other's existence), they developed a mutual, warm relationship, which relieved the suicidal identity's loneliness and gradually led her to allow the hand to regain its normal position. Finally, an integration of both states occurred, and the patient in her habitual state regained full control over the function of her right hand.

Suggestibility

The increased suggestibility of hysterical (dissociative disorder) patients, according to Janet (1907, Lecture 14), strongly relates to their absentmindedness, in which critical cognitive functions are suspended. To the extent that their fields of consciousness are retracted, these patients tend to forget all that is outside their present concerns and because of that may readily respond to a suggestion. As Janet (1894, 231–233) observed, this suggestibility does not depend on the induction of a hypnotic state, and it pertains to the "whole organism as well as the whole mind." Both negative (e.g., anesthesias, paralyses) and positive symptoms (e.g., pain in a limb) may be artificially induced in these patients with relative ease. Yet this suggestibility is a complex matter, as some hysterical patients are less suggestible than others and all resist suggestions at certain times. As Janet observed, it is extremely difficult to induce a suggestion in a person who has already received a suggestion or who has a fixed idea (powerful ideas that often are trauma-induced, discussed below). Thus, it is very difficult to use suggestion to change dissociative symptoms and traumatic memories (which depend on fixed ideas).

Is hysteria a result of suggestion, as some nineteenth-century and contemporary authors believe? Janet's observations were not consistent with this position. He observed that: (1) Patients, as a result of their restricted fields of consciousness, are often unaware of or indifferent to hysterical stigmata, which precludes an autosuggestive origin of the symptoms. (2) Hysterical stigmata occur in predictable forms and have remained the same since the Middle Ages in all countries in which they have been observed. And (3) although the disposition to suggestibility becomes more complete as the disorder progresses, mental stigmata show themselves very early (Janet 1894/1901, 357–358).

In summary, in his presentation of the mental stigmata, Janet showed that the synthetic function of personal consciousness can be disrupted. Sensations, perceptions of the environment, memories, affects, will and character traits may to a greater or lesser extent escape normal synthesis and assimilation into the habitual personality. What is lost is far from trivial, because the synthetic deficits are organized and directed according to subconscious fixed ideas. Thus, losses are consequences of subconscious phenomena, of dissociated systems of ideas and functions connected with a private sense of self, which also manifest themselves in those symptoms labeled mental accidents.

MENTAL ACCIDENTS:
POSITIVE DISSOCIATIVE SYMPTOMS

As stated above, the mental accidents are acute, transient features of hysteria (dissociative disorders) that tend to be intermittently present and are usually experienced as distressing or painful.

Subconscious Fixed Ideas and Hysterical Accidents

According to Janet (1894/1901), subconscious fixed ideas are thoughts or mental images that take on exaggerated proportions and have a high emotional charge. They are developed in an automatic manner, without the patient's conscious control or awareness. Unlike effects of hypnotic and other kinds of suggestions given by other people, these fixed ideas, according to Janet, are formed naturally under the influence of traumatic events, fatigue or severe illness.

To illustrate how subjectively traumatic experiences can induce fixed ideas, Janet discussed the case of Marie, who was blind in her left eye and anesthetic on the left side of her face (Janet 1889, 1894/1901). In the course of her treatment, Janet helped Marie to discover, by means of hypnosis, that she had developed these symptoms after having been forced, as a child, to sleep with another child who had mumps on the whole left side of her face. For several years and at the same time of the year, Marie subsequently developed patches of mumps that looked like those she had seen in the child, appearing on the same parts of the face. Ideas from this subjectively traumatic scene apparently had become fixed in her mind and then had been expressed through the dissociative symptoms. Using his substitution technique, Janet was able to help Marie get rid of these symptoms. Through hypnotic induction, he took her back to the child she feared and repeatedly made her reimagine the child as very nice and entirely without mumps.

As a rule, dissociative patients in their habitual personality state are unable to account clearly for the fixed idea that besets them (Janet 1894/1901, 279). Remaining in her habitual state, Marie was unaware of the ideas that formed the basis of her symptoms. Fixed ideas are present during waking hours, but may also be expressed during sleep and dissociative episodes in which trauma is reexperienced. These fixed ideas should not be regarded as simple subconscious thoughts, but as dissociated emotionally charged experiential states (Janet 1898; cf. van der Hart and Friedman 1989).

Dissociated identity states can be regarded as the carriers of these subconscious ideas. What Janet (1898) called *primary fixed ideas* are usually partial reexperiences of traumatic events, the type of representation of original events and responses that today might be called hallucinatory flashbacks. *Secondary fixed ideas* are derivatives of these primary fixed ideas. Some impress us as instances of generalization learning. Accordingly, the primary fixed idea "I am a little girl who is hurt by a man" (together with all related sensations, feelings and bodily manifestations) can generalize to "I still am this little girl, and all men will hurt me; I feel emotional and physical pain when any man comes close." Secondary fixed ideas also include *stratified fixed ideas*, which result from traumata in the patient's life history sustained prior to the one that caused the full-blown hysteria (dissociative disorder). This idea of "layers of trauma" has been elaborated both by Janet and more recent theorists (Janet 1898; van der Hart and Friedman 1989). *Accidental fixed ideas* are those newly produced by a recent event. In contrast to the other fixed ideas, they are easy to eradicate if treated immediately. For example, a patient currently in psychotherapy relived an incestuous rape during a session. Dominated by the idea "my brother was here [i.e., in the therapist's office] and raped me once more," she subsequently responded to this newly formed idea with general analgesia, anesthesia for touch, intense fear and immobility (freezing). This erroneous idea was corrected with relatively little therapeutic effort, and the related symptoms disappeared.

The reactivation of primary or stratified fixed ideas may occur through partial representations or much more inclusive representations of traumatic events and responses. Janet (1894/1901) labeled the former *hysterical accidents* and the latter *hysterical attacks* (discussed below). Whereas a partial reexperience of trauma leaves room for the appreciation of present circumstances ("I am in pain, but I know that I am an adult living in this current year"), during more or less total traumatic reexperiences the orientation to the present is lost. As the case of Marie shows, hysterical accidents include somatoform reactions and even quite peculiar ones ("mumps-like" skin alterations). In fact, (reactivated) fixed ideas may involve all sensory modalities and a wide range of other somatoform responses. Below we present a range of examples from Janet as well as contemporary clinical experience.

Dysesthesia   Dysesthesia is the presence of intrusive, often unpleasant sensations, which, while not painful, feel abnormal or uncomfortable. According to Janet, "Many hysterical (dissociative disorder) patients seem to have imperfect perceptions of the impressions which strike their senses" (1894/1901, 291). This can be a consequence of anesthesia. For example, in gustatory anesthesia, the expected taste of food is lost. Perceptual alterations may also relate to fixed ideas, as was evident in the case of Janet's patient Bertha, who found the color red repugnant because, as the color of blood, it reminded her of the tragic death of her father.

Hyperesthesia   Hyperesthesia is increased sensitivity to pain. Janet's patient Colinm., the victim of a railway accident, recovered completely from a serious abdominal wound; however, upon drinking alcohol, he reexperienced the accident and concomitant abdominal pain. He thus refrained from further alcohol consumption. Six years later, he experienced violent and terrible emotions related to the death of his wife and child, due to which he became morbidly sad and suffered intense abdominal pain. Pressing the scar would evoke reexperiences of the accident, in which context he would momentarily be distracted from his later troubles.

Many pain symptoms of dissociative patients are an expression of such subconscious fixed ideas. However, violent headaches may also be related to other causes, for example, dissociative state switches, or may accompany the synthesis of previously dissociated traumatic experiences (Janet 1898).

Audition   Auditory hallucinations of dissociative patients appear to stem from communications of dissociative states that are perceived as voices or a peculiar type of thoughts. The utterances of these dissociative (identity) states may reveal fixed ideas. A DID patient currently in therapy was often exposed to disturbing phrases (auditory pseudohallucinations), which, as it later appeared, were statements of a dissociative identity reproducing her highly sexually, physically and emotionally abusive mother's repetitive assertions, "You like it; you are just like me." In fact, these phrases were the essence of that state's identity.

The acuity of hearing may change, as clinically observed, under the influence of dissociative states. While in altered states, patients may lose hearing to withdraw from outer (traumatic) reality or, in contrast, become extremely perceptive of noises as part of hyperalertness to threats of danger.

Motor Disturbances   Janet (1907) stated that fixed ideas may also relate to motor disturbances, for instance, paralyses, contractures, problems of speech, tics and movements of chorea (tremors). Nondissociative psychiatric patients, like most people, deal with ambivalence consciously; dissociative patients, however, have usually found other ways of coping. Janet characterized this type of psychic life as dominated by state-dependent *monoideisms* (single fixed ideas) or *polyideisms* (limited sets of related fixed ideas), which direct thoughts, emotions, perceptions, sensations and actions (Janet 1894/1901, 1907). Thus various states may have widely diverging or even opposite ideas of themselves, other people, the world, time, place, preferred strategies of action, likes and dislikes. This fact led Kluft (see Chapter 11) to remark that multiple personality disorder (DID) patients suffer from multiple reality disorder. Due to divergent or contradictory monoideisms, struggles between dissociative states often ensue, and behaviors of all types may be postponed, prevented, undermined or abolished. A dissociative (identity) state may even interfere with an action of the habitual state of consciousness by paralyzing the related body part.

Nutrition Hysterical (dissociative disorder) patients often have problems with eating, which may relate to fixed ideas. Thus, Janet's patient Isabelle refused to eat anything for six weeks because of such a fixed idea (Janet 1894/1901, 288–290). She was not an ordinary case of anorexia, as she said: "I assure you that I am not at all possessed with the idea of not eating; it seems even that I should like to eat; but at the moment of beginning, the thought of it chokes me, disgusts me, and I cannot. Why? I don't know; despite my efforts to eat there is something that prevents me." During hysterical attacks, the reason for this "anorexia" became clearer. During an attack, Isabelle's deceased mother "appeared" and blamed her for a fault she had committed, telling her that she was not worthy to live and that she ought to join her (the mother) in heaven. To achieve this, her mother's "manifestation" ordered Isabelle not to eat. Janet subsequently discovered that the "fault" that Isabelle felt her mother was accusing her of related to a fixed (but erroneous) idea that she had murdered her sister (who in fact had died of natural causes).

HYSTERICAL ATTACKS:
REEXPERIENCES OF TRAUMATIC EVENTS

Janet (1907) observed that some hysterical (dissociative disorder) patients intermittently seem to lose consciousness and become unresponsive to external stimuli. During such episodes they may writhe with great, irregular, apparently meaningless movements (*emotional*, or *Briquet's attack*), become completely inert and immovable (*ecstasies*), or display combinations of both types (*complete,* or *Charcot's attack*). Janet conceptualized these various forms of *convulsive hysterical attacks* as inferior forms of somnambulisms. Somnambulisms (discussed below) are complete reactivations of dissociative identity states. Attacks are acute phenomena of relatively short duration (not lasting longer than a few hours at most), but they are repetitive in nature (tending to occur daily or even several times a day). They were estimated to present in about two-thirds of hysterical (dissociative disorder) patients (Pitres 1891).

Whereas in hysterical accidents single fixed ideas dominate only part of the experiential world, in hysterical attacks complex fixed ideas "affect the whole mind to the extent of destroying the consciousness the patient has of his own personality" (Janet 1894/1901, 366). Consequently, attacks are usually followed by dissociative amnesia for the contents of the experience. Even though during such attacks patients may appear to be unconscious, they are, in fact, "absorbed in an obsessing thought, which fills their small field of consciousness" (p. 387). "A fit of simple hysteria is nothing but the exact repetition of the disturbances by which vivid and painful moral impressions are manifested," Briquet (1859, 397) had already maintained. In the same vein, Janet concluded that hysterical attacks are complex, enlarged, disfigured and inferior expressions of emotions that have lost their intellectual aspect. They pertain to a "dream," to that complex of fixed ideas that constitutes a traumatic memory (Janet 1894/1901, 1898).

In great contrast with normal narrative memories, traumatic memories are predominantly expressed in a somatosensory way: The subject repeats acts and emotions as well as visual, kinesthetic, auditory and other somatoform perceptions pertaining to past trauma as if the event is unfolding in the present (Janet 1889, 1898, 1904, 1928; cf. van der Kolk and van der Hart 1989). Diverging from Briquet and from his own earlier observations, Janet (1932) later maintained that these traumatic memories need not entirely match historical facts, because they pertain to mental representations of these events, that is, impressions these events once evoked. These mental representations of trauma may, in addition to historical elements, also encompass curtailments (particular episodic aspects of a traumatic event may be lacking), elaborations (e.g., fantasies arising during trauma becoming part of the traumatic memory) and distortions (see Chapter 2).

During hysterical attacks (traumatic reexperiences), the dissociative identity states involved may experience pain, motor disturbances and other somatoform symptoms. To the extent that the habitual state of consciousness is activated, it experiences or suffers from them as well. Yet when a cognitive representation of the association between the traumatic event and the traumatic reactions does not reach or does not entirely reach this habitual state, the meaning of these symptoms may escape it (Janet 1894/1901). The habitual state may also fail to grasp what triggering events had set a particular attack in motion. However, this knowledge is usually accessible in one or more of the dissociative states.

Attacks—or fully reactivated traumatic memories, as we would now term them—are evoked by reminders of traumatizing events. These reminders include not only temporal data, daily life events and emotional and physiological states (van der Hart and Friedman 1992), but also what Charcot called *hysterogenic points*, the most frequently identified being in the lower side of the abdomen, also called the ovarian region. Pains in this area so often accompanied hysterical attacks that Janet wondered if this observation had led to Plato's theory linking these points to "an overexcited matrix which required satisfaction, which, if this satisfaction was not obtained, resulted in a hysterical fit" (p. 98). He went on to explain that in spite of appearances, these points and sensations are psychological, not physical in character. Today we might link them to the sensations accompanying sexual abuse.

A contemporary example of an attack presenting as a pseudoepileptic seizure was provided by a patient with DDNOS. A few times daily, this patient had acute pseudoseizures that generally lasted about fifteen minutes. Due to these seizures, she had painful and sometimes dangerous falls. No physical causes could be traced. In her normal state of consciousness, the patient was not aware of stimuli that triggered the attacks. However, while in one of her dissociative states, she was able to explain. Various stimuli reminded her of attempted suffocation by her father, incestuous paternal abuse, subsequent pregnancy and childbirth and the immediate forced separation from her child after birth. These stimuli reevoked a tremendous need to escape from associated traumatic memories. One such reminder related to physical sensations associated with pregnancy, such as having a full stomach. In her dissociative state, this patient was able to explain that the suffocation attempt had followed her refusal of her father's sexual advances. In the moments before losing consciousness, she had experienced pleasurable sensations and hallucinations, which were relived during one type of pseudoseizure. In another, less frequent type of attack, she threw herself upon the floor and, while moaning, crying, trembling and vigorously shaking and with uncontrolled movements of all limbs, she relived the sexual and homicidal assault.

SOMNAMBULISMS:
COMPLEX DISSOCIATIVE (IDENTITY) STATES

"It is a fact of popular observation that hystericals may at certain moments pass into abnormal psychological states, the first characteristic of which is to appear strange, extraordinary, very different from the normal psychological state of the subject," Janet (1894/1901, 413) remarked. These states were called *somnambulisms*: abnormal states, distinct from the normal life of the subject, "in which the patient possesses particular recollections, which he finds no longer when he returns to his normal state" (p. 415). These memories, which among others pertain to fixed ideas and traumatic recollections, tend to be rather directly available in these "second existences," which nowadays are often called dissociative identity states.

Somnambulisms differ from hysterical attacks in the following way. During a hysterical attack patients are absorbed in traumatic fixed ideas, while losing awareness of and adaptation to the current reality. In somnambulistic states they remain perceptive of the present and are able to adapt their behavior accordingly. Although less exclusively dominated by fixed ideas than hysterical attacks are, somnambulistic states are still organized around one main fixed idea (monoideism) or around a limited set of related fixed ideas (polyideism) directing thoughts, emotions, perceptions, sensations and actions (Janet 1894/1901, 1907). Thus, Janet described various types and degrees of complexity of somnambulism. For example, somnambulistic (dissociative identity) states vary in intellectual development, access to each other's memories, elaborateness, capacity to take control over consciousness and behavior and orientation to present realities.

Janet made many important observations regarding somatoform dissociation and these somnambulisms or dissociative identity states: Some patients, after switching to a complex dissociative state, could be free from symptoms such as anesthesias, amnesias and motor disturbances that were present in the habitual personality state. As remarked before, these body symptoms are state-dependent, mobile and contradictory. What is not sensed, perceived or controlled by one state of consciousness is processed by one or more other states. This produces a capricious symptomatic picture, which caused some to argue that hysteria is nothing but a condition of simulation and suggestion, notably Babinski (1901, 1909). Although somatoform symptoms may come and go for seemingly inexplicable reasons, they follow, in fact, rather consistent singular or complex ideas, which in many cases can only be discovered through direct contact and observation of patients in their various dissociative mental states (Janet 1894/1901).

DELIRIUMS:
DISSOCIATIVE PSYCHOTIC EPISODES

Some hysterical (dissociative disorder) patients tend to get caught in brief or more prolonged reactivations of somnambulistic states, in which they are poorly oriented to the present and are predominantly experiencing a hysterical attack. Such a condition, formerly called hysterical psychosis, is now termed *reactive dissociative psychosis* (Nijenhuis 1995; van der Hart, Witztum and Friedman 1993). Specific somatoform dissociative symptoms are manifested during such an episode. When patients are in such conditions, therapeutic interventions directed at reactivation of more healthy states (usually effective in other situations) often fail. The treatment of choice requires first joining the patient's alternate experiential world before using hypnotic suggestions to help the patient return to a less frightening world.

Janet (1898) presented various examples of such reactive dissociative psychotic episodes, among them his patient Achille (van der Hart, Witztum and Friedman 1993). One of our patients, Sonja, was diagnosed with dissociative disorder not otherwise specified, but also suffered from such intermittent reactive dissociative psychotic episodes. These episodes, which lasted for about two or three months, were the product of one or several dissociative child identity states, which fully determined the patient's psychological and somatoform condition. These child states reenacted trauma-related fixed ideas that totally filled her field of consciousness. For example, during one of them she behaved as if she had become a little girl obsessed with fear of hallucinated men in black suits. These images walked in the same way as her sexually abusive grandfather. He had also habitually worn a black suit. Meanwhile, the child state experienced pelvic and anal pains, intermittently assuming bodily postures that suggested that the patient was reexperiencing forcible rape. The dissociative child states could ordinarily be controlled by other dissociative states better oriented to the present, but during these dissociative psychotic episodes, healthier states could not be accessed. Sonja's psychotic spells could be broken when the dissociative child state was helped to symbolize the trauma-related affective and sensorimotor reactions. The child state needed to become able to transform these feelings and sensations into words.

In summary, although mental stigmata apparently involve functional losses, mental accidents can be regarded as positive symptoms pertaining to intrusions of more or less developed dissociative mental structures into the habitual state of consciousness. These intrusions stem from fixed ideas, dissociative relivings of traumatic events and responses (hysterical attacks), reactivations of dissociative identity states (somnambulisms) and dissociative psychotic states (deliriums). It thus may be said that *mental accidents are intrusions, reflecting manifestations of lost personal mental contents, that are dissociatively processed, stored and reactivated.*

Below we present a case example of a contemporary DID patient who manifested a multitude of somatoform dissociative symptoms that came to be understood as an integral part of her severely dissociative condition. Study of this patient's somatoform dissociative symptoms and their underlying fixed ideas may help therapists learn to recognize and map these connections in other dissociative disorder patients.

CASE EXAMPLE

History

When she was thirteen, Lisa (now age thirty-eight) finally felt strong enough to consult the family physician about somatic and psychological symptoms that had bothered her for years. That it took her so long, she said, was because her mother had forbidden her to complain, telling her that she was only making things up. More than twenty years after the event, Lisa related in psychotherapy how in her childhood her mother was indeed a figure to be feared. Lisa recalled severe and chronic sexual, physical and emotional abuse as well as emotional neglect, and she had been able to find documents and secure interviews with collateral informants that confirmed, or were consistent with, significant parts of her traumatic memories. For example, legal documents showed that when Lisa was age one, her parents were officially declared unfit. Shortly after this, her father died, and her mother remarried a man whom the authorities considered stable enough to provide a decent home for Lisa and her sister.

Sadly, this was not the case. As neighbors and others would later confirm, the mother continued to abuse the children emotionally and physically. Lisa's sister also described her mother's physical and emotional abuse. Both sisters reported sexual abuse by the stepfather. Lisa also recalled sexual abuse by other adults, both men and women, that had been initiated by her mother and allegedly involved child prostitution. Lisa (and other identity states) recalled memories of sexual abuse by a particular man living in her neighborhood. When she gained the personal strength to confront him in the presence of her husband and a friend, this alleged perpetrator admitted having abused Lisa for many years, starting at age twelve.

At age thirteen, Lisa had informed the police about the ongoing abuse at home. The police invited her parents and Lisa for joint questioning, during which the parents denied all abuse and Lisa felt forced to retract her accusations. Lisa very vaguely recalled that the police removed her from a block of flats, possibly because she was threatening to commit suicide. Subsequently she was transferred to a series of psychiatric institutions, where she remained for about a year and a half.

Lisa recalled being severely emotionally abused by staff members there, who subjected the girls to an authoritarian regime consisting of overuse of seclusion and medication and enforced senseless and repetitive activities. Lisa became blocked when trying to describe the former psychiatrist-in-chief and his house, which was situated on the premises.

Collateral data revealed that similar institutional abuse had been legally documented after complaints by several former patients (not including Lisa, who had lost all contact with other patients). These complainants accused the staff of emotional and physical abuse, and they additionally charged the psychiatrist-in-chief with sexual abuse, declaring that this man sexually abused them in his home. The psychiatrist subsequently was convicted and sentenced to several years of imprisonment.

During occasional leaves, as well as after her final release from this institution at age sixteen, Lisa's emotional, physical and sexual abuse continued at home, and she became impregnated by either her stepfather or another perpetrator.

Soon after, she met her future husband, who quickly, although far from completely, grasped Lisa's horrific circumstances. The couple decided to marry, which provided her escape from home. The husband proved to be a reliable, understanding and supportive partner, able to handle Lisa's complex psychiatric condition and to acquaint her with a more normal life. He helped raise Lisa's first child as his own and two more children were born.

Lisa had always been partially aware of the above traumatic events. However, in the course of psychotherapy she gained access to many more memories of abuse. Wishing to ascertain their validity, Lisa started to make inquiries into her past. Her mother responded by making telephone threats and physically attacking Lisa. As her investigation proceeded, Lisa's daughter was attacked by unknown men who threatened that inquiries about Lisa's past should stop.

SYMPTOMATOLOGY

Lisa's psychotherapist diagnosed her as suffering from DID. In addition to the psychological dissociative phenomena that justified this diagnosis, Lisa suffered a profusion of somatoform dissociation. Long before the DID diagnosis was made, both types of symptoms had been observed for many years by her husband and a close friend. These observations preclude explaining the symptoms as iatrogenic phenomena. Her somatic complaints included headaches, stomachaches and dizziness and also symptoms such as general analgesia, which are infrequently reported by normal individuals and nondissociative psychiatric patients. These more unusual symptoms (proper stigmata in Janet's terms) included the perception that parts of her body had disappeared and the intermittent inability to move. Lisa was continually surprised by these symptoms appearing "out of the blue" and disappearing unpredictably within minutes, hours or days.

Starting at age thirteen, Lisa frequented the family doctor at times as often as three times a week except when institutionalized. Although he paid careful attention to her case, he remained unable to make a suitable medical diagnosis. Medication proved ineffective. Although the consultations did not provide a cure or physical relief, Lisa valued his kind support. Yet increasingly feeling herself a nuisance, she began to avoid contacts with physicians. Lisa became aware that the course of her "real" somatic symptoms differed from that of the "strange" ones. The first were generally more stable in character and covered a longer time span, whereas the latter appeared intermittently, were of relatively short duration and could go away as unexpectedly as they had come. Finally she realized that these curious symptoms rarely lasted for more than two or three days, and she consequently decided that only when symptoms lasted longer than that span of time she would ask for medical help. Despite these precautions, she was repeatedly sent to medical specialists and hospitalized more than once. One of these referrals concerned her irregular menstruation. Sometimes she had periods three times a month and at other times once in three months. This irregularity could not be explained by pregnancy or anorexia.

If Janet was right in his opinion that mental stigmata and mental accidents are the true markers of hysteria (dissociative disorders), then (1) it should be possible to categorize Lisa's symptoms in terms of these and (2) this patient as a complex dissociative case should display most of these essential symptoms.

Lisa's Mental Stigmata: Negative Dissociative Symptoms

Anesthesias Lisa was aware of some anesthesias, but not of others. *Tactile anesthesia* was evidently present, since her body felt partly or completely numb at times. If anesthetic areas were touched, she would become aware of this only by looking, and even then she did not feel the touch. Lisa also had difficulty directing her own movements, due to the condition described above as *kinesthetic anesthesia*. Without looking at her limbs, Lisa had difficulty knowing their position in space or controlling their movements, as when knitting, sewing or writing. With eyes shut, she could not tell how firmly she was gripping the hand of the therapist. Occasionally she shut the door before her leg had cleared it. She broke lots of dishes and frequently placed objects inches away from the place she had in mind (*ataxia*). According to Lisa, the many scars and frequent bruises on her legs were a result of these insensibilities. She was annoyed with herself for repeatedly stumbling over objects that had been located in the same place for years.

The above symptoms already indicate the presence of *Lasègue's syndrome*. This disturbance could be further assessed using simple experiments. Upon eye closure, Lisa experienced her body as an assembly of unrelated and disconnected elements. Eyes closed, she was unable to touch her nose with her right hand; time and again the movement ended with her touching the right eye. However, as with most other somatoform symptoms, this condition was state-dependent. In one of her states the effect was consistently restricted to right-hand movements, in another state only left-hand movements were involved, and in still another the symptom was absent. Further, when we moved her arms while her eyes were closed, she was (in some of her dissociative states) unable to tell whether the arms had been moved, to mentally follow the direction of the movements, and/or to rate their final position. As with nineteenth-century hysterical patients, Lisa was able to become aware of these disturbances only via these examinations. In passing, we again point out, as Janet did, that these multiple and obscure symptoms cannot be understood simply as the result of simulation or self-suggestion.

It also happened that at times an arm, a leg or some other part of the body developed a thinglike quality. In this context, Lisa might also lose her sense of ownership of that limb or the entire body. At times, Lisa felt like a robot, a condition she also described as having no body, as being pulled into action by commands of unknown sources or as being a puppet on a string. This loss of control over movements accompanying the anesthesia can be understood as an intrusion phenomenon.

At other times, Lisa had the experience that the body, or a part of it, had vanished. This disappearance phenomenon affected most often her hands, breasts and pelvic area. She saw (*visual anesthesia*) and experienced (*organic anesthesia*) "holes" where those members should have been.

Visual anesthesia also presented in other forms. Lisa's visual acuity varied and occasionally she lost her eyesight entirely. This temporary blindness (*generalized visual anesthesia*) or blurring of vision occurred rarely and could generally be traced to anticipatory fear of perceiving a traumatic scene (e.g., when she felt socially obliged to watch the news or thrillers on television). She also noticed that at times familiar things around her would suddenly appear to be quite different than usual. Sometimes she described perceiving only parts of objects. At times she experienced tunnel vision (*retraction of visual field*). As mentioned, this partial visual loss was also a feature of those moments of kinesthetic loss when she could not see or feel parts of her own body.

The way in which Lisa visually apprehended her body was state-dependent. Each dissociative identity state experienced a divergent body schema, which systematically altered the visual and kinesthetic perception of herself. Her perceptions of actual body features, such as breasts, hairdo, color of hair and eyes, complexion, body height, weight and so on, were lost and then replaced by perceptions of features fitting the altered scheme.

Lisa reported short periods of deafness (*generalized auditory anesthesia*). Further exploration revealed that hearing acuity changed frequently, and at times sounds from nearby seemed to be coming from a great distance. It was also evident that her auditory perception varied with state. While in some states she consistently noticed the slightest sound of footsteps behind the door of the therapist's office (*systematized auditory hyperesthesia*), but in others she was seemingly oblivious to such sounds, even to loud outside noises that disturbed the therapist.

Once in a while, Lisa lost all sense of taste or smell (*gustatory and olfactory anesthesia*). Others might have to warn her that food was burning on the stove. More often than not, the loss of smell was paralleled by a loss of taste as well as a loss of emotion. It also might happen that all food and drinks tasted or smelled alike. In some states, she lost taste and smell preferences or aversions that she had had in others.

With Lisa, *analgesia* had been present in the context of previous self-mutilation, but also appeared at other times, especially when she felt threatened. Then it was often accompanied by concomitant stiffening of the body and inability to move. Lisa could also become analgesic on other occasions. For example, she once noticed by looking at her hands that she had sewn a finger to her needlework.

Genital anesthesia was another state-dependent phenomenon. She could have sexual contacts with her husband without physically or emotionally feeling a thing. However, one dissociative identity state, "Lady," was able to experience and enjoy genital and sexual sensations and emotions. In still another state, which until the second year of treatment remained unknown to Lisa and the therapist, she became instantly and completely passive and completely anesthetic upon the approach of one of her sexual abusers (this was the man she ultimately confronted). For some years this ongoing sexual relationship had been concealed by the identity shift and the amnesia that habitually followed the sexual contact.

Amnesia Lisa's dissociative amnesias affected both past and recent experience and involved autobiographical memory as well as implicit memory. Implicit memory loss manifested through state-dependent losses and gains of skills. For example, in her normal condition, Lisa was able to perform motor skills that, upon a transition to a child state, were instantaneously lost. In child states, she could neither write as an adult nor perform simple tasks such as using a door key. The execution of more complicated tasks, such as cooking meals and performing nursing tasks (her profession), was completely beyond her at these times. Adult movements might turn at any moment into childlike motion and adult speech into childlike talk as a wide array of psychological and somatoform capacities became inaccessible upon transition to younger identity states. In Lisa's case, amnesia was recognizable somatically long before we could map clearly the amnestic gaps in her psychic experience. These sharp fluctuations in motor skills could not be ascribed to fatigue, spells of laziness or lack of concentration, and seemed best explained as forgetting how to perform certain tasks.

In harmony with Janet's observations, we noted that changes in mental and motor skills also may vary between normal and dissociative states of comparable subjective age. Although she noticed the presence of her child, Lisa "had no child," she was "not the mother." She had amnesia for the birth of her abuse-conceived daughter and lacked childrearing motor skills. A dissociated female helper identity, called the "Helper," claimed to be the mother. In this state Lisa was able to provide a detailed account of the dramatic childbirth. The "Helper" also possessed the fine-tuned motor skills of holding and gently washing an infant, physically comforting an anxious schoolgirl and touching an adolescent daughter in an appropriate way. In other states these mothering skills were inaccessible. She no longer knew how to caress, and she washed her children far too roughly. We also noticed that her gaits were state-dependent. For example, while the "Lady" moved graciously and knew how to apply makeup, the "Helper" was more clumsy, walking briskly like a busy mother. These changes were accompanied by *modifications of character*, another mental stigma. The "Lady" showed interest in ladylike affairs. She enjoyed wearing stylish clothes, driving sports cars and attracting and receiving male attention. The "Lady" ignored the children, who were not hers, in her view, and often were in her way. In contrast, the "Helper" wore "efficient" coats with big pockets suited for carrying little bears and puppets and preferred a big car that could transport many children (she also took care of many child identity states).

Dissociations of autobiographical memory pertaining to the past and the present also involved the body. For example, the "forgetting" of certain body parts in some states seemed to coincide with amnestic gaps in those identity states for childhood adversities that had injured those parts of the body. The saying "out of sight, out of mind" was applicable here. Amnesia was an aspect of Lisa's shifts in body image. In child identity states, she lost awareness as well as ownership of her adult body features, which were replaced by childlike body images often further distorted by abuse-induced features (for example, one such identity state explained: "I have no mouth").

Motor Disturbances   Lisa's ataxia and Lasègue's syndrome have been described in the section on anesthesia. Other motor disturbances involved occasional immobility as a response to threat, paralyses and contractures. Lisa also experienced total loss of bodily control, as when overtaken by a dissociative state. Sometimes she described this as unknown forces directing her body, indicating the presence of intrusive subconscious fixed ideas (discussed below).

LISA'S MENTAL ACCIDENTS:
POSITIVE, OR INTRUSION, SYMPTOMS

Subconscious Fixed Ideas   Lisa's subconscious fixed ideas affected a wide range of senses, somatoform reactions and functions and emotions. These emotionally charged dissociated thoughts and images intruded into personal consciousness and on the awareness of other dissociative identity states. For example, they induced *dysesthesias*—intrusive, nonpainful sensations. For reasons that in her normal state she did not understand, Lisa at times experienced "things" or hands touching her body. Dissociative identity states understood these symptoms as related to experiences of rats crawling over her body and to scenes in which aggressive or sexually aroused men and women were grabbing at her body. Especially at nighttime, Lisa's mother habitually exiled her child to the barn or to an attic as "punishment." Both were rat infested. Other fixed ideas associated with dysesthesias included coldness (being exiled to the ice-cold barn), physical weakness (child states), strength (aggressive states) and feeling dirty (menstrual blood; see below). Since, as far as we can know now, these related to traumatic events rather than to secondary fantasies, they are classified as fixed ideas of the primary type.

Subconscious (primary) fixed ideas also led to *hyperesthesia* (pain). Lisa intermittently suffered from many localized pain symptoms relating to traumatic events, for instance, pain in the genitals, anus and abdominal region (sexual abuse). Sharply localized pains joined memories of physical abuse, for example, headaches (beatings around face and head), stomachaches (kicks in the stomach) and burning skin (due to having been "washed" by her mother with an abrasive). Explicit knowledge of associated traumatic events was often stored in the dissociative states experiencing painful responses. However, some states merely suffered a somatoform symptom without having an explanation for it. In these cases, closely related states that were not subjected to pain knew the reasons for the pain.

Fixed ideas might present as *pseudohallucinations*. For example, under the influence of a fearful child state, Lisa "saw" her mother in the office of the therapist. However, some visual disturbances did not seem to relate to fixed ideas, but to the reactivation of dissociative states in a more general sense. Lisa reported that double vision might go along with the copresence of dissociative states (coconsciousness). As she described it, then "two sets of eyes were watching simultaneously" or "someone else inside was using her eyes."

Lisa experienced seemingly inexplicable and sudden changes of taste and of related food preferences *(mobility of gustatory and olfactory symptoms)*. For example, a child state liked sweets, which Lisa despised. Lisa experienced cravings for sweet things that apparently stemmed from a "child inside." A "strange, disgustful" taste was dependent upon the reactivation of a dissociative state that reported having been forced to perform fellatio and to swallow sperm. Its fixed idea was that the penis of her abuser and his sperm were still in her mouth, which idea also induced nausea and choking sensations. The olfactory sense was also affected; for example, Lisa sometimes smelled gasoline, a substance that was part of a traumatic event.

Lisa demonstrated various *motor disturbances.* Symptoms related to fixed ideas caused intermittent inability or disability to act or move (partial or complete *catalepsy, contractures*), eat, swallow or speak *(aphonia, dysphonia)* as well as led to the uncontrolled performance of unintended motor acts. Here are some examples: (1) Approaching the door of the outpatient department, she found herself, to her astonishment and dismay, unable to move her hands and arms and so unable to open the door. Then "her legs walked the body to the car," upon which "the body took her home." Later a dissociative state claimed responsibility for this line of action: It had been opposed to the objective of the visit, which was to include a feared diagnostic evaluation. (2) At times, especially when she felt threatened or upon the reactivation of particular fearful child states, her body grew completely stiff or became totally immobile *(catalepsy/ecstasies/cataleptic somnambulism* [Janet 1894/1901]). When she entered unfamiliar or otherwise subjectively threatening situations, she might feel an urge to leave, but also feel unable to do so. At such times she might experience sudden inability to move or speak. Attempts at spoken language came out as mere noise. Afterward, she often experienced joint pain. (3) Tremors and uncontrollable defensive movements were occasionally present. These symptoms were traced to the fear or rage of dissociative child states (not those with a "freeze" response). (4) Lisa also experienced motor symptoms in relation to oppositions of *monoideisms* or *polyideisms* ("inner fights") between dissociative states, due to which acts could be postponed, prevented, interrupted or abolished.

Lisa's fixed ideas could have peculiar effects. We offer two examples: (1) Some of Lisa's dissociated identities feared blood, and they claimed the capacity to postpone menstruation or even to create a menstruation pause. Like some other DID patients we have observed, she reported that once menstruation began, the reactivation of child alters could induce an acute menstrual interruption. Their retreat allowed menses to recommence. (2) During her abuse-induced pregnancy, the "Helper" identity state felt she actualized wishes that the child had not been born by postponing the event. After ten months of pregnancy and in the absence of any signs of labor, she was admitted to a hospital, where, after considerable effort, birth was medically induced. The "Helper" had developed the idea that "it was put in my abdomen, so that's where it apparently belongs, so that's where it should stay."

Hysterical Attacks   Hysterical attacks accompanied many somatoform dissociative symptoms and related to the reactivation of traumatic memories and various fixed ideas. For example, when reliving exiles to the barn, Lisa shivered with cold (when the therapist was allowed to check, her skin temperature had indeed dropped) and became immobile. Once in a while, she suddenly would hit her body while "chasing" rats. Reliving childbirth, her body felt very enlarged, and she reexperienced abdominal cramps and pains. Reexperiencing sexual abuse, she froze. In some states she was in pain, in others she was analgesic. Lisa's traumatic memories thus were unlike typical narrative memories, since the traumata were expressed primarily as sensorimotor reexperiencing.

Somnambulisms: Complex Dissociative (Identity) States   Lisa's dissociative identity states, which showed all the characteristics of somnambulism, displayed intricate ties between psychological and somatoform functioning. For example, a particular dissociative identity state contained a lifetime of bad memories about menstruation. As a young girl, Lisa had not been allowed by her mother to use pads or bandages. Consequently, during her periods she had to stay away from school. At home, she tried to hide herself. Her mother appeared to take pleasure in showing any visitor what a "dreadful dirty daughter" she had by lifting Lisa's skirt. Later in life, when her monthly period was due, the state that felt "dirty" took control and bought excessive quantities of pads and new underwear. Until therapy, Lisa was amnestic for these behaviors. Time and again she was utterly confused at finding purchases she could not account for. The "somnambulistic" state shift and amnesia rendered Lisa "absent." On other occasions for "inexplicable" reasons she suffered intense menstrual pains and, feeling like a puppet on a string, could not resist compulsive and excessive washing. Some states claimed to have the ability to postpone menstruation. Behind all these phenomena, the *monoideism* was that she was dirty while menstruating.

Some of Lisa's dissociated identities, when reactivated in therapy, showed reasonable or even good adaptation to the actual surroundings, but others, at least initially, were so enmeshed in past behaviors and related psychological and somatoform responses that their reactivations had the qualities of a hysterical attack.

THE DEVELOPMENT AND THE CHARACTERISTICS OF
THE SOMATOFORM DISSOCIATION QUESTIONNAIRE (SDQ-20)

Lisa's case suggests that mental stigmata and mental accidents may be as characteristic of contemporary hysterical (dissociative disorder) patients as they were of the cases that Janet and some of his contemporary colleagues studied. Nijenhuis et al. (1996) developed a self-report questionnaire measuring somatoform dissociation. Using clinical observations of somatoform dissociation in cases such as Lisa's, a pool of seventy-seven items was formulated as a first step. Somatoform dissociation was defined as state-dependent somatoform responses suggesting a medical condition that had appeared in clinical settings upon the reactivation of particular dissociative states and that could not be medically explained. Six clinicians experienced in dealing with dissociative disorders judged the face validity of these items. As a result, two items were removed. The remaining seventy-five items were rated by fifty patients with dissociative disorders, who were diagnosed using the Structured Clinical Interview for DSM-IV Dissociative Disorders (SCID-D; Steinberg 1993; Steinberg, Rounsaville and Cichetti 1990, 1991; Steinberg et al. 1993). A control group included fifty psychiatric patients with other *DSM-IV* diagnoses.

The dissociative disorders group reached statistically significant higher scores on seventy-one items. Separate logistic analyses and determination of discriminant indices for each item revealed twenty items that best discriminated cases from noncases. Mokken analysis (Molenaar et al. 1994) showed that these twenty items are strongly scalable on a latent dimensional scale, which was interpreted as measuring somatoform dissociation. The items involve negative as well as positive dissociative symptoms. Reliability of the scale was high (Cronbach's alpha = 0.95). As our original and replication studies revealed (Nijenhuis et al. 1996, 1997, 1997b, 1998b), convergent validity was supported by high intercorrelations with self-reporting instruments measuring psychological dissociation (DIS-Q, Vanderlinden 1993; Vanderlinden et al. 1993; DES, Bernstein and Putnam 1986). Construct validity was supported by the finding that the SDQ-20 scores strongly discriminated between dissociative disorder and comparison patients, and that patients with DID obtained significantly higher SDQ-20 scores than patients with DDNOS or depersonalization disorder. Next, the degree of somatoform dissociation was correlated with reported trauma (Nijenhuis et al., 1998). The SDQ-20 also has very satisfactory criterion-related and discriminative validity: The scores were low in a mixed psychiatric group (which comprised mostly anxiety disorders, depression and adjustment disorders) and bipolar mood disorder; they were raised in a subgroup of eating disorder patients and were further raised in somatoform disorders, even higher in DDNOS, and were extreme in DID. All of these group differences remained statistically significant after controlling for general psychoneuroticism. The SDQ-20 is thus a scale of high psychometric quality for measuring somatoform dissociation.

From this initial instrument, the SDQ-20, a dissociative disorders screening version was derived (Nijenhuis et al. 1997, 1997b, 1998). Entering the items into a stepwise forward logistic regression analysis, a subset of five items (SDQ-5) was derived that as a group provided optimal discrimination between dissociative disorder patients and comparison patients. The symptoms include kinesthetic anesthesia ("It is as if my body or part of it has disappeared"), visual anesthesia, analgesia, loss of speech (negative dissociative symptoms) and a pain symptom ("pain while urinating," a positive dissociative symptom). Sensitivity (94 percent) and specificity (96 percent) of this SDQ-5 were high. The positive predictive value was 72 percent and negative predictive value 99 percent at an estimated prevalence rate of dissociative disorders of 10 percent. Two replication studies corroborated these first findings.

In summary, these data indicate that somatoform dissociative phenomena as measured by the SDQ-20 are very characteristic of dissociative disorder patients. The symptoms involve negative as well as positive somatoform dissociative phenomena, and they match the mental stigmata and mental accidents as described by Janet. The abbreviated screening version, the SDQ-5, is capable of detecting high rates of true positives and true negatives, meaning that these five items pertain to core symptoms of hysteria (dissociative disorders).

CONCLUSION

According to Janet, contemporary clinical observation and recent empirical research, pathological dissociation affects both soma and psyche. The findings from these various sources suggest that a lack of mental synthesis can result in a wide range of somatoform reactions and functions, as well as psychological reactions and functions that do not affect the body. In fact, the converging evidence suggests that somatoform dissociative phenomena belong to the essential symptoms of hysteria (dissociative disorders). Therefore, it is important to include this category of characteristic hysterical symptoms in modern views on dissociation, to elaborate the study of somatoform dissociation in *DSM-IV* dissociative disorders, to assess its prevalence and nature in various disorders that in the present diagnostic manual are classified as somatoform disorders and to reconsider the taxonomic classification of these disturbances. It is hoped that the availability of the SDQ-20 as an instrument for measuring somatoform dissociation will stimulate these developments.

The case examples and the results of our empirical investigations confirm Janet's observation that somatoform and psychological dissociation are highly intertwined phenomena, suggesting that both stem from a common source. Janet maintained that all dissociative phenomena result from a retraction of the field of consciousness and a lowering of the level of mental functioning, which favor the formation of dissociative mental structures. A phenomenological classification dichotomizing somatoform and psychological dissociation can be clarifying and serves to draw attention to the often overlooked somatoform dissociative phenomena. Nonetheless, we agree with Janet that this dichotomization is based on our cultural and psychological difficulties in dealing with what is in essence a unity.

Somatoform dissociative symptoms (as well as psychological dissociative symptoms) can also be described in terms of Janet's classificatory distinction between mental stigmata and mental accidents, or, as we have proposed to label these categories, negative and positive dissociative symptoms. These negative and positive symptoms impress us also as closely related phenomena. For example, localized anesthesias may be tied to fixed ideas (e.g., Lisa: "*I have no breasts*"). In the same vein, amnestic episodes represent shadows left by interruptions of normal consciousness by hysterical attacks and somnambulistic or dissociative psychotic states, and losses of motor control often seem related to reactivation of fixed ideas or more complex dissociative states. In combination, these losses and intrusions suggest parallel distribution of information processing by two or more mental states, causing the capricious and contradictory phenomenology of hysteria (dissociative disorders). Each state, no matter how weakly or strongly emancipated it is, seems to be endowed with a degree of consciousness encompassing a sense of identity. Although these nonsynthesized states have their own sense of self, they still are parts of the patient's mind. And although they may have their own body image and may function with different neurophysiological parameters, they still share the same body.

REFERENCES

American Psychiatric Association. (1987). *Diagnostic and statistical manual of mental disorders.* 3rd rev. ed. Washington, D.C.: American Psychiatric Association.

_____. (1994). *Diagnostic and statistical manual of mental disorders.* 4th ed. Washington, D.C.: American Psychiatric Association.

Babinski, J. (1901). Définition de l'hystérie. *Revue Neurologique* 9: 1074–1080.

_____. (1909). Démembrement de l'hystérie. *La Semaine Médicale* 9: 3–8.

Babinski, J., and Froment, J. (1918). Hystérie-pithiatisme et troubles nerveux d'ordre réflexe en neurologie de guerre (pp. 109–114). Paris: Masson.

Bernstein, E., and Putnam, F. W. (1986). Development, reliability, and validity of a dissociation scale. *Journal of Nervous and Mental Disease* 102: 280–286.

Bourru, H., and Burot, P. (1895). *La suggestion mentale et les variations de la personnalité.* Paris: J.-B. Baillière et Fils.

Bowman, E. S., and Markand, O. N. (1996). Psychodynamics and psychiatric diagnoses of pseudoseizure subjects. *American Journal of Psychiatry* 153: 57–63.

Breuer, J., and Freud, S. (1955). On the psychical mechanism of hysterical phenomena. In J. Strachey and A. Strachey, eds., *Standard edition of the complete psychological works of Sigmund Freud* (pp. 1–181). London: Hogarth.

Briquet, P. (1859). *Traité clinique et thérapeutique de l'hystérie.* Paris: J.-B. Baillière et Fils.

Charcot, J. M. (1887). *Leçons sur les maladies du système nerveux faites à la Salpétrière.* Vol. 3. Paris: Progrès Médical en A. Delahaye and E. Lecrosnie.

Crabtree, A. (1992). Dissociation and memory: A two-hundred-year perspective. *Dissociation* 5 (3): 150–154.

Edelman, G. (1992). *Bright air, brilliant fire: On the matter of mind.* New York: Basic Books.

Janet, P. (1886). Les actes inconscients et le dédoublement de la personnalité pendant le somnambulisme provoqué. *Revue Philosophique* 22: 212–223.

_____. (1889). *L'Automatisme psychologique.* Paris: Félix Alcan. Reprint: Société Pierre Janet, Paris, 1973.

_____. (1893). *L'Etat mental des hystériques: Les stigmates mentaux.* Paris: Rueff and Cie.

_____. (1894). *L'Etat mental des hystériques: Les accidents mentaux.* Paris: Rueff and Cie.

_____. (1898). *Névroses et idées fixes.* Vol. 1. Paris: Félix Alcan.

_____. (1901). *The mental state of hystericals.* New York: Putnam. Reprint: University Publications of America, Washington, D.C., 1977.

_____. (1904). L'Amnésie et la dissociation des souvenirs par l'émotion. *Journal de Psychologie*. 1: 417–453.

_____. (1907). *Major symptoms of hysteria*. London: Macmillan. Reprint: Hafner, New York, 1965.

_____. (1909). *Les névroses*. Paris: Flammarion.

_____. (1911). *L' Etat mental des hystériques*, 2d extended ed. Paris: Félix Alcan. Reprint: Lafitte Reprints, Marseille, 1983.

_____. (1928). *L'Evolution de la mémoire et de la notion du temps*. Paris: A. Chahine.

_____. (1932). Les croyances et les hallucinations. *Revue Philosophique* 113: 278–331.

Kihlstrom, J. F. (1992). Dissociative and conversion disorders. In D. J. Stein and J. E. Young, eds., *Cognitive science and clinical disorders* (pp. 248–270). San Diego: Academic Press.

_____. (1994). One hundred years of hysteria. In S. J. Lynn and J. W. Rhue, eds., *Dissociation: Clinical and theoretical perspectives* (pp. 365–394). New York: Guilford.

Krystal, J. H., Bennett, A. L., Bremner, J. D., Southwick, S. M., and Charney, D. S. (1995). Toward a cognitive neuroscience of dissociation and altered memory functions in post-traumatic stress disorder. In M. J. Friedman, D. S. Charney and A. Y. Deutch, eds., *Neurobiological and clinical consequences of stress: From normal adaptation to PTSD* (pp. 239–269). Philadelphia: Lippincott-Raven.

Loftus, E. F. (1993). The reality of repressed memories. *American Psychologist* 48: 518–537.

Molenaar, I. W., Debets, P., Sytsma, K., and Hemker, B. T. (1994). *Users manual MSP. A program for Mokken Scale analysis for polytomous items*. Version 3.0. Groningen: iec ProGAMMA.

Nijenhuis, E. R. S. (1990). Somatische equivalenten bij dissociatieve stoornissen [Somatic equivalents in dissociative disorders]. *Hypnotherapie* 12: 139–142.

_____. (1995). Dissociatie en leertheorie: trauma-geïnduceerde dissociatie als klassiek geconditioneerde defensie [Dissociation and learning theory: trauma-induced dissociation as classically conditioned defense]. In K. Jonker, J. Derksen and F. Donker, eds., *Dissociatie: een fenomeen opnieuw belicht [Dissociation: A phenomenon illuminated afresh]* (pp. 35–61). Houten: Bohn Stafleu Van Loghum.

Nijenhuis, E. R. S., Spinhoven, Ph., van Dyck, R., van der Hart, O., and Vanderlinden, J. (1996). The development and the psychometric characteristics of the Somatoform Dissociation Questionnaire (SDQ–20). *Journal of Nervous and Mental Disease* 184: 688–694.

_____. (1997). Somatoforme dissociatie: Wezenlijke kenmerken van somatoforme en dissociatieve stoornissen [Somatoform dissociation: Major symptoms of somatoform and dissociative disorders]. Presentation at the Conference on Somatic Complaints, Conversion, and Dissociation. Utrecht, Society of Psychosomatic Medicine, April 11.

_____. (1997b). The development of the Somatoform Dissociation Questionnaire (SDQ-5) as a screening instrument for dissociative disorders. *Acta Psychiatrica Scandinavica* 96: 311–318.

_____. (1998). Degree of somatoform and psychological dissociation is correlated with reported trauma. *Journal of Traumatic Stress* 11: 711–730.

_____. (1998b). Psychometric characteristics of the Somatoform Dissociation Questionnaire: A replication study. *Psychotherapy and Psychosomatics* 67: 17–23.

Pitres, A. (1891). *Leçons cliniques sur l'hystérie et l'hypnotisme*. Paris: Octave Doin.

Pribor, E. F., Yutzy, S. H., Dean, J. T., and Wetzel, R. D. (1993). Briquet's syndrome, dissociation, and abuse. *American Journal of Psychiatry* 150: 1507–1511.

Reed, G. (1979). Anomalies of recall and recognition. In J. F. Kihlstrom and F. J. Evans, eds., *Functional disorders of memory* (pp. 1–28). Hillsdale, N.J.: Erlbaum.

_____. (1988). *The psychology of anomalous experience*. Rev. ed. Buffalo, N.Y.: Prometheus. (Original work published in 1974.)

Ross, C. A., Heber, S., Norton, G. R., and Anderson, G. (1989). Somatic symptoms in multiple personality disorder. *Psychosomatics* 30: 154–160.

Sacks, O. (1984). *A leg to stand on*. London: Duckworth.

Saxe, G. N., Chinman, G., Berkowitz, R., Hall, K., Lieberg, G., Schwartz, J., and van der Kolk, B. A. (1994). Somatization in patients with dissociative disorders. *American Journal of Psychiatry* 151: 1329–1334.

Steinberg, M. (1993). *Structured Clinical Interview for DSM-IV Dissociative Disorders (SCID-D)*. Washington, D.C.: American Psychiatric Press.

Steinberg, M., Cichetti, D. V., Buchanan, J., Hall, P., and Rounsaville, B. (1993). Clinical assessment of dissociative symptoms and disorders: The Structured Clinical Interview for DSM-IV Dissociative Disorders. *Dissociation* 6: 3–16.

Steinberg, M., Rounsaville, B., and Cichetti, D. V. (1990). The Structured Clinical Interview for DSM-III-R Dissociative Disorders: Preliminary report on a new diagnostic instrument. *American Journal of Psychiatry* 147: 76–82.

_____. (1991). Detection of dissociative disorders in psychiatric patients by a screening instrument and a structured diagnostic interview. *American Journal of Psychiatry* 148: 1050–1054.

van der Hart, O., and Friedman, B. (1989). A reader's guide to Pierre Janet on dissociation: A neglected intellectual heritage. *Dissociation* 2 (1): 3–16.

_____. (1992). Trauma, dissociation and triggers: Their role in treatment and emergency psychiatry. In J. B. van Luyn et al., eds., *Emergency psychiatry today* (pp. 137–142). Amsterdam: Elsevier Science Publishers.

van der Hart, O., and Horst, R. (1989). The dissociation theory of Pierre Janet. *Journal of Traumatic Stress* 2: 397–412.

van der Hart, O., Nijenhuis, E. R. S., and van der Kolk, B. A. In preparation. Traumatic memories: Between reproductions and reconstructions.

van der Hart, O., and Op den Velde, W. (1991). Traumatische stoornissen [Trauma-induced disorders]. In O. van der Hart, ed., *Trauma, dissociatie en hypnose* [Trauma, dissociation and hypnosis] (pp. 71–90). Lisse: Swets and Zeitlinger.

van der Hart, O., Witztum, E., and Friedman, B. (1993). From hysterical psychosis to reactive dissociative psychosis. *Journal of Traumatic Stress* 6: 43–64.

van der Kolk, B. A., and van der Hart, O. (1989). Pierre Janet and the breakdown of adaptation in psychological trauma. *American Journal of Psychiatry* 146: 1530–1540.

Vanderlinden, J. (1993). *Dissociative experiences, trauma and hypnosis: Research findings and clinical applications in eating disorders.* Delft: Eburon.

Vanderlinden, J., van Dyck, R., Vandereycken, W., Vertommen, H., and Verkes, R. J. (1993). The dissociation questionnaire: Development and characteristics of a new self-reporting questionnaire. *Clinical Psychology and Psychotherapy* 1: 21–27.

Walker, E. A., Katon, W. J., Neraas, K., Jemelka, R. P., and Massoth, D. (1992). Dissociation in women with chronic pelvic pain. *American Journal of Psychiatry* 149: 534–537.

World Health Organization (1992). *The ICD–10 classification of mental and behavioural disorders: Clinical descriptions and diagnostic guidelines.* Geneva: World Health Organization.

PART II

Experiences
Body Image in Trauma

Everyone carries a room around inside him. . . . If one listens one can hear its mirror rattling.

Franz Kafka (1991, 1)

I don't have a face. I don't look in mirrors. I don't know what it is to have a boundary, to feel all the way out to the edges.

Patient in psychotherapy, unpublished

I feel my head is filled with garbage. . . . There's another skin beneath my skin and that skin is called Auschwitz.

Isabella L., witness (Langer 1991, 53)

One can direct one's inquiry to the body itself, no longer posited as a fact of nature, a constant and universal reality, but as an entirely problematic notion, a historical category, steeped in imagination.

J. P. Vernant (1989, 20)

If you could lick my heart, it would poison you.

Itzhak Zuckerman, leader of the Warsaw Ghetto Uprising (from the film *Shoah*)

River is not a bad name for the body.

Origen (Bynum 1995, 113)

The Body Silenced

*History's Dissociation
of the Speaking Body*

"Where does it hurt?"

[No response.]

"Does your head hurt, or your back, or your shoulders?"

[After a moment of silence.] "Ah, no, Madame, it does not hurt there."

"Then what is it that makes you ill?"

"It is my father who makes me ill."

Beizer (1994)

As we plunged deeper into our dialogue with the body, inarticulate as it first appeared, recurrent themes asserted themselves. D. Anzieu's wonderful book *The Skin Ego,* which, when we discovered it, seemed to constitute the very definition of a raid on the inarticulate (Eliot 1943), appeared in a most uncanny fashion in chapter after chapter sent by other contributors, who had discovered its treasures independently. Anzieu's eloquent description of the two types of anxiety commonly found in traumatized individuals is typical of the wisdom to be found in this book: "[In the first case] an instinctual excitation that is diffuse, constant, scattered, non-localizable, non-identifiable, unquenchable; when the psychical topography consists of a kernel without a shell. The individual seeks a substitute shell in physical pain or psychical anxiety. He wraps himself in suffering. In the second case the envelope exists but its continuity is broken into by holes. . . . Thoughts and memories leak away . . . a cause of considerable anxiety to have an interior which empties itself, especially of the aggression required for any kind of self-assertion" (1989, p. 102).

131

Anzieu's thoughts on the development and function of what he terms the "skin ego" inspired our first tentative explorations into the dark continent of the body. We were struck by the way in which assaults on the bodies of children—despite being silenced, altered, revised and ignored—somehow resurfaced in symptoms, their original truths intact but in code. So although silenced and excluded from ordinary discourse, a new and powerful language was being forged out of the body's struggle to remember and articulate the truth of personal experience.

In *Psychoanalysing Psychoanalysis,* Marie Balmary describes what we came to grasp about the paradox of the body silenced but speaking: "Those who have been sexually violated . . . have tried to express through hysteria, through the negations of sexuality . . . what they underwent. How would those whose thought and discourse have been violated tell what has been done to them if not through a condition where one no longer has either thought or speech? How would they try to escape if not by making use of a language that could not be understood, but which also could not be taken away from them?" (1982, p. 155).

So for a little over one hundred years, these signals, symptoms, codes have been examined, sometimes sensitively, sometimes not. Jean-Martin Charcot, at the Salpêtrière, reflected back to his hysterical patients a peculiar ambivalence. On the one hand, he rescued them from consignment to the limbo of their symptoms; on the other, he hardly ever listened to their words and literally overwrote their desperate and wordless statements by writing his own words on their bodies. The phenomenon of dermographism, or "writing on the skin" of the hysterical patient, is almost too apt a metaphor for the superimposition of the physician's narrative onto the patient's body. Beizer (1994) explains that today this phenomenon is understood as a form of physical urticaria whose outbreaks are provoked by a release of histamines. When the skin is touched, welts are raised that persevere for a time. The fascination with the possibility of this kind of writing on skin persists to the present. Beizer reports that two of the three physicians she spoke with maintained collections of dermographic photographs. This "fascination with the body's ability to bear meaning" constitutes an element of continuity over the past century; the meaning that was found, though, often reflected the physicians' own message rather than the unknown and possibly disruptive message that the body actually contains.

Nevertheless the interest, the study, the cataloguing of symptoms went on despite these glaring blind spots and survived to resurface in the last fifteen years in the rediscovery of dissociation. Perhaps most important for the future, Freud saw these patients too and learned much from Charcot. He carried the dialogue even further and, despite his misunderstandings, propelled the theory and practice of working with the symptomatic body/psyche to a new level. As Balmary states it so well: "Psychoanalysis has enabled us to pass . . . from the body to a relational system. From one's own body, to one's personal history, to one's family history, to one's relation to the Other; a great evolution that leaves no theory of mental life unchanged . . . regardless of how encompassing it may be" (1982, p. 1).

Looking back on what William James understood about these patients a century ago, it is hard to imagine a contemporary clinician having such grasp, mastery and depth of understanding: "In the wonderful explorations . . . of the subliminal consciousness of patients with hysteria, we have revealed to us whole systems of underground life, in the shape of memories of a painful sort which lead a parasitic existence, buried outside the primary fields of consciousness, and making irruptions thereunto with hallucinations, pains, convulsions, paralyses of feeling and of motion, and the whole procession of symptoms of hysteric disease of body and of mind" (James 1902, p. 230).

The ancients as well as nineteenth-century physicians posited the migrating womb as the cause of hysteria. Showalter (1985), writing in the context of twentieth-century feminism, sees the choked-off speech of the hysterical patient reappearing in coded bodily symptoms. One thinks of Anna O., who suffered from an elaborate sequence of speech disorders culminating in mutism. The treatment of the "talking cure," or perhaps more accurately the "cure through talking," rescued the symptom from the body and translated it into language. Hysterical discourse is remarkable for its silence and confusion, as in apnea or aphasia, as well as for its startling volubility: laughter, crying, speaking nonsense and animal sounds. Helene Cixous, quoted in Showalter's book *The Female Malady*, says: "Silence, silence is the mark of hysteria. The great hysterics have lost speech . . . their tongues are cut off and what talks isn't heard because it is the body that talks" (p. 161).

One of our patients who was struggling to find her creative voice revealed that she remembered her father persistently threatening to cut out her tongue if she told about abuse. He said this again to her while she was visiting him in a care facility. He was suffering from dementia, and when during one visit he suddenly turned to her and said, "I'm going to cut your tongue out," she knew that her recollection of the childhood scenes was true.

The persistent link between language and the confrontation with the hysterical body is reflected in contemporary therapists' attempts to grasp the array of symptoms presented by the traumatized patient. Balmary describes encountering the silenced patient speaking through the body: "Hysteria opened up the unconscious to psychoanalysis. It did so because hysteria is based not so much on a failure of language as on a disagreement with the father's language, in which the woman's body speaks the disagreement. The body joins in the conversation. Both hysteria and psychoanalysis deal with the borders of language, but they do so while standing on different sides: the hysteric resorts to the body to express her disagreement, the analyst reconverts the disagreement into the body of language" (1982, p. 1).

Charcot decoded some of this language, Janet went further, and Freud continued the process. In spite of stops and starts, losses and reversals, going down wrong roads for many years, losing some battles and winning others on the theoretical front, at last we have come again to the reconsideration of the traumatized body in relation to clinical practice.

When we began to look and listen, we found ourselves back in history with these early mystified but determined investigators, experiencing confusion and amazement. In one of our first conversations about this book, we discovered similar experiences with patients. We both had worked with patients who, as children, had been strangled in the course of sexual assaults and who, when those memories surfaced, displayed perfect red necklaces that persisted for days; in one case this circular mark would recur at widely spaced times whenever one of the many pieces of this event was brought to consciousness and integrated.

While doing trauma-based psychotherapy, we had both been confronted with atypical outbreaks of herpes, hives, rashes, inexplicable aches and pains, stuttering and mutism; patients reported convulsions, left-right splitting sensations in the body, loss or distortion of vision, spontaneous bodily contortions and bizarre sensations in the body such as broken glass in the stomach, insects in the abdomen, obstructions (like snakes) in the esophagus, holes in the heart and solar plexus and the feeling that the body was the wrong body, not their body. Piece by piece these fragmented symptoms of fragmented bodies began to make sense to us, and in the resulting dialogue we could see the gradual coalescing of this fragmentation into meaningful experiences for the patient.

The chapters in this section address the experience of trauma as it impacts body-image formation and ideation and the relationship between body image and sense of self. Mary Armsworth, Karin Stronck and Coleen Carlson (Chapter 5) concentrate on collecting data on body image and self-perception in women with incest histories. Here the test results supported clinical observations that abuse to the body may lead to negative body image and thence to violations or disruptions of a person's sense of being connected to self and others. Through these data we are able to grasp the clear connection between bodily trauma and negative body-image formation.

Chapter 6 on body-image distortions examines the relationship of sexual abuse to body image in modern psychoanalytic terms, tracing back each type of distortion to the traumatic moment and the child's imaginative efforts to comprehend and cope with the experience. Chapter 7, "Conversations with the Body," presents detailed clinical examples demonstrating the workings of the therapeutic conversation in exploring and bringing into language previously inarticulate experiences of body-image damage.

Valerie Sinason's Chapter 8 focuses on the self-image problems of children born with visible signs of devastating genetic illness or birth injury (Down's syndrome and cerebral palsy). She contends that even in these extreme conditions, body-image distortions can become equally or even more limiting than the catastrophic physical problem itself. This must be even more the case when the body's wounds are invisible, as in childhood maltreatment. Dr. Sinason's cases also provide instructive examples of conversations with the body and show how productive these can be with individuals of all chronological and mental ages. Sinason unravels some cases of compulsive masturbation by interpreting the behavior as an effort to find a mirror for the sexual aspects of the body.

The struggle to listen to and learn how to accurately decode the language of the body is at the heart of all of this work. The chapters in this section chronicle the struggle of each contributor to listen respectfully and to help the patient decode confusing bodily experiences. To this end are deployed our guile and experience, our research instruments, theoretical insights, psychotherapeutic techniques and metaphors from mythology and literature.

REFERENCES

Anzieu, D. (1989). *The skin ego.* New Haven: Yale University Press.

Balmary, M. (1982). *Psychoanalyzing psychoanalysis: Freud and the hidden fault of the father.* Trans. N. Lukacher. Baltimore: John Hopkins University Press.

Beizer, J. (1994). *Narratives of hysteria in nineteenth-century France.* Ithaca/London: Cornell University Press.

Bynum, C. W. (1995). *The resurrection of the body in Western Christianity, 200–1336.* New York: Columbia University Press.

Eliot, T. S. (1971). Four Quartets, East Coker in *The complete poems and plays, 1909–1950.* New York: Harcourt Brace Jovanovich.

Kafka, F. (1991). *The blue octavo notebooks.* Cambridge: Exact Change.

James, W. (1902). *The varieties of religious experience.* New York: Modern Library.

Langer, L. L. (1991). *Holocaust testimonies.* New Haven: Yale University Press.

Showalter, E. (1985) *The female malady: Women, madness, and English culture, 1830–1980.* New York: Penguin.

Vernant, J. P. (1989). Dim body, dazzling body. In M. Feher, *Fragments for a history of the human body,* Part 1 (pp. 19–47). New York: Urzone.

CHAPTER 5

Body Image and Self-Perception in Women with Histories of Incest

Mary Taylor Armsworth, Karin Stronck
and Colleen D. Carlson

Empirical and clinical reports describing the sequelae of unwanted sexual experiences in childhood point to a complex of disturbances in sense of self and body image resulting from the interplay of dissociative defenses and unmet developmental needs. This study investigated relationships between experiences of incest in childhood and disturbances in body image and self-perception, dissociation, difficulties with intimacy, feelings of self-worth and recognition of affect. A nonclinical sample of seventy-one women ($n = 36$ with a history of incest; $n = 35$ controls who were abuse-free) completed the Body Cathexis–Self Cathexis Scale (BC-SC), a measure of body and self-image; the Perceptual Alteration Scale (PAS) and the Dissociative Experiences Scale (DES), measures of dissociation; and selected ego functioning subscales from the Eating Disorders Inventory (EDI). Compared with the control group, women with a history of incest were found to have significantly greater body and self-dissatisfaction and higher levels of dissociation as measured with the PAS but not the DES. Negative body image was related to negative self-perceptions and, on EDI subscales, to not feeling in control and a general sense of worthlessness. Subscales on the EDI functioned differentially for the ethnic groups represented in this sample. Utility of the various instruments is presented as well as implications for practice and further research.

THEORETICAL BACKGROUND

Frequent references are made in the literature on sequelae of childhood incest to somatic symptoms as well as to long-term impacts on body image and self-functioning. With regard to changes in identity that result from prolonged or repeated trauma, Herman states, "All the structures of the self—the image of the body, the internalized images of others, and the values and ideals that lend a sense of coherence and purpose—are invaded and systematically broken down" (1992, 385).

Importance of the body in subsequent ego development was emphasized by Freud, who alluded to "a principle of internal differentiation and a containment principle" in his Project of 1895 (Anzieu 1989, 5). Fisher (1986) traces the literature on developmental aspects of body perception, citing numerous theorists. Among these are Jean Piaget, who described body movement as the "raw material of all intellectual and perceptual adaptation" and ascribed the organization of schemas to "the body interacting with objects" (Fisher 1986, 48). Werner saw the child's body experiences as a basis for all perceptions, providing a framework for defining self, organizing space and anchoring language in body images and feelings (Fisher 1986). Fisher concludes that the body plays a special role in the development of reality testing and cohesive identity formation and notes that a "fundamental dimension of the body image relates to how one experiences one's body boundaries" (1989, 54).

Childhood sexual abuse may have a deleterious effect on this developmental process. Fisher states: "Sexuality calls forth images of penetrating the body, gaining access to body openings, and heatedly merging one body with another. Sexuality means violating the boundary definitions characterizing almost all social interactions" (1989, 25). This experience of objects entering, crossing or merging with body boundaries may challenge the child's developing sense that there is a clear-cut "edge of me," leading to feelings of bodily vulnerability (Fisher 1989, 26).

Studies of the sequelae of sexual abuse have made frequent reference to disorders of body perception and body regulation, various forms of deliberate bodily injury and somatization processes. Recent reports have documented a high incidence of self-mutilation and suicide attempts (Goodwin 1982; Herman 1992; Turell and Armsworth 1992) and have demonstrated strong correlations between histories of early physical and sexual abuse and numerous self-destructive behaviors in adulthood (van der Kolk, Perry and

Herman 1991). Somatization disorders and alexithymic reactions appear frequently in populations who have reported sexual abuse in childhood (van
der Kolk et al. 1996). Somatic reactions (Rimsza, Berg and Locke 1988), psychobiological aspects of physical and emotional responses to trauma (van
der Kolk 1994) and difficulties related to embodiment (Young 1992) have
also been documented in sexually traumatized individuals. Difficulties with
embodiment following trauma seem to disrupt the development of cohesive
identity and body integrity (Armsworth 1992) and the management of ego
states. In addition, numerous authors have examined the impacts of sexual
or physical abuse on the developing body image, self-image and possible
connections between these disturbances and eating disorders (O'Brien 1987;
Oppenheimer et al. 1985; Sloan and Leichner 1986).

Although some authors have reported that the most serious long-term effects of early sexual traumatization result from highly intrusive or invasive
sexual abuse, such as oral, anal or vaginal penetration that includes forceful
or sadistic abuse (Elwell and Ephross 1987; Russell 1986), others (e.g., Grand
and Alpert 1993) argue that, regardless of associated variables of force or
penetration, the core disturbances resulting from incest derive from violations of the child's experience of being connected to others and disruptions
in his or her basic sense of physical-sensory continuities. Grand and Alpert
posit that these experiences result in a state of objectlessness with terror of
annihilation. Disruption in continuity of one's existence in time and space
creates incoherence and discontinuity, leading some authors (Kluft 1984,
cited in Goodwin 1985, 160) to delineate as one of the primary criteria for
childhood trauma the breaching or impairment of physical intactness
and/or clarity of consciousness. Young (1992, 91) summarizes core issues related to trauma to the body, stating:

> The experience of trauma also calls into question our relation to "having a
> body" and "living in a body," and makes profoundly troubling the centrality of
> the body in human existence and the body's claims upon us. It is this, the prob-
> lematic area of embodiment, which is so often overlooked or minimized in dis-
> cussions of sexual abuse and trauma. And yet it is undeniable that severe
> trauma is inscribed in and often on the bodies of survivors, leaving a mark that
> can perhaps be explained but never effaced.

The fourth edition of the *Diagnostic and Statistical Manual of Mental Disorders (DSM-IV)* of the American Psychiatric Association underscores the centrality of the body, requiring as an essential feature of posttraumatic stress

disorder (PTSD) "exposure to an extreme traumatic stressor involving direct personal experience of an event that involves actual or threatened death or serious injury, or other threat to one's physical integrity" (1994, 424).

Although a literature on body involvement in trauma has begun to accumulate, to date there is little empirical work or research instrumentation for systematic examination of this area of human development and behavior. What we have are numerous theoretical references to the centrality of the body in human existence that might inform studies investigating how traumatic events could impact on the development of self-image. Questions remain about how to operationalize these ideas into testable research designs.

D. W. Winnicott (1945, 1965) emphasizes embodiment, or "indwelling," as a core constituent of cohesive selfhood. In his view, infants only become integrated and personalized, or "called into existence," as they come to experience linkages between self and body and body functions. The skin serves as a limiting membrane, the division between "what is me versus what is not me." Anzieu (1989) focuses on the "skin ego" as a psychic structure providing containment and enabling definition and protection of psychic functions. In the absence of containment, disturbances in reality functioning related to "what is inside me" versus "what is outside me" develop, setting the stage for projective identification and identity disturbances (Bick 1968). Krueger (1989) proposes that when the body does not serve as a "container," individuals may rely instead on the body as a "regulator." For instance, a person may use external body behaviors such as bingeing, purging or self-mutilation to control or regulate internal subjective states. Stolorow and Atwood (1992) emphasize that the failure to achieve indwelling results in extreme states of disconnection of mind and body, leaving individuals vulnerable to states of depersonalization, mind-body disintegration or disidentification with the body. With specific reference to childhood sexual abuse, they believe that a separation between mind and body may serve as a form of defensive disidentification ensuring psychic survival in the face of unbearable conflicts and bodily experiences.

The current research investigated the relation between incest and body image, self-image, dissociation and ego functioning in a culturally diverse, nonclinical sample of women and men with histories of incest compared with a control group. In addition, this research examined the utility of a number of instruments for future research and clinical applications.

METHOD

Participants

Seventy-one women from a community college population in a Southern metropolitan area participated in this research to examine the relation between a history of incest and body image, self-image, dissociation and ego functioning. Subjects were 36 women with self-reported histories of incest and a control group of 35 women. Subjects were drawn from a larger community college sample of males and females who reported the presence or absence of various abuse experiences (sexual, incestuous, physical and physiological). The overall study yielded a return of 606 completed packets of data from approximately 800 distributed; of this sample, 226 were males and 380 were females. The abuse group was determined by selecting all female subjects who endorsed specific items related to sexual experiences with a family member or surrogate family member in which there was a clear power or dependency differential and at least a five-year age difference. Control subjects were drawn from the pool of female subjects who reported no incest experiences or other abuse categories, with groups balanced for age and race.

The mean age of the female incest group was 30.33 years (*SD* = 10.61) and 30.70 years in the control group (*SD* = 10.20). The combined sample (*n* = 71) consisted of 2 Asian Americans, 19 African Americans, 17 Hispanics and 33 Caucasians. An examination of the incest experiences reported by females were as follows: fondling of subjects' genitals, 67 percent; fondling subjects' breasts, 50 percent; being kissed, 33 percent; fondling perpetrators' genitals, 28 percent; intercourse, 25 percent; attempted intercourse, 19 percent; perpetrator masturbated in front of victim, 14 percent; oral-genital contact, 10 percent; anal penetration, 3 percent; and mutual masturbation, 3 percent. The categories overlap, resulting in totals greater than 100 percent. Incest perpetrators reported by this sample (percentages rounded) were: male cousins (38 percent); brothers (19 percent); fathers and uncles (each 14 percent); grandfathers (11 percent); stepfathers (6 percent); and mothers, aunts, female cousins, stepbrothers and foster fathers (each 3 percent). (Totals are greater than 100 percent, because some subjects described multiple perpetrators.)

Frequency of occurrence (percentages rounded) of incest experiences were: 1 occurrence (n = 14; 39 percent); 2–3 occurrences (n = 9; 25 percent); 4–5 occurrences (n = 7; 19 percent); 6 or more occurrences (n = 6; 17 percent). Seven women (19 percent) told someone of the incest and two women (6

TABLE 5.1

Frequency of Psychological Conditions in Childhood, Adolescence, and Adulthood and Frequency of Adult Victimization Experiences Reported by Abused (n = 36) and Nonabused (n = 35) Women

Condition	Frequency for Abuse Group (%)	Frequency for Nonabused Group (%)
Depression as child or adolescent	27	3
Depression as adult	76	27
Anxiety as child or adolescent	30	6
Anxiety as adult	36	19
Hospitalized for psychological problems	13	0
Suicidal thoughts	45	19
Suicide attempts	7	3
Anorexia	11	6
Obesity	33	6
Bulimia	11	0
Adult Victimization Experiences		
Attempted stranger rape	22	7
Stranger rape	7	3
Attempted acquaintance rape	11	3
Acquaintance rape	3	3
Attempted date rape	25	3
Date rape	8	0
Attempted mate rape	14	3
Battered by date	11	8
Battered by mate	19	8

percent) stated that the incest was reported to authorities. Forty-four percent of respondents (n = 16) reported that the incest was extremely upsetting to them; 42 percent (n = 15) reported it as moderately upsetting; and 14 percent (n = 5) reported it as not upsetting. Forty-four percent (n = 16) reported the incest experiences as extremely damaging; 31 percent (n = 11) as moderately damaging; and 25 percent (n = 9) as not damaging.

Table 5.1 presents additional information from the demographic questionnaire, including summaries of psychological conditions in childhood, adolescence and adulthood reported by the abused and control group and a summary of adult victimization experiences for both groups. The clustering with incest of childhood and adult emotional, self-abusive and victimization problems suggests that this nonclinical sample may be comparable to other published samples, including those drawn from clinical populations.

Subjects were recruited through community college classes and given extra credit by instructors for returning a sealed research packet completed anonymously. Completion of the packet was not a requirement for extra credit but returning it was. Packets were distributed and retrieved by trained research assistants from the project. The research packet consisted of the Lifetime Stress Events Questionnaire (Armsworth 1989), a 300-item self-report instrument devised to collect quantitative information from participants on frequency, intensity and duration of family stresses and abusive experiences (physical, emotional, sexual and physiological). The abuse categories are endorsed on a Likert-type scale from 0 (never) to 7 (continuously in childhood and adolescence). In addition, demographic information and questions related to health, pregnancy and psychological functioning are included.

Body image and self-image were assessed using the Body Cathexis–Self Cathexis Scale (BC-SC), Form D (Secord and Jourard 1953), which consists of two 40-item scales. According to the authors, the basic assumptions of this instrument are that negative feelings about the body are associated with undue concern about pain, disease and bodily injury and with feelings of insecurity involving the self. The Body Cathexis Scale (BC) measures the degree of satisfaction with body image and various parts and processes of the body. Body image, as measured by the BC-SC, has been shown to be significantly related to global self-esteem (Secord and Jourard 1953). The Self Cathexis Scale (SC) measures satisfaction with the self. Items on Form D of the BC-SC measure are endorsed on a scale ranging from 1 (have strong positive feelings) to 5 (have strong negative feelings), with 3 indicating no feelings one way or the other. Since the body is the most tangible and visible component of the self, the body is the anchoring point for a more inclusive concept of the self. Body cathexis is related to self-image, although it is a separate part of it. Secord and Jourard reported split-half reliabilities of 0.83 on the BC and 0.92 on the SC for females. Balogun (1986) reported alpha ranges from 0.81 to 0.87.

Dissociation was assessed with the Perceptual Alteration Scale (PAS; Sanders 1986) and the Dissociative Experiences Scale (DES; Bernstein and Putnam 1986). The PAS is a self-report questionnaire consisting of 60 items endorsed on a scale with a response range from 1 (never) to 4 (almost always). Sanders reported a Cronbach alpha of 0.95. The DES is a brief, self-report measure of frequency of dissociative experiences. It was designed to serve as a screening instrument for dissociative disorders and in determining the contribution of dissociation to various psychiatric disorders. A 0 to 10 response scale is used to quantify experiences for each item to reflect a wider range of dissociative symptomatology. Test-retest reliabilities reported a range from 0.79 to 0.96.

The Eating Disorders Inventory (EDI; Garner and Olmsted 1984) was constructed to assess a number of psychological and behavioral traits commonly found in individuals with eating disorders. It consists of 146 items endorsed on a Likert-type scale from 0 (always) to 6 (never). The EDI consists of eight subscales. Higher scores on the EDI subscales indicate stronger ego functioning. For the current study, three subscales composing measures of serious ego deficits (Ineffectiveness, Interpersonal Distrust and Interoceptive Awareness) were examined. These subscales were selected because they measure constructs frequently mentioned in the literature on trauma and abuse, and few alternative instruments tapping these dimensions are available.

The Ineffectiveness subscale assesses feelings of general inadequacy, insecurity, worthlessness and not being in control of one's life. Garner and Olmsted suggest that the concept of ineffectiveness also includes a negative self-evaluation (self-concept component). Sample items from the Ineffectiveness subscale are: (a) "I feel empty inside (emotionally)"; (b) "I have a low opinion of myself"; and (c) "I wish I were someone else." The Interpersonal Distrust subscale assesses a sense of alienation and a general reluctance to form close relationships. It relates to an inability to feel comfortable expressing emotions toward others. Sample items from this subscale are: (a) "I am open about my feelings" (the distrustful are not); (b) "I need to keep people at a certain distance" (some feel uncomfortable if someone tries to get too close); and (c) "I have close relationships" (those with trust problems may answer "never"). The Interoceptive Awareness subscale reflects one's lack of confidence in recognizing and accurately identifying emotions and visceral sensations of hunger or satiety. Sample items from this subscale are: (a) "I worry my feelings will get out of control"; (b) "I get frightened when my feelings are too strong"; and (c) "When I am upset, I don't know if I am sad, frightened or angry."

RESULTS

The measures used in this study were found to have highly acceptable reliability estimates, indicating high levels of internal consistency. The Body

Cathexis Scale yielded an alpha of 0.95; Self Cathexis Scale yielded an alpha of 0.97; and the Perceptual Alteration Scale yielded an alpha of 0.90. The Body Cathexis and Self Cathexis Scales are positively correlated ($r = 0.72$, $p < 0.0001$). This indicates that a more negative view of one's body is related to a more negative self-concept. Negative body cathexis was also found to be related to feelings of not being in control and a general sense of worthlessness as reported on the Ineffectiveness subscale of the EDI ($r = -0.31$, $p < 0.02$). Negative body cathexis was also related to higher dissociation as reported on the DES ($r = 0.32$, $p < 0.007$) and the PAS ($r = 0.57$, $p < 0.0001$), indicating that as negative feelings about the body increase, so does dissociation. The Self Cathexis Scale was also found to be negatively correlated with the Ineffectiveness subscale of the EDI ($r = -0.44$, $p < 0.001$). This indicates that those who have a positive self-concept tend to feel more secure, worthwhile and in control of their lives. In addition, a more negative view of the self was related to higher dissociation (DES; $r = 0.33$, $p < 0.002$; and PAS, $r = 0.45$, $p < .0001$). Correlation between the DES and the PAS was 0.53 ($p < 0.0001$).

The Body Cathexis and Self Cathexis Scales were found to significantly discriminate the incest from the abuse-free group (F [1, 69] = 23.30, $p < 0.0001$ and F [1, 69] = 11.63, $p < 0.001$, respectively), with the women in the incest group reporting greater dissatisfaction with their bodies and their view of themselves (see Table 5.2). In addition to group comparisons, a descriptive analysis of mean item scores was performed to yield further understanding of differences on specific items on the Body Cathexis–Self Cathexis Scale (see Table 5.3). In examining the Body Cathexis scores that fell above a mean score of 3.0 for both groups (scores of 1 indicate strong positive feelings; 2 indicates moderate positive feelings), the abuse-free group had no items in this range. For the women with histories of incest, the following items had mean scores greater than 3: appetite, waist, body build, profile, arms, chest, hips, feet, knees, posture, weight and sex activities. Likewise, an examination of mean scores of 3 or greater on the Self Cathexis Scale indicated that the abuse-free group had no items in this range. The abused group reported mean item scores of 3 or greater on the following items: procrastination, self-assertiveness, love life, sex appeal, fears, tolerance and will power. (See Table 5.4 for comparison of all item mean scores by group.)

The Perceptual Alteration Scale significantly discriminated between the abused and abuse-free group with the abused group reporting higher dissociative symptoms (F (1, 69) = 6. 58, $p < 0.01$). The level of dissociation re-

TABLE 5.2

Mean Group Differences on Measures of Body Cathexis-Self Cathexis, Dissociation, and Selected Subscales of the Eating Disorders Inventory (N = 71; n = 36 abused; n = 35 nonabused)

		Mean	SD	F value	P value
Body Cathexis	Control	83.9	22.9	23.30	0.0001
	Abused	110.8	23.9		
Self Cathexis	Control	81.0	27.9	11.63	0.001
	Abused	103.9	28.6		
Perceptual Alteration Scale	Control	105.7	15.7	6.58	0.01
	Abused	115.1	15.6		
Dissociative Experiences Scale	Control	1.32	1.16	0.23	0.63 n.s.
	Abused	1.19	1.12		

Eating Disorder Inventory Scales			Mean	SD		F value	P value
Ineffectiveness	Control	Afr.-Am.	43.5	5.8	Group	4.81	0.03
Subscale		Caucasian	47.1	7.4	Race	0.70	0.50
(Higher scores		Hispanic	38.6	9.1	Group	4.09	0.02
indicate					Race		
effectiveness)	Abused	Afr.-Am.	34.7	8.2			
		Caucasian	37.1	10.7			
		Hispanic	44.0	7.5			
Interpersonal	Control	Afr.-Am.	24.7	6.0	Group	0.19	0.66
Distrust		Caucasian	33.6	3.8	Race	4.17	0.02
Subscale		Hispanic	23.6	6.4	Group	5.76	0.006
(Higher scores					Race		
indicate trust)	Abused	Afr.-Am.	24.7	6.2			
		Caucasian	26.9	6.2			
		Hispanic	30.4	4.8			
Interoceptive	Control	Afr.-Am.	36.7	8.3	Group	3.32	0.07
Awareness		Caucasian	49.3	5.6	Race	5.48	0.007
Subscale		Hispanic	35.2	8.0	Group	4.44	0.02
					Race		
	Abused	Afr.-Am.	32.2	9.4			
		Caucasian	38.0	8.2			
		Hispanic	41.3	10.0			

TABLE 5.3

Mean Item Scores for Abused (n = 36) and Nonabused (n = 35) Women on Body-Cathexis Items   (1 = Strong positive feelings; 2 = Moderate positive feelings; 3 = Have no feelings one way or another; 4 = Have moderate negative feelings; 5 = Have strong negative feelings)

Item	*Abused Group*	*Nonabused Group*
Hair	2.4	2.1
Facial complexion	2.5	2.1
Appetite	3.3	2.7
Hands	2.7	2.0
Distribution of hair over body	2.8	2.3
Nose	2.9	2.2
Physical stamina	2.8	2.0
Elimination	2.9	2.5
Muscular strength	2.7	2.3
Waist	3.3	2.4
Energy level	2.7	2.3
Back	2.8	2.5
Ears	2.4	1.9
Age	2.3	1.7
Chin	2.7	2.0
Body build	3.3	2.1
Profile	3.2	2.0
Height	2.2	2.0
Keenness of senses	2.2	1.6
Tolerance for pain	2.5	2.4
Width of shoulders	2.6	2.1
Arms	3.0	2.0
Chest (or breasts)	3.1	2.1
Appearance	2.8	1.9
Digestion	2.7	2.5
Hips	3.6	2.6
Resistance to illness	2.4	2.0
Legs	2.9	2.1
Appearance of teeth	2.7	1.8
Sex drive	2.9	1.9
Feet	3.2	2.3
Sleep	2.5	1.9
Voice	2.2	1.9
Health	2.2	2.0
Knees	3.1	2.2
Posture	3.1	1.9
Weight	3.7	2.6
Sex activities	3.1	2.0
Face	2.4	1.8
Sex organs	2.7	1.8

Table 5.4

Mean Item Scores for Abused (n = 36) and Nonabused (n = 35) Women on Self Cathexis Items   (1 = Strong positive feelings; 2 = Moderate positive feelings; 3 = Have no feelings one way or another; 4 = Have moderate negative feelings; 5 = Have strong negative feelings)

Item	Abused Group	Nonabused Group
Sense of humor	2.0	1.7
Independence	2.1	1.9
Temper	2.6	2.5
Ability to express self	2.5	2.2
Self-understanding	2.4	1.7
Artistic talents	2.7	2.4
Tolerance	3.0	2.0
Moods	2.8	2.4
General knowledge	2.4	1.7
Imagination	2.4	1.9
Popularity	2.4	2.2
Self-confidence	2.9	1.9
Ability to accept criticism	2.9	2.4
Capacity to work	1.8	1.4
Ability to meet people	2.3	1.6
Personality	2.3	1.6
Ability to concentrate	2.7	2.1
Procrastination	3.6	2.7
Self-assertiveness	3.1	2.4
Ability to express sympathy	2.4	1.7
Sensitivity	2.0	1.4
Ability to lead	2.7	2.2
Impulses	2.4	2.2
Intelligence	1.9	1.9
Athletic skills	2.9	2.5
Happiness	2.7	1.9
Creativeness	2.3	2.0
Love life	3.6	2.1
Sex appeal	3.1	2.1
Skill with hands	2.4	2.2
Gracefulness	2.8	2.1
Fear	3.5	1.4
Memory	2.7	2.1
Vocabulary	2.3	2.1
Thriftiness	2.4	2.2
Self-discipline	2.9	2.0
Suggestibility	2.6	2.1
Will power	3.0	1.9
Ability to make decisions	2.7	1.8
Self-consciousness	2.9	2.0

ported by the control group falls within one *SD* of the mean reported for university students by Sanders (1986, 97). The DES, on the other hand, did not significantly discriminate the abused from the control group (F [1, 67] = 0.23, $p < 0.63$).

ETHNICITY OF SUBJECTS

No significant ethnic differences were found for the BC-SC scales or the dissociation measures. However, the three subscales of the EDI did show ethnic differences. Of the three subscales of the EDI, the Ineffectiveness subscale significantly discriminated the incest group from the control group for African Americans and Caucasian women, but not for Hispanic women. On the Interpersonal Distrust subscale, the abuse-free Caucasian group differed significantly from the abuse-free Hispanic group, with the Caucasian group reporting higher distrust than Hispanics. The abuse-free Caucasian women differed significantly from the Caucasian women with histories of incest on distrust, with the abused group reporting lower distrust. However, Hispanic women with histories of abuse reported higher interpersonal trust compared to the Hispanic control group. African American abused and abuse-free women did not differ significantly on Interpersonal Distrust or the Interoceptive Awareness subscales. Of the three ethnic groups, only the Caucasian women with incest histories differed significantly from the Caucasian abuse-free group on the Interoceptive Awareness subscale, with the abused group reporting lower awareness of their emotions and bodily sensations. Within the control group, African Americans and Hispanics differed significantly from Caucasian nonabused females, with the latter reporting higher self-awareness. The three scales of EDI function differentially across the ethnic groups; validity of this measure needs to be investigated for differences in functioning for ethnic groups other than Caucasian women. However, looking only at the Anglo-American women, the abused group differed as expected, showing more ineffectiveness, more interpersonal distrust and less interoceptive awareness.

DISCUSSION

This research examined body image and self-perceptions in a sample of incestuously abused and abuse-free subjects and found support for a number of theoretical observations about the impact of trauma on body concepts.

The results of this study indicated that dissatisfaction with one's body is significantly higher in the abused sample, and this is related to negative self-image, less perceived control over one's life and higher dissociative symptomatology. Additionally, Caucasian abused females were significantly less aware of body cues and bodily processes as compared to nonabused Caucasian females. Dissatisfaction with one's body may lead Caucasian abused women to pay less attention to their bodily processes and ignore or split off bodily cues. However, Hispanic and African American abused females did not differ significantly from nonabused Hispanic and African American females on this measure. There were significant ethnic differences within the nonabused control group. As mentioned earlier, the EDI needs further investigation regarding validity across ethnic groups.

This study appears to lend support to the theoretical and clinical observations that abuse to the body, in this case incestuous abuse, may lead to violations or disruptions of a person's sense of being connected to self and others through negative body and self-perceptions, insecurity about the functioning of body and self and lowered awareness of body cues and processes. The elevations noted in dissociative phenomena in the sexual-abuse group are indicative of a traumatic disruption in continuity of one's existence in time and space that breaches or impairs a sense of physical intactness and clarity of consciousness (Kluft 1984, cited in Goodwin 1985) and engenders ongoing episodes of incoherence and discontinuity (Grand and Alpert 1993). The fact that this research employed a nonclinical sample and found significant levels of negative impact of incest on body image and satisfaction may lend support to the position of Grand and Alpert (1993) that disturbances to body image and continuity are likely to occur regardless of force or penetration.

With regard to instruments used in this research, all appear to have utility in clinical settings as well as in future research. The Body Cathexis–Self Cathexis Scale could offer greater utility by inclusion of specific items related to sexual organs and functions for further understanding of a person's sexual self. The scale, as it exists, however, is a useful tool for examining clients' or subjects' perceived body image and self-image.

Both measures of dissociation, the DES and the PAS, offer utility in research and clinical examination of dissociative phenomena in individuals with histories of abuse. The DES, as stated by Bernstein and Putnam (1986), is intended for use with clinical samples and is likely to yield more striking results there than in the current nonclinical sample. The PAS has not yet been developed psychometrically to the extent of the DES; it warrants further exploration, especially in use with normal adults and less disturbed clinical populations.

The three ego-deficit subscales from the EDI were used in this study to assess feelings of lack of control over one's life and other aspects of disconnection and discontinuity of experience. The subscale items may provide valuable information in clinical situations to aid clients in further understanding their own issues of control, intimacy and awareness of internal states. However, because of the possibility that ethnic differences may overwhelm other effects, these measures may not be ideal for research involving small multiethnic samples.

Future research that continues to explore and incorporate the interaction between bodily, affective and cognitive experiences and research on somatization processes and disorders is likely to yield valuable information on the perplexing and complex issues related to the effects of trauma to the body.

REFERENCES

American Psychiatric Association (1994). *Diagnostic and statistical manual of mental disorders.* 4th ed. Washington, D.C.: American Psychiatric Association.

Anzieu, D. (1989). *The skin ego: A psychoanalytic approach to the self.* New Haven: Yale University Press.

Armsworth, M. W. (1992). Role of body and physical self in development of cohesive sense of identity and body integrity. Paper presented as part of a workshop entitled, "Advanced Issues in Treating Incest," L. McCann, Chair, at the Eighth Annual Meeting of the International Society for Traumatic Stress Studies, Los Angeles, Calif.

_____. (1993). Lifetime Stress Events Questionnaire. 3rd ed. Unpublished instrument. University of Houston, Houston, Tex.

Balogun, J. A. (1986). Reliability and construct validity of the body cathexis scale. *Perceptual and Motor Skills* 62: 927–935.

Bernstein, E. M., and Putnam, F. W. (1986). Development, reliability, and validity of a dissociation scale. *Journal of Nervous and Mental Disease* 174: 727–735.

Bick, E. (1968). The experience of the skin in early object relations. *International Journal of Psycho-Analysis* 49: 484–486.

Elwell, M. E., and Ephross, P. H. (1987). Initial reactions of sexually abused children. *Social Casework* 68: 109–116.

Fisher, S. (1989). *Sexual images of the self: The psychology of erotic sensations and illusions.* Hillsdale, N.J.: Erlbaum.

_____. (1986). *Development and structure of the body image.* Vol. 1. Hillsdale, N.J.: Erlbaum.

Garner, D. M., and Olmsted, M. P. (1984). *Eating disorder inventory manual*. Odessa, Fla.: Psychological Assessment Resources.

Goodwin, J. (1982). Suicide attempts: A preventable complication of incest. In J. Goodwin, ed., *Incest victims and their families* (pp. 109–116). Boston: Wright PSG.

_____. (1985). Post-traumatic symptoms in incest victims. In S. Eth and R. Pynoos, eds., *Post-traumatic stress disorder in children*. Washington, D.C.: American Psychiatric Press.

Grand, S., and Alpert, J. L. (1993). The core trauma of incest: An object relations view. *Professional Psychology: Research and Practice* 24: 330–334.

Herman, J. L. (1992). Complex PTSD: A syndrome in survivors of prolonged and repeated trauma. *Journal of Traumatic Stress* 5: 377–391.

Krueger, D. W. (1989). *Body self and psychological self*. New York: Brunner/Mazel.

O'Brien, J. D. (1987). The effects of incest on female adolescent development. *Journal of the American Academy of Psychoanalysis* 15: 83–92.

Oppenheimer, R., Howells, K., Palmer, L., and Chaloner, D. A. (1985). Adverse sexual experience in childhood and clinical eating disorders: A preliminary description. *Journal of Psychiatric Research* 19: 357–361.

Rimsza, M. E., Berg, R. A., and Locke, C. (1988). Sexual abuse: Somatic and emotional reactions. *Child Abuse and Neglect* 12: 201–208.

Russell, D. E. H. (1986). *The secret trauma*. New York: Basic Books.

Sanders, S. (1986). The Perceptual Alteration Scale: A scale measuring dissociation. *American Journal of Clinical Hypnosis* 29: 95–102.

Secord, P. F., and Jourard, M. (1953). The appraisal of body-cathexis: Body-cathexis and the self. *Journal of Consulting Psychology* 17: 343–347.

Sloan, G., and Leichner, P. (1986). Is there a relationship between sexual abuse or incest and eating disorders? *Canadian Journal of Psychiatry* 31: 656–660.

Stolorow, R. D., and Atwood, G. E. (1992). *Contexts of being: The intersubjective foundations of psychological life*. Hillsdale, N.J.: The Analytic Press.

Turell, S., and Armsworth, M. W. (1992). Self-mutilation behavior in incest survivors. Paper presented as part of a symposium entitled "Trauma and Victimization in the Lives of Adults," M. W. Armsworth, Chair, at the 38th Annual Meeting of the Southwestern Psychological Association, Austin, Texas.

van der Kolk, B. A. (1994). The body keeps score: Memory and the evolving psychobiology of posttraumatic stress. *Harvard Review of Psychiatry* 1: 253–265.

van der Kolk, B. A., Pelcovitz, D., Roth, S., Mandel, F. S., McFarlane, A., and Herman, J. (1996). Dissociation, somatization, and affect dysregulation: The complexity of adaptation to trauma. *American Journal of Psychiatry*, Festschrift Supplement 153: 83–93.

van der Kolk, B. A., Perry, J. C., and Herman, J. L. (1991). Childhood origins of self-destructive behavior. *American Journal of Psychiatry* 148: 1665–1671.

Winnicott, D. W. (1945/1975). Primitive emotional development. In *Collected papers: Through paediatrics to psychoanalysis* (pp. 145–156). New York: Basic Books.

_____. (1965). Ego integration in child development. In D. W. Winnicott, *The Maturational processes and the facilitating environment* (pp. 56–63). New York: International Universities Press.

Young, L. (1992). Sexual abuse and the problem of embodiment. *Child Abuse and Neglect* 16: 89–100.

CHAPTER 6

Body-Image Distortion and Childhood Sexual Abuse

Reina Attias and Jean Goodwin

This chapter reviews concepts of body image and body ego in order to provide a theoretical framework for those body-related pathologies that may coincide with the presence of dissociative symptoms and histories of sexual abuse.

Normal development of body image and body ego is necessary for self-cohesion, emotional containment, physical coordination, bodily pleasure, accurate reality testing and the overarching achievement of effectiveness, including self-mastery (Fisher and Cleveland 1958). Bodily symptoms reported after sexual abuse include disordered eating and other self-injury syndromes, sexual and somatization spectrum disorders, depersonalization syndromes in which the body image develops gaps or disappears and the multiple body images and body egos that characterize dissociative identity disorder (DID).

Internal shifts in body image may underlie these body problems and often can be traced back to children's ways of understanding their sexual abuse. These constructs include: (1) incorporation experiences in which garbage, vermin, inanimate objects, body parts of the abuser, fantasized pregnancies, parent figures or other victims or their ghosts are felt as internal presences; (2) loss experiences including fragmentation, mutilations, amputations, holes or gaps, invisibility or transparency, soul-loss, disembodiment or emptiness; or (3) distortions including genital changes, dehumanization and size or age changes. We will use clinical examples to illustrate how these fantasies arise during childhood sexual abuse, how they become elaborated into symptoms and how they can be addressed in psychotherapy.

Linking to body image such symptoms as self-mutilation, somatic pain, disordered eating, helplessness and self-denigration and then further linking the body-image changes to the child's experience of sexual abuse give therapist and patient a way to context these symptoms and intervene (see Parts III and IV, this volume).

Techniques that permit communication and resolution of body-image material are described and include talking about the body, body symptoms and body images and noting consistent and recurring themes. Adjunctive techniques include imaging the body in sandtray and art therapy. These interventions clarify childhood beliefs about bodily harm and defective body image and help the patient express fantasies of incorporation, dissolution and distortion and resolve these into images of transformation, growth, repair and reconstruction.

NORMAL DEVELOPMENT OF BODY IMAGE

The concept of body image is complex and can be traced back to Freud. The following contemporary definition conveys the multiple psychological mechanisms summarized by the term: "Body image . . . refers to the body as a psychological experience, and focuses on the individual's feelings and attitudes toward his own body. It is concerned with the individual's subjective experiences with his body and the manner in which he has organized these experiences" (Fisher and Cleveland 1958, 7).

Normally body image develops out of three types of experience: the mother's mirroring of the infant through physical touch and emotional response, the infant's experience of his or her own behavior and its effects, and the infant's beginning experience of his or her own internal bodily sensations. According to Freud (1923/1961, 26), the body ego develops before the psychological ego. "The ego is first and foremost a bodily ego; it is not merely a surface entity but it is itself the projection of a surface." This leads to one of the fundamental tenets of psychoanalysis: that every psychical phenomenon develops in constant reference to bodily experience.

A major marker of body-image development is the mirror stage, which begins in the second year of life, when infants develop an interest in their own mirror image, and is completed when they realize fully that the image is of their own body (Lacan 1977). This early body image is consolidated in the oedipal stage and then must be reworked at puberty around new body changes. Krueger (1989, 26) provides a concise summary of this process:

> The developmental experiences of the body self that become represented as body image begin in the first awareness through the mirroring self-object, evolving in healthy development into a cohesive, distinct, accurate and consistent, evocative image of one's body and its relationship to its physical surroundings. The body image must evolve accurately as one's physical body matures, and be integrated in the development of the psychological self.

As early as 1955, Linn observed that "the body image must have a developmental history" (39).

The body ego has been described as a kind of skin with functions that include shielding against overstimulation or physical attack, containing feelings and sensations and receiving and communicating information (Anzieu 1989). The body ego thus maintains the holding functions of the mother of infancy while also conferring a sense of boundaried individuality. This "skin" functions as a kind of envelope that gives the self a sense of unity and cohesion despite disparate sensory inputs. Defects in this function lead to an experience of body fragmentation. Pleasure and sexuality are also mediated through this "skin."

Preverbal and nonverbal memories may be contained in this layer of the ego and may be experienced here, literally or symbolically, as wounds or sores. Just as the psychological ego can turn against itself, becoming self-critical and self-depriving, so the body ego may turn on itself destructively either in conscious, or "accidental," self-harm or psychosomatically. Both phenomena are seen in cases of severe unresolved trauma (van der Kolk, Perry and Herman 1991).

It is important for the psychological ego to contain accurate information both about body image and the body. This allows the development of physical coordination and grace, bodily pleasure, ego integration and reality testing. Peto explains the connection with reality testing as follows: "Finding and evaluating external reality is to a great extent determined by refinding one's own body in the environment. Thus the body image is of decisive importance in grasping the world around us" (1959, 225).

The experience of "effectiveness" is a fundamental bodily experience that is the core of self-esteem and reality testing. Effectiveness begins with the infant's capacity to affect the mother's emotional response and is solidified by motility, which allows the infant to affect other objects in the environment. Finally, the evolving capacity to control or shift emotional experiences or states brings effectiveness to a higher, abstract level of self-mastery.

Traumatic bodily experiences by definition are those that cannot be mastered by the developing self/body. Such experiences may produce anaclitic depression, learned helplessness and overwhelming anxiety, further interfering with each step in the development of effectiveness and culminating in the deficits in self-soothing and the ability to change states that characterize posttraumatic syndromes.

Cause and effect begins as an experience of one's body having an effect before it becomes a cognitive map for explaining problems and solving them. Werner (1957) hypothesized that many other cognitive functions are rooted in body experience: space perception, numerical concepts and language. Erikson speaks of experience as anchored in the ground plan of the body: "Children find first in their bodies what they will later encounter in the world" (1950, 108).

When bodily experiences are altered in infancy, lasting effects are seen in ego functioning. For example, in the congenital defect of esophageal atresia, tube feeding into the stomach replaces sucking at the breast. Developmentally one observes delays in the infant's capacity to register hunger and satiety, decreases in motility and exploration and muting of the intensity of maternal attachment. Monica, who survived esophageal atresia in infancy, as a child was observed bottle-feeding her doll and decades later her own normal infant with the baby lying flat in a position that would have been more suitable for gastric tube feeding (Engel 1962; Engel et al. 1985). Other early environmental insults such as tactile overstimulation or inadequate feeding have been linked to chronically disordered response patterns; for example, some children of depressed mothers give up trying to signal or interact with the mother and develop instead self-soothing rituals like rocking or come to rely on painful self-stimulations like hair-pulling (Lichtenberg 1978; Novick and Novick 1996). These observations point to strong links between bodily experiences and ego adaptations.

Fisher and Cleveland summarize the implications of these findings: "The theoretical importance of this line of thought is great because it suggests the idea that various basic skills and capacities may be dependent upon a well-organized body image. It raises the question whether body image may not be a fundamental substratum which is necessary in order to build up other response systems of the individual" (1958, 8).

THE IMPACT OF SEXUAL ABUSE ON BODY IMAGE

It makes intuitive sense that sexual abuse occurring during the development of body image or even after would have disruptive effects at many levels. Research on patients with histories of sexual abuse describes an array of symptoms that reflect body image disturbances: eating disorders (Goodwin and Attias 1993; Waler, Ruddock and Cureton 1995; Byram and Wagner 1995; Vanderlinden and Vandereycken 1996), somatic complaints (Goodwin 1993a; Dubowitz et al. 1993), conversion disorders affecting sensation and perception (Goodwin 1989; Bychowski 1943), depersonalization (Galdston 1947), boundary problems (Herman 1992) and fragmentation into multiple psychological and body egos in DID (Goodwin 1993b; Chapter 11, this volume). The frequent disturbances in sexual function are accompanied by problems of embodiment, hatred of the body and a sense of not owning the body (Westerlund 1992; Galdston 1947; Young 1992). In some examples (deYoung 1982) over half of sexually abused women report deliberately injuring the body, often the breasts and genital areas.

In the *DSM-IV* (*Diagnostic and Statistical Manual of Mental Disorders*, fourth edition) field trial of 100 women with somatization disorder (Pribor et al. 1993), over 90 percent reported some kind of abuse, while 80 percent reported sexual abuse. Body symptoms seem inextricably linked with posttraumatic phenomena. Van der Kolk and coworkers (1996) found in the *DSM-IV* field trial of more than 500 traumatized subjects that elevations of somatization were found in 87 percent of subjects with current posttraumatic stress disorder (PTSD), 75 percent of subjects with past PTSD and only 34 percent of subjects who had never had PTSD.

The experience and pain of sexual abuse may be understood by the child as a betrayal by the body at many levels. The bodily discomfort itself makes the body feel out of control and unintegratable and creates shame. Physical pain is overwhelming and extremely disorganizing and may trigger dissociation. The pain may become an enduring structure of the sexually abused child's body image (Biven 1982). The abuser, especially if this is a loved person and especially if there is bodily penetration, may be experienced as an extension or appendage to the child's not yet fully boundaried body. So the actions of the abuser, too, may feel like a betrayal by the body. The intense emotions triggered by the abuse may also be experienced as largely physio-logical insults, an additional assault by the body on the child-self.

The child's developmental capacity to fend off these insults is minimal and archaic, as Peto points out: "The early ego integrates or tries to inte-grate, the internal and external onslaught of stimuli into the body image. At this age the body image or parts of it become identical with the earliest ob-jects. The body image symbolizes in a magic archaic way the objects, object relationships, feelings and the complexity of 'good' and 'bad' situations" (1959, 224).

Insofar as the abuse leads to a parent loss (either of an abuser or of a par-ent who the child feels is unable to perceive or protect), the child is deprived of a holding environment and becomes more reliant on the already strained body image to provide containment and a sense of cohesion and reality. One consequence may be that the psychological ego begins to assume some of the functions of the body ego in providing a protective shield of words and fantasies. Given the failure of bodily effectiveness, such fantasies may be magical and regressive and contain a core of hopelessness, surrender and even suicidality, as the body and its actions come to be seen as inessential and peripheral to the now omnipotently defined self (Winnicott 1989).

Symptoms developing in the wake of body-image disruption secondary to sexual abuse can be understood in three ways: extrusion, expression and restitution. Insofar as the body is experienced as defective and a betrayer, even as an extension of the abuser's body, there may be attempts to shed this skin, now experienced as destructive and alien. This parallels the mytholog-ical story of Hercules and the poison skin, in which Hercules struggles to di-vest himself of a poisonous cloak given to him by his angry wife and discovers that the cloak has adhered to his skin. He realizes that he cannot get rid of it without tearing his own flesh. Folk ideas and rituals about exor-cism may be understood as efforts at extrusion (Goodwin, Hill and Attias 1990).

Symptoms also function as an expression of the child's sense of gaps, de-fects or breaks in the integrity of the body image. Self-mutilation, for exam-ple, may be experienced as the reproduction of psychic wounds, creating tangible evidence of the abuser's iniquity, which, if shown to the abuser, would paralyze the abuser with shame, just as Perseus was able to immobi-lize the Medusa by reflecting back her own image in his shield. Another way to understand self-mutilation is to return to the list of basic functions of the body ego now impaired by abuse. The self-harm symptom can paradoxically act to shield the individual from overstimulation or attack (by putting the self in control of the infliction of pain) while containing emotions and affects (substituting physical pain for emotional pain) and communicating (by disrupting dissociative numbing) missing summarization of sensation and feedback about the body as a cohesive unit.

There is also great pressure to conceal these expressions of the abuse in compliance with the injunctions and threats from the abuser, which are merged with internal injunctions. In part because of complex boundary problems, there is severe confusion, and patients may experience their own wounded self as fatally toxic if seen (like Medusa) and the reality of the abuse as a fatal image that must be concealed. They may try desperately to conceal their bodily symptoms, such as vomiting, and their own expressions of rage, terror or sadness for fear that these would be lethal if witnessed.

Body symptoms may also function in a restitutive way by supplying a new skin or body image that often has magical qualities or powers like those conferred by the magic capes of mythology or like Achilles' magically invulnerable skin.

Anzieu (1989) describes a different type of restitution in which people wrap themselves in suffering. It is as if, after too many disappointments in childhood, they have given up hope of using the body as a source of pleasure and competence. But the body in pain has come to seem a powerful retaliatory and regulatory weapon that makes them feel special, in control and still alive (Novick and Novick 1996).

CASE MATERIAL

The child's experience of the body as defective is a direct result of the body's inability to ward off the traumatic assault. The body has been overwhelmed and is therefore experienced as bad or monstrous. When the defense of depersonalization or dissociative identity confusion accompanies the traumatic assaults, this may further alienate the child from his or her own bodily environment and come to interfere in an ongoing way with the healthy development of bodily ego.

The following cases describe moments in treatment when material about defective body image was disclosed, how this material was handled therapeutically, and the impact of this therapeutic work on beginning the restoration of bodily ego and subsequent healthy ego functioning.

CASE 1: INCORPORATION OF THE ABUSER'S BODY OR BODY PARTS

A thirty-two-year-old woman had been severely and sadistically sexually abused by her brother from age three. After two years of psychotherapy she was prepared to utilize art-therapy techniques. During a session she created a long phallic-appearing object and exclaimed in surprise that this was the object she had felt in her esophagus as far back as she could remember, causing a feeling of suffocation and blocking the expression of certain feelings and thoughts. We continued to explore this through art-therapy techniques and ceremony until she was able to feel that this object had been "removed" and her "own throat" restored. At this point there was a dramatic improvement in her ability to use words to describe her feelings and body sensations and to link these to the abuse; there was also a noticeable improvement in assertiveness at work and in her relationships.

CASE 2: EXTRUSION OF A BODY PART AS NOT-ME

A thirty-year-old professional woman had compulsively mutilated her right wrist and forearm for ten years. When she remembered sexual abuse at age six, she also remembered that the neighbor had held out his hand and that she had clasped it in her own. He had then led her to a bedroom where the sexual abuse took place. Her childhood fantasy that the hand had betrayed her and she could have cut it off and thus saved herself from the abuse had been enacted in the self-cutting. She was able seek plastic surgery to repair her extensive scars following her reconstruction of these events as a narrative sequence.

CASE 3: INVISIBILITY EXPERIENCES

An eighteen-year-old student caught sight of a reflection in a subway window and thought, "I wonder who that person is. She looks like a concentration-camp victim." She then realized with a shock that it was her own reflection. The experience of sudden connection to her body was instrumental in causing her to seek treatment for her previously denied anorexia. It was not until years later that she recovered memory of severe sadistic sexual abuse starting at two and a half and ending at fourteen. During psychotherapy her enduring illusion of invisibility, her sense of her body as magically invulnerable and her neglect of her real body through the anorexia were interpreted as defensive against experiencing the body memories these symptoms contained, which finally allowed her to reconstruct the sadistic abuse. Only after a long process of integrating the lost sense of her own real body was she able to begin to act visibly and concretely as a "real person" in the world.

Case 4: Experiencing Gaps in the Chest Cavity Around the Heart

A thirty-three-year-old artist with a long history of anorexia had been sexually abused by her father from early childhood to age eleven. She constructed an image of her heart showing most of the surface eroded away and patched together as if with solder, with the blood showing through here and there. She felt she was constructing a literal representation of her heart, and in making and discussing this piece in therapy she felt sadness for the first time about what had happened to her and was able to reconnect the abuse to her feelings in an integrative way.

Case 5: Experiencing a Gap in the Skin and a Distortion in the Knee Joint

A thirty-six-year-old professional woman entered therapy because of anxiety and fear that she might be an incest victim. In treatment she revealed a chronic frightening symptom. At times she would experience her knee opening to reveal twisted bones, ligaments and blood. Although she was aware that this was not an actual event, this awareness was not sufficient to prevent extreme panic. When she had reconstructed a narrative describing severe sexual abuse in childhood by a family friend, her symptom could be linked to a bathroom rape at age five during which the perpetrator violently wrenched and twisted her leg in the process. When this connection was made through therapy, reconstructive narrative and the use of collage, the symptom was no longer so intrusive and gradually disappeared.

DISCUSSION

Techniques for working with body image include (1) careful verbal inquiry allowing the patient to realize with relief that the therapist is aware of thoughts and images about the body-self the patient may have believed were "crazy" and (2) reconstructive narrative. Art-therapy and sandtray techniques seem to be most useful in the diagnostic phase and later in finalizing and concretizing the body-image reconstructions, reparations and insights.

Play therapy can quickly locate children's damaged sense of body. Madge Bray (1992) recounts a case of a five-year-old child beautifully illustrating the beginnings of body-image problems. In this instance the sexual abuse became manifest as introjected garbage and contamination. The child reported the presence of "spider disease." She said to the therapist, "You've got to help the little girl. She has the spider disease. And there are poisonous spiders in her tummy. And it's full of, full of poisonous spiders, and soon her tummy is going to burst open and the poisonous spiders will fly out everywhere and poison every human in the land." She later revealed the origins of spider disease: "Well, it comes in a hole in your mouth and in your tummy, and the naughty Daddy put it in there with the white stuff." The healing of spider disease required an operation on her dolly with the mother present. The patient directed the therapist in the operation in which the stomach was opened, the spiders removed, and the heart removed so it would not get contaminated. Then all was cleaned out, the heart replaced and the dolly sewed back up. This operation led to the gradual reconstitution of the relationship with the mother (who was very supportive) and the termination of therapy.

The dissociation, internal confusion, externally imposed secrecy following the abuse and the shame, both about the assault and the symptoms, often leave victims without the necessary language or concepts to connect the distorted body experiences with other symptoms and with the abuse. In addition, the patients may be so terrified that the damage to the body is permanent that they are reluctant to reveal these thoughts, feelings or images. Therefore, it is important for the therapist to screen specifically for bizarre bodily sensations and fears centered around the body-self and help patients relate these early disruptions of the healthy formation of body image to the abuse. The very fact that the therapist is willing to discuss the body in all of its secret and frightening aspects reassures patients that the damage may be reparable and that the body is included in the therapeutic work. For the therapist to take seriously the suffering connected with body-image distortion is generally experienced as enhancing patients' sense of empathic connection and therapeutic alliance.

When the distorted body image is understood, it becomes possible to work on correcting the body image and providing a foundation for the restoration of healthy ego functions.

REFERENCES

Anzieu, D. (1989). *The skin ego.* New Haven: Yale University Press.

Biven, B. (1982). The role of skin in normal and abnormal development with a note on the poet Sylvia Plath. *International Review of Psycho-Analysis* 9: 205–228.

Bray, M. (1992). *Poppies on the rubbish heap: Sexual abuse: The child's voice.* London: Canongate.

Bychowski, G. (1943). Disorders in the body image in the clinical pictures of psychosis. *Journal of Nervous and Mental Disorders* 97: 310–334.

Byram, V., and Wagner, H. L. (1995). Sexual abuse and body image distortion: Brief communication. *Child Abuse and Neglect* 19 (4): 507–510.

deYoung, M. (1982). Self-injurious behavior in incest victims: A research note. *Child Welfare* 87: 577–584.

Dubowitz, H., Black, M., Harrington, D., and Verschoore, A. (1993). A follow-up study of behavior problems associated with child sexual abuse. *Child Abuse and Neglect* 17: 743–754.

Engel, G. L. (1962). *Psychological development in health and disease.* Philadelphia: Saunders.

Engel, G. L., Reichsman, F., Harway, V. T., and Hess, D. W. (1985). Monica: Infant feeding behavior of a mother gastric fistula-fed as an infant: A 30-year longitudinal study of enduring effects. In E. J. Anthony and G. H. Pollock, eds., *Parental influences in health and disease* (pp. 29–90). Boston: Little, Brown.

Erikson, E. (1950) *Childhood and society.* New York: Norton.

Fisher, S., and Cleveland, S. (1958). *Body image and personality.* Princeton, N.J.: Van Nostrand.

Freud, S. (1923/1961). The ego and the id. In J. Strachey, ed. and trans., *The standard edition of the complete psychological works of Sigmund Freud.* Vol. 19 (pp. 3–66). London: Hogarth Press.

Galdston, I. (1947). On the etiology of depersonalization. *Journal of Nervous and Mental Disease* 105: 25–39.

Goodwin, J. (1989). *Sexual abuse: Incest victims and their families.* 2d ed. Chicago: Mosby/Yearbook.

———. (1993a). Childhood sexual abuse and non-epileptic seizures. In J. Rowan and J. R. Gages, eds., *Non-epileptic seizures* (pp. 181–1992). New York: Butterworth.

———. (1993b). *Rediscovering childhood trauma.* Washington, D.C.: American Psychiatric Press.

Goodwin, J., and Attias, R. (1993). Eating disorders in survivors of multimodal childhood abuse. In R. Kluft and C. Fine, eds., *Clinical perspectives on multiple personality disorder* (pp. 327–341). Washington, D.C.: American Psychiatric Press.

Goodwin, J., Hill, S., and Attias, R. (1990). Historical and folkloric techniques of exorcism: Applications to the treatment of dissociative disorders. *Dissociation* 3: 94–101.

Herman J. (1992). *Trauma and recovery.* New York: Basic Books.

Krueger, D. W. (1989). *Body self and psychological self.* New York: Brunner/Mazel.

Lacan, J. (1977). *Ecrits: A selection.* Trans. A. Sheridan. New York: Norton.

Lichtenberg, J. (1978). The testing of reality from the standpoint of the body self. *Journal of the American Psychoanalytic Asso*ciation 26: 357–385.

Linn, L. (1955). Some developmental aspects of body image. *The International Journal of Psycho-analysis* 36: 36–42.

Novick, J., and Novick, K. K. (1996). *Fearful symmetry: The development and treatment of sado-masochism.* Northvale, N.J.: Aronson.

Peto, A. (1959). Body image and archaic thinking. *International Journal of Psychoanalysis* 40: 223–231.

Pribor, E. F., Yutzy, S. H., Dean, J. T., and Wetzel, R. D. (1993). Briquet's syndrome dissociation and abuse. *American Journal of Psychiatry* 150: 1507–1511.

van der Kolk, B., Pelcovitz, D., Roth, S., Mandel, F., McFarlane, A., and Herman, J. (1996). Dissociation, somatization and affect regulation: The complexity of adaptation to trauma. *American Journal of Psychia*try (Festschrift Supplement) 153: 83–93.

van der Kolk, B. A., Perry, B., and Herman, J. L. (1991). Childhood origins of self-destructive behavior. *American Journal of Psychiatry* 148: 1665–1671.

Vanderlinden, J., and Vandereycken, W. (1996). Is sexual abuse a risk factor for developing an eating disorder? In M. Schwarta and L. Cohn, eds., *Sexual abuse and eating disorders* (pp. 17–22). New York: Brunner/Mazel.

Waler, G., Ruddock, A., and Cureton, S. (1995). Cognitive correlates of reported sexual abuse in eating disordered women. *Journal of Interpersonal Violence* 10 (2): 176–187.

Werner, H. (1957). *Comparative psychology of mental development.* New York: International Universities Press.

Westerlund, E. (1992). *Women's sexuality after childhood incest.* New York: Norton.

Winnicott, D. W. (1989). On the basis for self in body. In C. Winnicott, R. Shepherd and M. Davis, eds., *Psychoanalytic explorations* (pp. 261–283). Cambridge, Mass.: Harvard University Press.

Young, L. (1992). Sexual abuse and the problem of embodiment. *Child Abuse and Neglect* 16: 89–100.

CHAPTER 7

Conversations with the Body

Psychotherapeutic Approaches
to Body Image and Body Ego

Jean Goodwin and Reina Attias

Whenever patients in psychotherapy tell us about the self or the history of the self, they are also telling us about the body and its history. When the personal history involves childhood trauma, it is a history about pain in the body, about distorted images of the body and about a body-self whose functioning has been disrupted by trauma.

Some patients with a history of childhood trauma come into treatment with a litany of bodily symptoms and disturbances of bodily sensations. These patients tell us about headaches, stomachaches and other unexplained pain (Chapperon 1996); anesthesias; sexual and self-harm impulses; and sleep and eating disturbances (Goodwin and Attias 1993). However, in other clinical situations, such as those discussed in this chapter, it is not apparent at the beginning of treatment that there is a sense of damage in the bodily sphere that must be addressed. Patients like those discussed here generally present with a desire to improve ego functioning. They sense a lack of personal cohesion. It is sometimes difficult for them to organize their emotions, their narratives or the world around them. They feel ineffective in the world and in relationships, which never seem to reach the level of intimacy they desire.

As these patients tell us in more detail about the way they think about themselves, they demonstrate a fundamental difficulty in identifying the self with the body. Their image of the body may be highly inaccurate, leading to unwarranted self-criticisms or unrealistic expectations for the self to function in a disembodied or superhuman way (Kreuger 1989).

Anzieu (1989) describes these problems as body-ego deficits, defects in the "skin ego," which shields against overstimulation, contains feelings and sensations and receives and communicates information at nonverbal levels. Freud told us that the ego is "first and foremost a bodily ego" (1923/1961, 26), and Jung uncharacteristically agreed, saying, "The ego is the psychological expression of the firmly associated combination of all body sensations" (1960, 40).

If therapists follow Anzieu's line of reasoning and try to connect the patient's ego problems to the image of the body and to bodily sensations, the patient will often reveal a body image that is disorganized, fragmented, dismembered, multiple or riddled with gaps or intrusions. At this point the patient may disclose previously concealed, ignored or disconnected body symptoms. As these symptoms and body-image distortions (see Chapters 6 and 13, this volume) come to be understood as communications from the body requiring decoding, previously absent disorganized or fragmented autobiographical narratives often begin to be restored, becoming more cohesive and coherent (Klepner 1987/1993; Klopstech 1993; Galdston 1947).

Many obstacles must be overcome for this kind of therapeutic work to proceed. Little training is provided to therapists about how to navigate in the bodily sphere. The feeling that this is terra incognita combines with fears of harming the patient and with hopes that a specialist with more expertise—perhaps a physician or an adjunctive therapist—could handle this aspect of the work with greater effectiveness. Therapists' own therapy may never have addressed this area of connecting body sensations, body image and body-ego functioning with conscious ego skills, leaving them with no personal compass to guide the work (Jacobs 1994).

This chapter outlines three approaches psychotherapists can use in bringing the body into the therapeutic conversation. First, we give examples of how the therapist's cognitive focus and development of a new vocabulary can overcome barriers to the inclusion of the world of the body. As Aaron Beck has written: "Another essential component of the self-concept is the 'bodily self,' 'somatic self,' or 'body image.' . . . This conception of bodily state may be more crucial than actual physical condition in determining feelings and sensations" (1979, 204). Much can be learned simply by routinely inquiring into this area.

Second, we describe ways in which nonverbal and paraverbal channels of communication and symbol-making capacities can be developed within the therapy. These avenues involve attention to basic bodily functions in a way that reestablishes in therapy the holding functions of the mother of infancy (Winnicott 1965; Anzieu 1989). Important symbolic exchanges involve the use of physical objects that have often remained substitutes for human objects in the relational life of the deprived child. Such objects sometimes persist into adulthood as "cherished and loved special possessions which bring comfort and solace and act as integrators of body parts" (Kestenberg and Weinstein 1978, 76). Transitional objects have continued importance in the lives of traumatized individuals because they help to reestablish the defective boundaries of the "skin ego," providing self-soothing and a sense of self-possession and, in addition, preserving the traumatized child's hopefulness about the capacity to create and discover goodness in the world.

Some traumatized individuals have not been able to discover this transitional way of using physical objects, and do so for the first time in psychotherapy. Any and all physical elements of the therapy space can come to be used in this way. With such individuals, the use of play therapy, art therapy and other adjunctive therapies involving material objects can become central to the work. The therapist also serves as a significant transitional object, helping the patient to rebuild the scattered body-self. As Kestenberg notes: "The transitional object is an external aid in the integration of body parts, rhythms and shapes into a three-dimensional image of the body" (Kestenberg and Weinstein 1978, 76–77).

The third step for the therapist is to become proficient enough in this body conversation with the patient to enable the translation of bodily communications into verbal narratives (Klepner 1987/1993). Feelings, fantasies and childhood scenes that have been locked inside the body are no longer disowned and denied, but are transformed into personal history. Levine (1991) has noted that the psychophysiological freeze response often crowds out other body memories about the traumatic moment, depriving the survivor of somatic reminders of the body-self's efforts toward fight or flight. A technique he terms *somatic bridging* is used during retelling of traumatic episodes so that these active self-protective elements can be reclaimed. Levine's work is of interest because it provides a theoretical explanation for the repeated clinical observation that such processing often leads to bodily reexperiencing (once termed *abreactive crisis*) and may have the effect of resolving long-standing feelings of hopelessness and helplessness in the face of the trauma (see also Chapter 2, this volume).

In this chapter we will discuss barriers to conversing with the body and the process of developing nonverbal channels of communication. Then two detailed case reports illustrate this communicative process as it takes place in early and later phases of psychotherapy.

INCLUDING THE BODY IN VERBAL PSYCHOTHERAPY: OVERCOMING BARRIERS

Psychotherapy is designed to provide repeated opportunities to experience and develop effectiveness and autonomy. Because of body-mind dualism, the therapist may forget that the patient's body as well as the patient's mind is participating in these exercises. In a particular session such expressions may include changes in pulse, blood pressure, skin conductance or respiratory rate; facial expressions and gestures; laughter and weeping; moaning, sighing, humming or other prosodic linguistic phenomena; experiences within the hour or descriptions of occurrences outside therapy of pains, anesthesia, drowsiness, hunger or sexual sensations; bodily experiences of emotions; mimicry of important people or events; or changes in body posture or position (Donald 1991). As Siegel has pointed out: "I have found that the nonverbal actions of the patient on the couch often open the door to memories otherwise hidden. This is true especially of very early or very traumatic experiences, such as incest" (1996, 25).

In trauma therapy, these reactions are heightened when the patient experiences bodily flashbacks. At the opposite pole, the traumatized patient may be completely dissociated from bodily reactions. Sometimes therapists may find themselves experiencing the patient's disowned body sensations—trying to contain in their own body the patient's tears or the restless tension of the impulse to flee (Siegel 1996). Such moments are ripe for therapeutic error. Therapists must refrain from either acting impulsively on the basis of such sensations or fleeing from or denying them, as if they constituted catastrophic error. The therapeutic task is to recognize the sensations as the patient's lost property and hold it in such a way that it can be reclaimed. Because these bodily phenomena are so volatile and unconscious, trauma therapists must provide many opportunities for recognizing and expressing them. Talking directly about the body combats depersonalization, clarifies traumatic regression and challenges fears that the body is too damaged to be included in the recovery process. As Aldous Huxley wrote, "The body possesses one enormous merit; it is indubitably *there*, whereas the personality as a mental structure may be all in bits" (1936, 110).

Because the body-ego self has largely been excluded from the teaching of both the theory and technique of psychotherapy, the therapist may have difficulty finding a way to talk directly about the patient's bodily experiences without perpetuating the "normal" dissociation of such experiences that occurs so commonly in Western society. It can be useful for therapists to become aware of personal anxieties and fears that arise in the course of these conversations with the body. Discomfort, shame, panic and helplessness in the therapist may arise not only in response to narrative, but also to the patient's nonverbal communications in the bodily movements or facial expressions that accompany flashbacks (Simonds 1994).

Familiarity and eventual comfort with these personal reactions allow therapists to ask routinely, "What is happening in your body right now?" At this point the patient can begin to integrate the bodily aspects of the current therapeutic experience and also can start to clarify how the bodily experience as a child was excluded from the family language or distorted in various ways. While the abuser may have ignored the immediate bodily expressions of the child's physical and emotional pain, other caretakers may have ignored more subtle or delayed nonverbal expressions of distress. Thus, respectful verbal inclusion of the patient's body experience in the therapeutic conversation underlines the possibility for a new kind of experience in therapy, one that is not a compulsive repetition of victim-perpetrator interactions.

Once therapists have dealt with their own alarms about this kind of inquiry, they can begin to address the patient's fears. One source of such fears is the belief that if dissociative barriers between body and mind are breached, the victim will have to experience unbearable and overwhelming pain and tension. Therapists should not minimize the potential for painful bodily sensations and flashbacks, but can remind the patient that the conditions for therapeutic reexperiencing are quite different from the original traumatic situation and are in the service of healing the trauma. This helps the patient to become less disorganized and panicked around the pain, which can lead to greater control of pain-triggered anxiety and dissociation, thus strengthening the body ego and the ego's sense of mastery.

Another source of the patient's fear about bringing the body into psychotherapy is the belief that the real body, like the distorted body image, has been utterly smashed and destroyed beyond any possibility of healing or repair. Consistent and firm containment (Winnicott 1949/1958) by the therapist is helpful here along with cognitive therapy. As Beck says, "By correcting erroneous beliefs, we can damp down or alter excessive, inappropriate emotional reactions" (1979, 214). The bodily suffering is not as endless or as shameful as the patient's traumatic cognitions have constructed it. The therapist's calm in the face of the patient's catastrophizing together with the boundaried reliable containment of the therapeutic space allows the patient to rediscover a middle ground between complete dissociation from the body and unbearable suffering inside the hurt body. In this framework the patient has an opportunity to experience bodily sensations in a new and nontraumatic way, while simultaneously being helped to imagine the body and embodiment differently. Sometimes at this point a thorough physical examination is necessary to help the patient distinguish between physical damage to the real body and psychic damage to the body image. The patient may also engage in spontaneous mirror work, an activity usually characteristic of two year olds, in an effort to establish similarities and differences between the real body and the body image (Lacan 1977).

Some patients may object to including the body in treatment because they experience the body as a betrayer or enemy, at times even as a part of the abuser's body. The disorganizing and fragmenting effects of pain itself lead to alienation from the body and "contain not only the feeling that the body hurts but that the body hurts *me*. . . . This sometimes becomes visible when a young child or an animal, in the first moments of acute distress, takes maddening flight, fleeing from its own body as though it were a part of the environment that could be left behind" (Scarry 1985, 47).

Our patients, who cannot physically flee the body, do so psychologically by means of dissociation. This depersonalization has its roots in the childhood trauma: "During their travail they sometimes had to give up ownership of their bodies in a regressive way in order to survive psychologically" (Siegel 1996, 25). Therapists experienced in treating dissociative identity disorder (DID) will realize that the disowning, rejection, condemnation, denial and flight from the body parallels conflicts with child ego states that contain messages about childhood pain. At times the dissociated patient must be helped to listen to and negotiate with the body just as with alter ego states. As Klepner points out: "By making the body-self an 'it' and relegating the 'I' . . . to the mind, our body in a sense becomes the disowned self. . . . Despite the fact that we disown them they are constantly seeking expression" (1987/1993, 69).

DEVELOPING NONVERBAL AND PARAVERBAL CHANNELS OF COMMUNICATION AND SYMBOL-MAKING CAPACITIES

Twentieth-century psychotherapy has perhaps been overly focused on verbal communication, sometimes to the exclusion of the body. Unfortunately, verbal narrative is the channel most often blocked or damaged by death threat, bodily pain or traumatic anxiety that overwhelms the ego (see Chapter 1, this volume). However, the human brain is not restricted to Wernicke's area of the left cortex for the perception, registration, remembering, symbolic manipulation and transformation of experience. We have already outlined the ways in which mimetic expression can become part of verbal psychotherapy.

Written language, which also involves somewhat different brain areas than speech, can become a communicative pathway, accessible through list making, letter writing, journaling and creative writing, which may bypass prohibitions on speech or blocks to articulation (Pennebaker, Hughes and O'Heeron 1987; Donald 1991). Exercises in writing or drawing about feelings and bodily sensations can help patients access their own body-ego material, thereby recovering from the inarticulate spaces of pain experiences that can then be named, discriminated and integrated.

Patients with multilingual skills may find their disclosures of abuse emerging first in an adopted language or American Sign Language. Profound integrative emotional work takes place as these stories are retranslated back into the patient's native tongue.

Traumatized individuals often have complex and meaningful relationships with inanimate objects. There may be family photographs, childhood transitional objects, boxes of school papers and drawings that have been saved for years, often in unconscious preparation for therapeutic reworking. Sometimes it may be necessary to inquire about the existence of such materials. For patients whose families were chaotic and disorganized, the finding and reclaiming of such objects may become a prolonged quest that in itself illuminates the devastating realities of their childhood history. Working with these materials in psychotherapy brings the childhood body into the work.

Adjunctive therapies (which by definition are always adjuncts to verbal psychotherapy) can be used productively not only to bypass the trauma-related difficulties with verbal expression, but also to enter this rather inarticulate world of the body and especially the word-shattering experience of body pain. Adjunctive treatments must be tailored carefully both to the individual patient and to the stage of treatment (Goodwin and Talwar 1989; Hoppmann 1992; Kluft 1993; Chapter 9, this volume). They include body work, including exercise programs, massage, martial arts and techniques like rolfing and acupuncture; relaxation and meditation disciplines like yoga; movement and music therapies; psychodrama; wilderness therapy; sex therapy; and the art therapies, including use of drawing, sculpture and clay work, mask making, collage and sandtray work (which includes some elements from play therapy). All of these adjunctive modalities can lead to body flashbacks that must then be brought into the verbal therapy and translated and worked through at that level.

Sandtray work (Kalff 1980) allows the production of graphic representations of the "inside" of the body, reflecting the patient's fantasies and fears about bodily damage. Helping the patient to see these fears and name them can bring them into ego consciousness. Because of the symbol-shattering nature of pain, it is helpful initially for patients to be able to choose images from the therapist's wide array of sandtray toys rather than having to produce their own symbols; the analogy is to the picture boards used long ago by the nonspeaking hearing impaired that allowed them to substitute mimetic and kinetic behaviors for the blocked skills of verbal symbol making. Once the body-image fantasies have been externalized, the patient can begin to link body-image distortions to particular aspects of the trauma, as well as to bodily symptoms and deficits in body-ego capacities that have affected the experiencing and manipulating of the body in real space and time.

Physical objects can also be used by the psychotherapist in more free-form ways. Sometimes a sandtray object that has become particularly meaningful for the patient will be taken home. Photographs may also be taken of the sandtray depictions and given to the patient together with notes suggesting ways to work with the figures in psychodramatic dialogue or journaling. Some patients will copy or tape notes from the therapist into their own journals. Once the principle of transitional objects is grasped, individual therapists will be prompted to devise many creative modes of exchanging objects with patients. The patients' creativity is engaged in turn, as they experience greater freedom in the use of the physical objects than is possible with the therapist alone.

For trauma patients who refuse or are not ready to utilize these adjunctive approaches, the body can be involved in the therapeutic conversation in other ways. At the most fundamental level, the therapist can focus attention on basic bodily functions—eating, sleeping, elimination, self-care. At higher levels, this evolves into interventions around self-protection: escaping abusive relationships, sexual self-protection, finding ways to support oneself financially and developing a reliable network of caregivers. This acknowledging at a cognitive level of the necessity to experience bodily needs as reality is a prelude to the patients' allowing themselves to relinquish depersonalization and reconnect to bodily sensations and feelings (Lineham 1993).

CASE MATERIAL:
TRANSLATING THE BODY'S MESSAGES INTO NARRATIVE

The following cases illustrate how both verbal and nonverbal interventions were employed to further the body-image integration and body-ego functioning in two patients. The first case involves an account of intrafamilial sadistic abuse and a diagnosis of atypical dissociative disorder, and the second case involves multimodal abuse and complex posttraumatic stress disorder (PTSD). The first case provides a window into the first two years of psychotherapeutic work during which a language about the body and its suffering was being developed and nonverbal and paraverbal channels of communication were being established. The second case illustrates the therapeutic process at a much later phase in the work, when most of the patient's bodily manifestations could begin to be expressed and discussed at the level of verbal narrative.

In both cases the struggle to find words for the more profound pain still continues. As Winnicott so wisely observed: "Out of several years' intensive work it is notoriously difficult to choose a detail; nevertheless, I include this fragment in order to show that what I am putting forward is very much a part of daily practice with patients" (1958, 248).

Case 1

A forty-five-year-old woman sought psychotherapy because of feelings of internal fragmentation and a sense that she was once again being exploited in a relationship. Although she was quite functional, she felt she had never realized her true potential. Previously she had worked for seven years with two different therapists. She had always had clear memory of sexual abuse between ages five and thirteen by a cousin. However, this had not been a focus in her previous psychotherapy, and she had never seen it as a serious problem.

Her memories of childhood were exceedingly fragmented, which was compounded by the fact that her father's occupation required the family to move almost every two years. She was aware of and disturbed by confused feelings of anger, fear and terror concerning her mother, who was dead. She was extremely intelligent and was acutely sensitive to her own fragmentation of memory and the lack of self-cohesion, which became intense and disorganizing whenever she tried to describe those childhood years.

Early on she began to bring in drawings of disorganized houses with doorless rooms and staircases that led nowhere. She found these upsetting and was anxious about their meaning.

One of her earliest sandtray efforts depicted her body-image and body-ego condition (see Chapter 13 for a more comprehensive discussion of this material). She had purchased fourteen tiny girl dolls (they looked like trapeze artists) and pulled them apart in the sandtray along with eight baby dolls, also dismembered. The final picture in the sandtray showed legs, arms and heads partially buried in the sand. While she was working on this sandtray, she became very agitated and started to cry. "How will I ever get them back together again? It's impossible." This first sandtray was useful in giving us a picture of the patient's feeling world and sense of body-self structure. The sandtray work proceeded in several different ways: At times it tended toward redirection and self-soothing, at other times it tended toward interpretation in order to achieve emotional distance and at still other times it became abreactive work (Sobol and Schneider 1996; Sachs 1993).

This session opened a door that allowed body-ego experiences linked to traumatic memory slowly to begin to surface. Over the next few months the patient would bring out the box of dismembered dolls as she narrated painful scenes with her mother, sometimes holding or covering a doll with a blanket as if it were her hurt child-self.

The next breakthrough came with writing. She discovered that she was able to allow the flood of buried words (like the buried body parts) to appear on pages and pages of letters and journals, often in childlike printing and syntax, which she would bring weekly to the therapist. These letters would be carefully attended to during the sessions and each memory discussed. Gradually more and more self states would contribute written memories or feelings, and the story of the abuses began to emerge. She also spontaneously brought in family photographs that raised many questions for her.

As her narrative became more coherent, work with the dismembered dolls tapered off. She also began to have lower-abdominal pains when narrating in sessions as well as outside of sessions when triggered by reminders of the abuse.

One day she brought in a drawing of a honey stick and asked the therapist, "What is this?" In the next session she created a sandtray depicting a mother doll sticking something into a girl doll's bottom. Only several sessions later was she able to begin hesitatingly to verbally describe this scene. We slowly pieced together sadistic abuse by her mother, which had begun in her preschool years. This series of abuse images hadn't been narrativized or sequenced and needed to be laboriously absorbed and then reworked in the light of other simultaneous abusive contexts.

The somatic flashbacks during sessions were intensely painful. While the somatic flashback was in progress, careful gentle inquiry by the therapist sometimes could elicit a verbal description of the childhood scene that seemed to be contained in the bodily pain. The patient felt that both her narrative capacity and her body-self would slowly come together and then would fly apart again when she reexperienced the reality of her remembered pain. She began to grasp that as the memories and the body pain were recovered, this process itself became the re-*membering,* the collecting of the dismembered parts of herself first depicted in sandtray.

Ultimately she depicted this predicament in drawings of a patchwork body image in which certain body parts were connected to memory, physical pain and emotion, but other parts were still anesthetic and amnesic. Rendering visible this body-image fragmentation helped make available for therapeutic work her ego fragmentation around this traumatic material.

She was able at times to deploy her adult skills to narrate and integrate the multiple abusive experiences. At other times this would collapse as she returned to her previous mode of distrusting and abandoning both her body sensations and her childhood memories, attempting to function again in a disembodied way. Although the bodily flashbacks were extremely painful, she realized that working in this way was a necessary step toward reclaiming body sensations connected to pleasure. The simple awareness of the feeling of wind on her face was a new experience.

After two years she was able to use several therapeutic sessions to prepare herself for a pelvic examination. Previously such examinations had been accompanied by anesthesia and amnesia. This time, however, she was able to discuss her fears during sessions and express her anxiety about discovering serious internal damage. During the examination she told the physician about her sexual abuse and about her fears about the examination. The physician responded by acknowledging her need for an especially sensitive and gentle approach. She was very pleased both with her capacity to remain present and with the results of the examination, which were normal.

In this case the ego seemed to contain in itself the traumatic experiences. Very few symptoms appeared emotionally or behaviorally, except general flattened affect and somewhat diminished functioning. Extreme body pain emerged only during flashbacks related to the trauma therapy. In this early phase of the clinical work, it was necessary for the therapist to be available between sessions to help the patient decode remembered pain. Since memories were lodged primarily in the body ego, body metaphors became the route to reconstruction and integration.

CASE 2

A thirty-five-year-old attorney sought treatment because of low self-esteem and problems with intimacy. He had not connected these problems with remembered sexual abuse by a grade-school coach; the patient's report at the time had led to the discovery of other victims and the coach's dismissal.

The patient remembered, however, that even long before that incident, he felt that something was wrong with his body, as if perhaps something had been taken out of his chest, leaving him stooped over. This was the position he assumed in therapy, bent over, with forehead resting on his palm. In childhood he had believed as well that something had been removed from his genitals. His sexual history consisted of brief, often consensually sado-masochistic affairs, sometimes with prostitutes. His sadomasochistic interests centered on the use of excretions. However, he had to bolster himself with alcohol to participate and was at times amnesic.

Preoccupations with the body were also evident in his work and creative adaptations. Specializing in personal injury cases allowed him to surround himself with clients he saw as even more wounded and damaged than himself. His hobby of doodling had since adolescence produced image after image of dismembered body parts, merged monstrous chimeras and dead children, often with weeping mothers bent over them.

Therapeutic work was primarily verbal, although often focused on the patient's body position and sensation and on his out-of-therapy body experiences and impromptu sketches. He found himself devising his own exercise and weight-loss regime and for the first time in his adulthood allowed himself to have a mirror in his home. In the first six months of therapy, he lost thirty pounds as his body habitus became more muscular and masculine-appearing. He also acquired a new age-appropriate wardrobe. Repeatedly he noted the discrepancy between the mirror image and his body image.

He traced the overweight, hunched-over figure in his imagination first to his toddler's body cowering against the wall during his mother's beatings and then to his latency body curled on a mat masturbating a male molester but too ashamed to look up. The image contained, too, a revenge wish about kneeing the molester in the genitals and watching him double over with pain. At another level the body image that so disgusted him was that of his often depressed, overweight mother. His fantasy of bodily fusion with his mother allowed imaginary comfort from her, escape from the victim role and fantasy opportunities to punish and control her by mistreating his own body. In therapy, once he became able to weep, the bent-over posture seemed more natural, even facilitative, and once a crying spell was exhausted, he could arise from it seemingly taller and expanded.

The sadomasochistic practices bridged emotionally to anger, but more to the dread and confusion he felt during the molestation, because he had no idea what would happen next and felt, when the molester ejaculated, that he must be urinating or that perhaps someone was bleeding.

As treatment proceeded, the patient was able to involve himself in an intimate long-term sexual relationship that still involved reenactments, but of less terrorizing aspects of the traumatic scenes. For example, only when he brought the partner into his exercise regimen did he realize that this included many specific aspects of the molester's coaching regimen. When he was able to weep about this in the presence of the partner, anxiety was relieved. It was as if the child's body, with its feelings and desires, could now be present in the relationship, and he experienced sexual contact, for the first time, in a fully embodied way. Previously, his risk-taking sexuality had been in the service of counterphobic defenses against fears, memories and sadness about the childhood molestation.

In this case the self-image was distorted by a sense of gap or mutilation, as if the loss of vital body parts had somehow drained away his own self or soul substance (Shengold 1989). The childhood conviction of genital damage was multidetermined by psychodynamic and regressive conflicts, but its traumatic antecedents probably included the childhood cremasteric reflex (the retraction of the testicles into the body cavity under extreme stress), which may have occurred during his earliest panic reactions (Bell 1965).

Mutilation fantasies were balanced by incorporation fantasies. Body-image gaps were imaginatively filled by introjections of elements of the abuse and of both abusers. His merger with mother is reminiscent of the "one body for two" problem as described by Joyce McDougall in *Theaters of the Body* (1989). This can also be understood as a bodily manifestation of identification with the aggressor. This fusion with an adult female no doubt contributed to his worries about his genitals. The patient's doodles may have functioned to extrude symbolically these introjected figures, so they could be moved out of his own imaginary insides and into concrete, visible external images, thus achieving a kind of exorcism. Similarly, these images externalized his sense of woundedness and mutilation. The creation of imaginary playmates or dissociative identities often achieves similar extrusions of painful traumatic material.

The sadomasochistic practices allowed a posttraumatic play (Terr 1994) solution to the intense anxiety triggered by sexual situations. By becoming the initiator of hurtful practices and the controller of pain and fear, the patient's anxiety was somewhat reduced and the ever threatening sadness and tears were kept at bay. Although in female victims anger often seems the most blocked affect, for this male patient hurt and grief were the principal affects locked into the body and inaccessible for direct expression. Tears were crucial. As Henry Maudsley observed long ago, "The sorrow that has no vent in tears, makes other organs weep" (McDougall 1989, 139).

SUMMARY

Exploration of body-image and body-ego functioning proceeds in the ordinary course of good psychotherapy. However, the more aware trauma therapists can be of how fundamental the body ego is to the healthy functioning of the ego, the more creative they will be in devising and being alert for therapeutic opportunities for conversations with the body-self. We still are at the beginning of understanding the relationship of body ego to the conscious ego and the role of body image and body ego in storing traumatic experiences. One could hypothesize that it is when explicit memory is lost or unformed and traumatic experience exists primarily as implicit or behavioral memory that body image and body ego will be most affected. In these cases psychotherapy may need to focus more on nonverbal or mimetic communications (Terr 1994; Donald 1991) and on helping the patient to translate these into verbal narratives that then become part of conscious history.

REFERENCES

Anzieu, D. (1989). *The skin ego*. New Haven: Yale University Press.

Beck, A. T. (1979). *Cognitive therapy and the emotional disorders*. New York: Meridian, Penguin Books.

Bell, A. (1965). Significance of scrotal sac and testicles on the prepubertal male. *Psychoanalytic Quart*erly 34: 182–206.

Chapperon, J. A. (1996). Chronic memories: Chronic body pain disorders as undiagnosed, untreated dissociated trauma. Presented at the 12th annual ISSD conference, San Francisco.

Donald, M. (1991). *Origins of the modern mind: Three stages in the evolution of culture and cognition*. Cambridge, Mass.: Harvard University Press.

Freud, S. (1923/1961). The ego and the id. In J. Strachey, ed. and trans., *The standard edition of the complete psychological works of Sigmund Freud*. Vol. 19 (pp. 3–66). London: Hogarth Press.

Galdston, I. (1947). On the etiology of depersonalization. *Journal of Nervous and Mental Disease* 105: 25–39.

Goodwin, J., and Attias, R. (1993). Eating disorders in survivors of multimodal child abuse. In R. Kluft and C. Fine, eds., *Clinical perspectives on multiple personality disorder* (pp. 327–341). Washington, D.C.: American Psychiatric Press.

Goodwin, J., and Talwar, N. (1989). Group psychotherapy for incest victims. *Psychiatric Clinics of North America* 12: 279–293.

Hoppman, W. H. (1992). *The case of facial armoring: The place of body therapy in the treatment of dissociative disorders*. Paper presented at the Ninth Annual Conference of ISSD, Chicago, Illinois.

Huxley, A. (1936). *Eyeless in Gaza*. London: Carroll and Graf.

Jacobs, T. J. (1994). Nonverbal communications: Some reflections on their role in the psychoanalytic education. *Journal of the American Psychoanalytic Association* 41 (3): 741–762.

Jung, C. (1960). *The psychogenesis of mental disease*. Bollingen Series 20. Vol. 3. Princeton, N.J.: Princeton University Press.

Kalff, D. M. (1980). *Sandplay*. Boston: Sigo.

Kestenberg, J. S., and Weinstein, J. (1978). Transitional objects and body-image formation. In S. A. Grolnick and L. Barkin, eds., *Between reality and fantasy: Transitional objects and phenomena*. New York: Aronson.

Klepner, J. I. (1987/1993). *Body process: Working with the body in psychotherapy*. San Francisco: Jossey-Bass.

Klopstech, A. (1993). Sexual abuse: The body remembers even when the mind does not. *Journal of the International Institute for Bioenergetic Analysis* 5 (2): 36–44.

Kluft, E. S. (1993). *Expressive and functional therapies in the treatment of multiple personality disorder*. Springfield, Ill.: Charles Thomas.

Krueger, D. W. (1989). *Body self and psychological self*. New York: Brunner/Mazel.

Lacan, J. (1977). *Ecrits: A selection*. New York: Norton.

Levine, P. D. (1990–91). The body as healer: A revisioning of trauma and anxiety. *Somatics* 8 (1): 18–27.

Linehan, M. M. (1993). *Cognitive-behavioral treatment of borderline personality disorder*. New York: Guilford.

McDougall, J. (1989). *Theaters of the body*. New York: Norton.

Pennebaker, J. W., Hughes, C. F., and O'Heeron, R. C. (1987). The psycho-physiology of confession: Linking inhibitory and psychosomatic processes. *Journal of Personality and Social Psychology* 52: 781–793.

Sachs, R. G. (1993). Use of sandtrays in the beginning treatment of a patient with dissociative disorder. In R. P. Kluft and C. G. Fine, eds., *Clinical perspectives on multiple personality disorder* (pp. 301–310). Washington, D.C.: American Psychiatric Press.

Scarry, E. (1985). *The body in pain: The making and unmaking of the world*. New York: Oxford University Press.

Shengold, L. (1989). *Soul-murder: The effects of childhood abuse and deprivation*. New Haven: Yale University Press.

Siegel, E. V. (1996). *Transformations: Countertransferences during the psychoanalytic treatment of incest, real and imagined*. Hillsdale, N.J.: Analytic Press.

Simonds, S. L. (1994). *Bridging the silence: Non-verbal modalities in the treatment of adult survivors of childhood sexual abuse*. New York: Norton.

Sobol, B., and Schneider, K. (1996). Art as adjunctive therapy in the treatment of children who dissociate. In J. Silberg, ed., *The dissociative child* (pp. 191–218). Lutherville, Md.: Sidran.

Terr, L. (1994). *Unchained memories: True stories of traumatic memories, lost and found*. New York: Basic Books.

Winnicott, D. W. (1949/1958). Mind and its relation to the psyche-soma. In *Through pediatrics to psychoanalysis* (pp. 243–254). New York: Basic Books.

_____. (1965). Ego integration in child development. *The maturational process and the facilitating environment*. New York: International Universities Press.

CHAPTER 8

Challenged Bodies, Wounded Body Images

Richard III and Hephaestus

Valerie Sinason

This chapter examines the emotional impact that noticeable signs of brain injury or chromosomal disorder have on physically challenged or learning-disabled children and adults.

All children and adolescents have conscious and unconscious fantasies about their bodies. Klein (1932) theorizes that the child's early fears about the dangerousness of the mother's body and the child's own body often develop from fantasies about mutual attacks. In adolescence in particular, girls and boys often look in the mirror wondering how this outside picture might match their inner picture of themselves. Worries about sexuality and the development of sexual characteristics are often displaced to the face—to the nose, that sticks out, to spots, to strands of hair that are felt to destroy the whole sense of self. It can be a painful time when "face" values can overtake more integrated ideas about the worth of what is behind a face, inside a person.

It is much harder to deal with these issues when there is something permanent that shows on the face or in the speech, when there is some physical sign that marks the individual as noticeably different. At the most primitive level, such difference can be experienced as due to sexual damage. The connection between noticeable physical and mental differences and sexuality is a painful one. At the root there is unresolved anger and fear that some flaw or wrongness in the sexual and procreative connection between a man and a woman could lead to damaged offspring. In the same way that the illegitimate have had to carry social and cultural fantasies about wild, unlawful sexuality, so the congenitally different carry, stamped on their bodies, the mark of what is feared as unnatural and destructive sexuality. This may become part of the fantasy life of both the parents and the child.

MIRROR, MIRROR ON THE WALL

CASE 1

Carole, a thirteen-year-old girl with Down's syndrome, sat in my therapy room and picked up a toy mirror. She looked at her face carefully. Then she put on a toy crown and looked at her face. She took the crown off. Then she put a necklace on and looked in the mirror. She took it off. She was frowning. I said she did not look pleased with what she saw in the mirror. Deep in her own thoughts, she did not appear to hear me. Then she picked up a black veil and wound it round her head. She took it off; then she covered her face with it so that she looked mummified. She took it off; then she covered the mirror with the veil. Her eyes filled with tears. Then she threw the mirror. It was unbreakable and held in a plastic frame. Otherwise it would have broken, the way she felt broken at that moment. She sat and cried.

I said she did not think she could look at herself without adding on something: a crown, a necklace, a veil. Perhaps she did not think I would care for her unless she was a princess or a queen. But then that was no good, because she felt like a useless princess. She wished she could cover her face up to hide her Down's syndrome or throw it away.

"Why doesn't my Down's syndrome go away?" she asked. "Why is it here? Each time I look in the mirror it is still here."

CASE 2

Joan, a twelve-year-old with Down's syndrome, was referred because of her public masturbating and hair pulling. Behavioral treatment, social-skills lessons and sanctions had failed to make any impact, and part of her head was now bald. When I entered the therapy room, she sat opposite me violently masturbating, with her legs wide open.

"I wonder why you want me to look between your legs," I said. "The medical word is *vagina*," I added (many learning-disabled children and adults have not been given the vocabulary necessary to frame their sexual questions). My question had no impact. She continued masturbating. I continued with more questions. "Is it a feeling you are wondering about? . . . Is it a picture in your head? . . . Are you wondering if you are the same as me?"

Suddenly she stopped masturbating, looked at me with great alertness and asked, "Has my vagina got Down's syndrome?"

I said, "What an intelligent question." Because her face looked different, how could she know if the other parts of her body might not be different too. We were then able to explore her fears about difference, and as that exploration continued, the driven, destructive nature of her masturbation was ameliorated.

In another session Joan made a male doll and female doll kiss. She looked at the kiss carefully from every angle. When I commented that perhaps she was wondering how her mom and dad made her and what had happened, she lifted the female doll's hair and felt it down to the root. "Gone wrong," she said, "right to the root." Exploring her sense of being made wrong right from the beginning was another step toward relieving her compulsive self-injury.

COMMENTS: THERAPEUTIC RESOLUTIONS

Carole's and Joan's experiences illustrate the significance of mirrors. Carole and Joan were asking in therapy the questions children ask of mirrors. The first mirror, as Winnicott (1967/1971) has pointed out, is the mother's eyes. Babies look up into the eyes of their primary caregiver and in that shiny mirror see how they are loved. We become the reflection we see looking at us.

This mirror is not passive. It actively sends messages to the child, projecting the first and deepest internal self-representation. When a child is unwanted, there is no gleaming light or twinkle that says "You are lovable"; there is coldness, hurt, shame, hate, fear, anger. "[Children] look and do not see themselves," says Winnicott (1967/1971, 112). "There are consequences." That unloving mirror actively projects into the vulnerable child the message that he or she is not wanted. Blind children cannot see the look in their parents' eyes, but they can hear the tone of their voices and feel the response of their bodies, receiving images of worth or worthlessness in these ways (Fraiberg 1975).

In 1977 eighteen profoundly retarded men were tested for mirror and photographic memory and recognition of themselves (Harris 1977). Nine were given mirror training, but there was no improvement in recognition. I wonder whether there was such terrible narcissistic injury from not looking like their own families, and from having suffered so many unloving reflective responses from human mirrors, that it was easier to give up altogether trying to find the self in the mirror. As Winnicott wrote: "If the mother's face is unresponsive, then a mirror is a thing to be looked at but not to be looked into" (1967/1971, 112).

In their work on perinatal bereavement at the Tavistock Clinic, psychoanalysts Sandy Bourne and Emmanuel Lewis (1991) found that adult ideas about the reason for a malformed baby link up with unconscious memories of childhood fantasies about how babies are made and unmade or destroyed and stir up feelings of shame (1989, 938). It takes time in treatment to deal adequately with these issues, which have their origins in the deepest layers of the psyche.

In a psychotherapy group I ran for severely learning-disabled adults, a young woman shyly mentioned that Simon Weston, a badly burned and facially disfigured British veteran of the Falklands war, had gotten married. Movingly, the whole group then showed their knowledge of this young man's history and the painful impact of his disfigured face. For them, it became clear that his face represented a hopeful icon, one that said it was possible to wear disfigurement as a badge of honor and not be shamed by it. However, it was only after the group had been ongoing for four years that they could experience me, the representation in the transference of their nondisabled parents, as someone who could find them lovable despite their visible differences.

At this point in the group's life a physically challenged and learning-disabled young woman came in triumphantly. "Boys on my estate teased me. They threw stones at me and called me a spastic. I said I was a spastic and they were lucky they weren't, but they were rude boys and I was not rude." We all, including myself and my cotherapist, applauded her. She understood the nature of her difference and the fear it evoked and could elucidate for the nominally "normal" boys the ugly process they were involved in.

The heroism of some gifted individuals imprisoned in damaged bodies has been satisfyingly documented in the last few years in a number of star-studded films, plays, books and television shows. Notable examples include Daniel Day Lewis as Christy Brown in *My Left Foot* and John Hurt in *Elephant Man*. This trend has helped create a more inclusive emotional climate. It should be borne in mind, however, that not only are the majority of physically challenged people no more emotionally or intellectually gifted than anyone else, but that those who are multiply challenged have very few chances and little encouragement to develop their gifts.

Recognizing and tolerating difference is a complex task in most cultures. Not being average, not being in the majority, whether due to race, religion, class, economic status, educational position or physical or mental difference, can make people feel very isolated. However, within the United Kingdom alone nearly 6.5 million children and adults have some kind of disability. Within the United Kingdom there are 360,000 children who were born with some serious congenital problem. Worldwide, over 1 percent of all new babies born will have some kind of disability.

In trying to understand patterns of adolescent and adult male difficulty in coping with physical and mental differences, I have found it useful to study in detail Shakespeare's characterization of Richard III as well as the injured but creative Greek divinity Hephaestus.

RICHARD III: CROOKED BODY, CROOKED MIND

> *Then, since the heavens have shap'd my body so,*
> *Let hell make crook'd my mind to answer it.*
> *I have no brother, I am like no brother;*
> *And this word "love," which greybeards call divine,*
> *Be resident in men like one another*
> *And not in me. I am myself alone.*
>
> **Richard, in Shakespeare's *Henry VI*, Part III, Act V, Sc. 6**

> *But I, that am not shap'd for sportive tricks,*
> *Nor made to court an amorous looking-glass;*
> *I, that am rudely stamp'd, and want love's majesty*
> *To strut before a wanton ambling nymph;*
> *I, that am curtail'd of this fair proportion,*
> *Cheated of feature by dissembling nature,*
> *Deform'd, unfinish'd, sent before my time*
> *Into this breathing world, scarce half made up . . .*
>
> **Richard, in Shakespeare's *Richard III*, Act I, Sc. 1**

Unlike most of the physically challenged, Richard III is of royal birth and educated. Nevertheless, his response to his visible bodily difference addresses universal human problems faced by individuals in similar positions. Richard has objectively quantifiable organic damage. As portrayed by Shakespeare and chronicled by Sir Thomas More (1557), Richard, born prematurely, was lame and hunchbacked. That, as with any organic condition, adds an extra burden to the normal difficulties of life. However, as we have

seen, what can be far more crucial to the ultimate quality of life is the meaning made of the bodily problem. Hatred at the difference between the
wounded, injured self and other "normal" people ("I am like no brother")
may create secondary problems (Sinason 1988) that can cause even greater
human distress and destruction than the original condition. I see these secondary problems as the result of the complex, exaggerated defensive
processes undertaken to hide the pain of the actual physical problem.

Shakespeare's portrayal of Richard III reveals how the bearers of congenital injuries feel rudely stamped by the sexual act that created them.
Whereas normal children often try to deny that their existence is due to their
parents' lovemaking (or at best might have come from one deviation, necessary in order to create them, in an otherwise spotless celibate life), children
born with a handicap feel inextricably linked to the procreative act. The hatred of parental sexuality may then be transferred to others. Shakespeare's
Richard speaks of "wanton ambling nymph[s]," projecting his own warped
sexual feelings onto the court women by seeing them as wanton and revealing his jealousy of their unfettered capacity to amble. They have the luxury
of normal limbs. Richard's raw hatred of the parental couple includes envy
and fear of their bodily intactness and their sexual capacities as well as rage-
ful jealousy at feeling forever excluded from their relations.

According to Thomas More (1557), on June 13, 1483, as part of his cam-
paign to seize the crown, Richard accused his mother, the queen, and the late
king's mistress, Jane Shore, of trying to murder him by witchcraft. Regardless of historical truth, the emotional truth represented by Thomas More's
account is important:

> "Ye shall see in what wise that sorceress and that other witch of her counsel,
> Shore's wife, with their affinity, have by their sorcery and witchcraft wasted my
> body." And therewith he plucked up his doublet-sleeve to his elbow, upon his
> left arm, where he shewed a withered arm and small, as it was never other [sic:
> as it had always been]. And thereupon every man's mind sore misgave him,
> well perceiving that this matter was but a quarrel for well they wist that the
> Queen was too wise to go about any such folly. And also, if she would, yet
> would she of all folk least make Shore's wife of her counsel, whom of all women
> she most hated as that concubine whom the King her husband had most loved.

The disgust and fear of the parental sexual coupling that had produced
him extended to all the sexual relations of his parents. Luckily, Richard's
emotionally based linking together of mistress and wife was seen by those

around him as irrational. Other madmen with power who invoked witch-craft have been able to cause many deaths.

HEPHAESTUS: THE REJECTED BODY RETALIATES

Hephaestus was the only Greek god who was not perfectly formed. He was ill-made and lame in both legs (Burkert 1985). His stumbling gait made the gods laugh. Hera, ashamed of his ugliness and imperfections, tried to hide him from the immortals. She cast him from Olympus into the sea, where he was looked after by Thetis, but spent nine years hidden away.

This story is painfully familiar—the shock of having a handicapped child so often leads to abandonment and rejection of the child. Hephaestus grows up to become a blacksmith and superb craftsman. He is linked with fire. To punish his mother for her cruelty, he sent her a golden throne, which, when she sat on it, gripped her with invisible hands so she could not extricate her-self. Physical force, symbolized by the god of war, Ares, could not move her.

When Dionysus made Hephaestus drunk, he agreed to free his mother in exchange for a beautiful bride. He was given Aphrodite, goddess of love, fertility and seafaring, the physically perfect woman so often imagined by lonely, isolated and frustrated men. Aphrodite is unfaithful to him, and he deals with his humiliation by snaring her and her lover, Ares, in a magic couch he invented so that they are exposed to the gods, who laugh at them just as they had once laughed at him. Hephaestus makes the gods laugh on another occasion when he mimics the beautiful youth Ganymede and hob-bles around a banquet pouring out wine. He built palaces for the gods and lived in a dwelling of glittering bronze. Most of the time he could be found by the hot furnaces, poking the fire.

Hephaestus and the myths about him make us aware of the secondary de-fense of laughter to control the public humiliation of being physically differ-ent. Both situations in which he evoked the laughter of the gods involved displacing sexual humiliation onto others—in both cases onto splendidly beautiful others. The fear of being seen as ugly and sexually distasteful is widespread among those with physical disabilities. It seems that if the in-fant's first mirror, mother's eye, registers distaste, as Hera's did and as those of many parents do when initially faced with the shock of an injured child, a sense gradually grows of not being the wanted, beautiful, healthy child. Hephaestus has to ensnare the most beautiful and desirable goddess,

Aphrodite, and the swift and powerful Ares and become the mocker as a means of capturing those qualities for himself.

Physically different children or adults may feel they have somehow caused the powerful destruction they see in the damaged body. The alternative—feeling the victim of powerful, destructive forces—is even less comfortable. This can result in continuous reparative attempts by demonstrating special talents. The superb skills Hephaestus develops can be seen (Klein 1932) as a struggle to atone for the damage, which succeeds only to a point. It was Freud (1909) who, through his conversations with four-year-old Hans and his parents, first understood the childhood fantasy that babies came from the anus and that an aspect of children's interest in their feces was the fantasy of fecal babies. Hephaestus, deprived of feeling himself the product of a normal marital relationship, needed to remain at work in the dark, hot furnace area of anality, manufacturing golden robotlike women. So many of the developmental burdens on physically different children hinder the resolution of oedipal issues; this type of retreat is not uncommon.

Although Hephaestus later protects his mother from his father's wrath, his retaliation against her with the golden throne mocks her sexuality, I believe, in that she is stuck down by her bottom. For those forced into wheelchairs by the nature of their handicap there is further meaning. Nature has not let them separate and walk away; they have to remain stuck down. To rise courageously above this requires good nurturance and constitutional gifts. Not surprisingly, people will often respond to this frustration by becoming even more immobilized and immobilizing than the realities of their situation require.

CASE STUDY: HOWARD/HEPHAESTUS

Howard is an eighteen-year-old handicapped young man who lives in a hostel, as he had proved unmanageable at home. There is certainly an increased family burden for the parents of a handicapped child (Friedrich and Friedrich 1981) and the divorce rate for such parents is three times the average (Sternlicht and Deutsch 1972). His parents had been in foster care themselves as children and the blow of his birth injury ("I knew he wasn't right at birth"), which was formally recognized when Howard was two as cerebral palsy and severe learning impairment, was too much for them. Howard's increasing violence made it all the harder for them to manage.

He was referred by his hostel because of his head banging, masturbating in public and furious attacks on staff because they "weren't giving him a woman." Art therapist Simon Cregeen (1988), who works with such young men on sexual issues, commented that they experience almost perpetual frustration toward staff for not providing them with sexual partners. The staff, themselves only a few years older than Howard, were struggling with their own social and sexual attitudes toward Howard as a physically and mentally challenged peer. On the one hand, there was a feeling that because of his difficulties, he had a right to sexual gratification regardless of any emotional relationship. On the other hand, there was concern that his negative behavior and attitudes might automatically doom any link with another person. He agreed to consider therapy, I later learned, only because of the enticement, offered by his workers, that the assessment might help him have a relationship with a woman.

The first time I saw Howard, he was wearing a short-sleeved T-shirt that revealed his well-proportioned torso. He held his head at an angle to try to hide the side that showed the effects of his brain injury. He fixed his eyes on mine strongly, as if to prevent me from seeing his wasted legs in the wheelchair.

I introduced myself to Howard and his worker, but then Howard dismissed the worker sneeringly: "Go now." The worker turned and left. It was clear that Howard saw the worker only as legs, as nothing more than despised appendages that helped him get about. The worker felt guilty for having legs and being able to push the young man in the wheelchair and was therefore accepting his contempt without comment. Feelings of guilt for being normal are a heavy burden for those who work with disabled young people. There is also an urge to deny the painful envy and even hatred that wheelchair-bound people may feel for their caretakers.

I explained to Howard that his workers had referred him to me because they felt he was unhappy about himself and becoming violent because of it, and that not having a girlfriend seemed a part of his unhappiness. "Crap. Crap. Talk, talk." I said it was very easy to turn talk to crap. "Crap, crap," he repeated, an uncertain echo of himself. I said maybe he wished some talk did not turn to crap. He was quiet for a moment and then said, "Talk. Talk. I can talk. I don't need talk." I said he could talk and he couldn't walk, and it seemed he was hurting the area he could manage in—talking—because being unable to walk pained him so, and at the moment too it felt painful because he didn't have a girlfriend.

"I don't want the ugly ones. That's all I get. The ugly ones no one wants. The ones in the wheelchairs, the ones with no proper faces. The ones that can't speak. What are you going to do for me? Kiss my arse?" I said he had come to see a woman to talk about his problems, and not only was she a Mrs., but she was physically intact too. And I told him as long as he saw close contact only as something to do with kissing arses and crap, he would not be able to enjoy the relationship of love whatever his physical problems were. He was quiet again. "I can go." I agreed he could. There was a long silence. "I'm stuck in the chair." I said he was stuck in the wheelchair because of his disability, but he had the freedom, with the help of that chair, to move in or out of the room. However, I went on to say, maybe it was deeply hurtful that he could get that freedom only because of the chair.

"I'm thick." I said we knew he had learning problems as well, but that maybe he was using that rude term about himself just now by way of an apology to the chair and me for accusing us of restricting his freedom, when it had been his own mixed feelings that made him feel so stuck.

"I don't want a girl thicker than me." I said he seemed to be worrying that I expected him to. "And if she is in a chair and not as thick as me, how will we do it?" There was a long silence. I said that was an important thing to think about. It might indeed be physically hard to make love; he might need help. It might not be possible. But it seemed as if fear of needing help or being humiliated had made him avoid all the steps for actually meeting and learning to care about someone. "I did meet someone. She couldn't use her arms and I had to do all her lifting." He looked ruefully at his strong arms. "It went on and on." I said he did have strong arms and maybe he was proud they could do strong work, but he did not want to have to use them all the time.

"No." Long silence.

I said it was almost time to stop and we could have another exploration next week to see if he would like to come and meet me regularly. "Talk. Crap," he said, girding himself up for the outside. "I'm leaving now." I said I would write. He did not turn his head around, but whizzed his wheelchair out, almost knocking over the young man who brought him.

I wrote a letter offering a second appointment if he wanted one, but he did not. I have not heard from him since. However, that one meeting made clear to me that the painful self-assessments all adolescents have to go through are terribly heightened for those struggling with a wounded self-image connected to physical or mental differences.

DISCUSSION

For Howard, as for Richard III, the relationship of love had turned into a degraded sexuality. The wounded self-image and secondary psychological complications stemming from his physical imperfections meant that his sadism, envy and destructive feelings had found a home in a distorted image of love. His hurt at his nonworking legs and, to a lesser extent, his mind was assuaged when he attacked what was healthy in himself and in others.

These secondary sequelae and the travestied images he had created protected him from the unbearable awareness of his own bodily difference. He could only bear to touch on it a few times. "I don't want the ugly ones. That's all I get." Every adolescent is aware of the hierarchy of selection caused by levels of attractiveness. Howard could not accept his disadvantages due to bodily difference, and his self-hatred was then directed against other people in the same situation, especially young women.

His oedipal struggle for his mother was made harder by the fact that she was not physically challenged. As Robinson and Robinson (1976) point out, a particular source of psychopathology in some congenitally injured individuals is the slowness of their passage through and their poor resolution of the stages of psychosexual development. Emotional fixation at early stages of development perpetuates already immature defense mechanisms.

Like Hephaestus, Howard had strong arms to help him take on restitutive work, but it seemed as if using this power to tackle big tasks made him still more aware of the destruction he feared he had caused. Therefore he fearfully inhibited even what he could do.

Adolescence, as we know, is painful, but it is even more so for young people, like Howard, who realize how acutely different they are from peers and how uniquely difficult will be their struggle for a marital partner and a successful career.

For Hephaestus not to entrap the beautiful and swift, for Richard not to use his hunchback to escalate his hatred means resisting the siren call that some cannot bear not to follow. That is the call that takes them back to the womb, unhurt yet by the congenital condition that will afflict them. It means resisting regression to an autoerotic state (finding sexual pleasure only in one's own body). Giving that up means looking into the mirror and truly facing the actual physical reality. But the ultimate reward of this dialogue with the mirror is the possibility of real relationships, both sexual and emotional.

REFERENCES

Bourne, S., and Lewis, E. Perinatal bereavement. (1995). *British Medical Journal* 302: 1167–1168.

Burkert, W. (1985). *Greek religion*. Trans. J. Raffan. Oxford: Blackwell.

Cregeen, S. (1988). The sexual needs of handicapped people. Paper given at the British Institute for Learning Disability, Barnsley, September 26.

Fraiberg, S. (1975). The development of human attachments in infants blind from birth. *Merrill-Palmer Quarterly* 21: 315–344.

Freeman, R. D. (1970). Psychiatric problems in adolescents with cerebral palsy. *Developmental Medicine and Child Neurology* 12: 64–70.

Freud, S. (1909/1961). Notes upon a case of obsessional neurosis. In J. Strachey, ed. and trans. *The Complete Psychological Works of Sigmund Freud*, vol. 10. (pp. 153–318). London: Hogarth Press.

Friedrich, W. N., and Friedrich, W. L. (1981). Psychosocial aspects of parents of handicapped and non-handicapped children. *American Journal of Ortho-Psychiatry* 46: 580–590.

Harris, L. P. (1977). Self-recognition among institutionalised, profoundly retarded males. *University of Texas Bulletin of the Psychonomic Society* 3 (4): 229–239.

Klein, M. (1932). *The psycho-analysis of children*. London: Hogarth Press.

More, Sir Thomas (1557/1986). In P. Johnson, ed., *The Oxford book of political anecdotes*. Oxford: Oxford University Press.

Robinson, H. B., and Robinson, H. (1976). *The mentally retarded child*. New York: McGraw-Hill.

Sinason, V. (1988). Richard III, Hephaestos and Echo: Sexuality and mental/multiple handicap. *Journal of Child Psychotherapy* 14: 93–105.

Sternlicht, M., and Deutsch, M. (1972). *Personality and social behaviour in the mentally retarded*. Lexington, Mass.: Lexington Books.

Winnicott, D. W. (1967/1971). Mirror-role of mother and family in child development. In *Playing and reality* (pp. 111–118). London: Tavistock.

PART III

Psychotherapy
The Traumatized Body in Treatment

Canst thou not ... pluck from the memory a rooted sorrow ... and with some sweet oblivious antidote cleanse the stuft bosom of that perilous stuff which weighs upon the heart?

Shakespeare, *Macbeth*, IV, iii

I have another self ... weltering in tears. ... I carry it deep inside me like a wound.

M. Tournier (1972, 21)

It is easier to fall ill than learn the truth. ... So take care of your maladies. ... They always have something to tell you.

M. Pavic (1990, 68)

When the mother is missing, we spend our whole life wandering, without a body, lights lost in the night, hearts that beat aimlessly, blood that goes on circulating without rhyme or reason ...

A. Savinio (1988, 297)

It was a great tree, beautiful and strong. I knew it was what I was looking for. ... It seemed it had always been there though I had only just discovered it.

Analysand's report of a dream (Scott 1951, 262)

The most important part of the integration of a personality is to make peace with one's own body.

Elvin Semrad (Rako and Mazer 1983, 23)

The Body in the Mirror
The Body and the Self

When the body begins to tell us about itself in psychotherapy, it does so in metaphor and parable. If we expect to hear about symptom complexes, anatomical body parts or the natural history of disease, we will be disappointed. What we hear instead are stories—stories and dreams about trees, trees that may turn out to mark the Garden of Eden; stories about talking mirrors, magical capes that confer invulnerability or gorgeous dresses that have the power to inspire love; stories about princes and princesses in distress who use great cunning and wizardly helpers to survive; and stories about beasts who inhabit vast, dark castles where vital secret knowledge is stored.

Communicating by means of these metaphors often provides immense relief to patients, who tell us they never wanted to have a body in the first place, much less talk to us about it, and who describe how every aspect of their bodily living—gender, eating, sleeping, elimination, sexuality—has been for them a source of grief and anxiety, never of pleasure.

The patients' need to speak in parables is often difficult for therapists to accept. They long for an image of the body-self that would resemble their idea of a biological organism; some imagine that if this troublesome idea of the psyche could only be jettisoned, we could navigate much better with only a body and a brain. What patients bring to therapists is a much less portable idea of the self; it is something more like an entire gypsy caravan than anything the biologists are prepared to deal with. And assembling the entire tarot deck and collected Grimms' fairy tales of their patients' psyches is in some ways the least of the problem. They must also round up all their fingers and toes, the heart and all its neighboring internal parts and connectors, the voice,

197

the shadow, the genitals, the face. It is not a straightforward task. As Becker wrote, "Man's body is a problem . . . that has not been explained. Not only his body is strange, but also its inner landscape, the memories and dreams. Man's very insides . . . are foreign" (1973, 51). So in this section you will hear stories not about brain and body, but about strange inner landscapes.

Barry Cohen and Anne Mills begin with a review of their studies of the tree drawings of suicidal and dissociative individuals, drawings that reveal swiftly and forcefully otherwise hidden body-self conditions (Chapter 9). How is it that the tree drawing can become such a useful mirror for this inarticulate self? Like the body-self, the tree has roots, a trunk, arms and a crown. Like the standing human being, the tree connects earth and sky and derives nourishment from both realms. The tree has bark, which, like skin, can become damaged or be bored into. Like the psyche, the tree grows and heals itself from deep inside its core. Even when it seems certainly and indubitably dead, the tree can burst into life again with returning spring. At the very impenetrable center of the tree is the heartwood; surrounding this are the tree's rings—its memory.

The tree is also like the mother's body, supplying protection, shade, nurturing fruit, rootedness and stability (Jung 1967). This identification with the body and with the mother's body reappears in myth and fairy tales. Daphne chooses to become a tree rather than succumb to Apollo's sexual pursuit; the princess in the Indian tale discussed in Chapter 13 also learns to transform herself into a tree. Many other fairy-tale princesses take refuge in tree branches in otherwise dark and fearsome forests. In the Grimms' tale "Thousandfurs," the princess, disguised in furs and fleeing her incestuous father, crawls inside a tree for shelter, using it as a kind of substitute skin. We will return to this ancient story about sexual abuse later when we discuss magical garments.

Cohen and Mills also discuss the drawing paper itself as a signifier of skin or "skin ego" and the ways in which both childhood assaults on the skin and recent self-mutilative attacks can be represented and reenacted using drawing paper. Writing paper, too, can serve this function. Kafka (1911/1976) described a "yearning to write all my anxiety entirely out of me, write it into the depths of the paper just as it comes of the depths of me, write it down in such a way that I could draw what I had written back into me completely." A sexual-abuse survivor who took up papermaking as a hobby used every step in the process to repair functions of the skin ego. The mashing and pressing of the pulp came to signify protectively crushing her abusers into liquefaction; the reek of the preparation helped her remember the rottenness of her childhood environment. The color, texture, luminescence and shape of each sheet as well as the message conveyed were carefully tailored to the intended recipient, as if a patch for that person's skin.

The idea of patches for damaged ego skin also comes up when patients make collages in which images of happy families or strong and beautiful bodies are mixed with images of horror, with carefully overlapped margins so as to leave no gaps. One is reminded of Frida Kahlo, physically shattered by polio and a terrible bus accident, who used collage to decorate the corsets that held together her "body in many pieces." Like emotionally shattered patients, she used collage as a mode of self-repair.

These images are patches, but they are also multifaceted mirrors. What we are searching for is a good mirror, a just mirror, one that will reflect every aspect of the self—the pain, despair, sexuality, excitement, the undistorted goodness and the eagerness to love. Journals of writings and drawings often become such a mirror, a mirror that can grow and change. Bad mirrors, like those in Hans Christian Andersen's "The Snow Queen," are a frequent legacy of childhood deprivation and chaos. Such a mirror "enlarges whatever is ugly and shrinks almost to nothing whatever is good and beautiful" (La Belle 1988, 37). Growing up with such a mirror has consequences. Partners may be chosen who continue to mirror and reinforce the familiar bad self-image. Positive feedback becomes easy to discount: "If they only knew the real me ... " The quest for a better mirror for one's sexuality, in sexual abuse one of the most wounded aspects of the body image, may turn into compulsive promiscuity or exhibitionism, always in the end reflecting the original negative image.

Such bad mirroring has its origins in the externalizations that emotionally damaged parents displace onto children. As in "Snow White," the mother splits off her own helplessness and need for connection and imagines these exist only in the child. Thus when she looks into her mirror, she sees only the omnipotent queen, untouched by such vulnerabilities. It is only when the child becomes able to see that this monstrous, distorted image, the ugly witch, is part of the other, not of herself, that she can escape it and begin to become acquainted with her own real body and its useful sensory equipment, which can then provide in an ongoing way more accurate views of herself, others and the rest of the world.

Chapters 10 and 11 take us into this world of the fun-house mirror. We describe one group of patients who look into the mirror and see pain and disease that doctors cannot locate in the body; a second group of patients look into the mirror and see either nothing—no body to worry about or attend to—or an invulnerable body, which likewise requires no nurture or care. Kluft describes dissociative patients who look into the mirror and see a panoply of characters, each of whom figures in a restitutive fantasy about how the trauma could have been prevented, muted or healed. Kluft's longest case also involves the use of clothing as a marker for transformation and growth.

This brings us back to the magical garments in fairy tales and the story of "Thousandfurs." Much of that heroine's weaponry in defense against her father's incestuous propositions involves her wardrobe. She asks for three dresses—as beautiful as the sun, the moon and the stars—and then for a coat made from the fur of a thousand animals. Ultimately, she will fit all three dresses into a nutshell and use the fur to disguise herself as an unknown beast for her escape into the forest. We understand now why the dresses fit into such a tiny container—the body image lives in the imagination and is therefore supremely portable, but it does need to be held within an intact boundary, the nutshell, which can preserve the good body image against traumatic damage. We also understand that the thousand furs signify the thousand pieces into which the body image can be shattered by trauma. The princess also takes with her tiny golden charms—a ring, a wheel and a spindle—which will end up in her true love's soup, an indicator perhaps that they represent internal qualities that might appropriately be swallowed and belong inside the body. Again, these self aspects are represented as golden and thus uncontaminated, as completed circles and thus intact. It is important to the story that the prince is sensitive enough to recognize and attend to these minute, golden ornaments in the midst of the princess's vociferous and insistent posttraumatic career as a blackened beast. His capacity to appreciate not only her gorgeous dresses, but also these delicate inside treasures qualifies him as an adequate mirror, the kind of mirror we strive to become as therapists.

Great art is the ultimate mirror, reflecting the totality of the human condition, including those elements that history may not choose to record. Even when science loses track of the body in the ebb and flow of its latest preoccupations, art will always find it again. "Art," said Kafka (1976, 134), "is a way to dazzle with the truth." Psychotherapy can sometimes dazzle too, when it achieves that perfect mirroring that brings hidden but long-known facts to the white heat of reality.

What amazed us as we began to explore Kafka (Chapter 12) is that he seemed to have mapped, in the absence of therapy, this entire metaphorical landscape—trees, mirrors, beasts and all. Kafka tells us about houses whose hidden staircases climb to secret rooms inhabited by mirror-image doubles we never imagined existed. There is a fearlessness in the way Kafka did not flee from these images but, as Alice Miller says, "thought them through to their bitter end." Another child-abuse victim, Virginia Woolf, saw in dreams a beast looking back at her from the mirror (La Belle 1988, 69) and wrote a novel from the viewpoint of a dog (*All That Summer She Was Mad*).

Kafka is most eloquently the poet laureate of the body as beast, reminding us that all the beasts in fairy tales are at some level the body's proxies. This is the beast-body we imagine we could escape from or trick or live without. Sometimes, like Beauty in "Beauty and the Beast," we order it to go somewhere else to eat and do all the other "disgusting" things it does. When we glimpse the beast in the mirror, we imagine it is somehow other than our self and that we do not have to keep the promises we have made to it. Much of adolescent development hinges on the recognition of the princely powers, passions and delights contained within the castle-body of this beast. Those who reject the beast, as did the Samsa family and Beauty's father, end up living in a world that must always feel impoverished and diminished to anyone who has glimpsed the vast dimensions of the beast's castle, which provides height and breadth and depth enough for real transcendence and transformation to take place.

REFERENCES

Becker, E. (1973). *The denial of death*. New York: Free Press.

Jung, C. G. (1967/1976). The philosophical tree. In *Collected works of C. G. Jung. Alchemical studies*. Trans. R. F. C. Hull. Bollingen Series 20. Vol. 13 (pp. 251–341). Princeton, N.J.: Princeton University Press.

Kafka, F. (1976). *The diaries: 1910–1923*. Ed. M. Brod. New York: Schocken Press.

La Belle, J. (1988). *Herself beheld: The literature of the looking glass*. Ithaca, N.Y. and London: Cornell University Press.

Pavic, M. (1990). *Landscape painted with tea*. Trans. Christina Pribicevic-Zoric. New York: Knopf.

Rako, S., and Mazer, H. (1983). *Semrad: The heart of a therapist*. New York: Aronson.

Savinio, A. (1988). *Operatic lives*. Marlboro, Vt.: The Marlboro Press.

Scott, R. D. (1951). The psychology of body image. *British Journal of Medical Psychiatry* 24: 254–266.

Tournier M. (1972). *The ogre*. New York: Pantheon.

CHAPTER 9

Skin/Paper/Bark

*Body Image, Trauma and
the Diagnostic Drawing Series*

Barry M. Cohen and Anne Mills

Therefore the tree is the image of our condition.

Andreas Alciatus, 1538

According to artist Paul Klee, "Art does not render what is visible; it renders visible." Although he was not referring to the use of drawings in psychological assessment, Klee's comment is nonetheless apt in a clinical context. For the severely traumatized dissociative client, making art to communicate thoughts, experiences and self-perceptions is not only functionally beneficial, but cognitively necessary. This is because traumatic experiences are so disruptive that they are unlikely to be transferred to memory in lexical terms (Horowitz 1970) and must be stored as sensory or iconic schemas. Such schemas are typically inflexible and remain unavailable to the adult client in verbal therapy. For this reason, art provides a schema-based process by which severely traumatized clients can render these inner experiences visible isomorphically (Cohen 1996).

Isomorphism is the central concept in the psychology of art and the expressive arts therapies. It refers to the similarity in structure between a person's internal state and its outward expression (Arnheim 1974). Isomorphism allows clients to externalize deeply personal experiences or sensations through the strategies and styles in their art, conveyed by lines, shapes and colors (Cohen and Cox 1995). It is isomorphism as well that allows therapist-viewers to assume they can develop useful hypotheses regarding the mind state of those clients from the clients' artwork.

Cohen (1996) has elsewhere described in detail the similarities between the qualities inherent in the visual arts and those that characterize dissociative reality. Briefly, these include bisociation (pairing or associating incompatible elements), plasticity (malleability of form, time and space) and multileveledness (several distinct levels of meaning can be apprehended in a single work of art, with no hierarchy of importance among these levels). Because these elements are found in both the creative process and the phenomenon of dissociation, dissociative clients can communicate their reality well using visual art, in some cases better than in any other modality, including talking. This helps explain why images by highly dissociative clients are often visually compelling, therapeutically invaluable and diagnostically informative.

ART, DISTORTED BODY IMAGE AND SELF-HARM

For psychotherapy to be complete and successful for individuals with posttraumatic disorders, it is necessary to investigate body image. The goal of this aspect of treatment is to have clients feel that they live in their bodies, exercise some authority over them and yet are dependent on them. "To live in a body and to see it as essential to one's identity, is, for the trauma survivor, both dangerous and crazy. On the other hand, to deny the body and its centrality to both personal and social identity is to deny oneself the rights, substance, and 'location' of personhood" (Young 1992, 95).

There are many obstacles to talking about body image. When clients believe there is something deeply wrong with their body, they might also need to defend against this belief by dissociating (the mind is *me*, the body is *not-me*). They may repress knowledge of bodily phenomena, especially in the therapist's presence. Or they may rationalize that the topic does not need to be raised, since they believe what is wrong with their body would be apparent to anyone who sees them. They may also avoid the subject due to shame or fear.

Art is an excellent means to evaluate distorted body image. Drawings, paintings and sculpture made in art therapy can reveal distorted body image and introduce it into the therapeutic conversation in a way that clients can tolerate.

It is theorized that childhood experiences of sexual abuse, physical neglect or repeated, intrusive medical procedures are linked to disruption in the development of normal body image. This disruption translates into distortions in body image and, isomorphically, into distortions in art imagery.

Art reveals body-image problems in the same way that projections show psychological disturbance. In both cases, the amount of fragmentation and distortion has a direct relationship to the degree of disorder and often to the severity of the trauma (Mills and Cohen, in press).

Distorted body image may also be profitably discussed in connection with chronic, low-lethality self-harm. Like certain imagery and structure in the art-making process, it is an observable manifestation of the distorted body image. Theory and clinical observation suggest that distorted body image is a necessary precondition for the syndrome of deliberate self-harm (Pattison and Kahan 1983).

Very briefly, self-harm is in part an attempt to find satisfactory solutions to dilemmas that are often body-based (for example, derealization, depersonalization, bodily fusion or misattributing body agency or ownership). This includes the self-harm that can occur when using the body in aesthetic enactments that publicly explore questions of violence, ritual, gender or privacy (as in the work of artists Gina Pane, Vito Acconci or Chris Burden). Self-injury may also result from attempts at self-care, for example, seeking the kind of calm found in the physiological response to pain or pursuing erotic pleasure that is associated with pain (Kafka 1969; Pao 1969; van der Kolk 1996).

The practice of chronic, low-lethality, direct self-harm, such as cutting, is usually concealed by the client. Yet at the same time there is internal pressure to reveal it. Displaying this activity and ideation to the therapist through art maintains an appropriate boundary, yet garners the caring witness's gaze.

Certain types of self-harm seem to be expressed frequently in therapeutic art. Skin-related self-injury images, such as those of the opening of wounds or, to a lesser degree, of burning or biting, are relatively common. The depiction of blood is highly valued; blood seems to signify life, death, pain and abuse simultaneously. Forms of chronic self-harm not directly related to skin (head banging, overdosing, harmful regimens) appear rarely. It is not clear, however, whether wound imagery correlates with the artist's actual behaviors or simply his or her impulses or fantasies.

Whereas a psychologically healthy person can be seen as "subject" (self) in relationship to "objects" (others), the object of the self-mutilating subject is the self. That is, persons objectify themselves by acting out on themselves, just as perpetrators of abuse transform their victim from a person into a thing at the

moment of abuse (Spiegel 1991). For self-mutilators, one of the inherently curative aspects of using art is that it provides them with a concrete external object that can stand in for themselves. "What is seen as self-abuse by others . . .
is not experienced as self-abuse by many trauma survivors. . . . Their abuse is
heaped on the same hated 'other' (their bodies, which are not them) as was
the abuse of their tormentors" (Young 1992, 98–99).

The drawing page is, however, neutral. It is passively receptive, containing and nonretaliatory, yet open to projections of all sorts by the maker. It is
an ideal toward which many analysts strive.

Skin and Paper

Why is skin frequently the site of the self-injuries we see in therapeutic art?
Skin is our largest organ, one that has become softer and less hirsute through
evolution. It is our largest physical boundary, distinguishing the *me* from the
not-me, and contains autoimmune defenses. Its hues, textures and smells have
social value and can show membership in a group. Skin senses both inwardly
as well as outwardly, participating in both subjective and objective reality.
Skin has pockets and cavities where sense organs of taste, smell, hearing and
vision are located. The sense of touch is, of course, located in skin. Skin can
even speak—by blushing (shame) and exhibiting gooseflesh (fear).

In trying to depict the things they see, artists engage in a kind of rapprochement with surfaces, volumes and colors—sometimes detached, other
times merging (Milner 1950/1981). They are exploring the space between
themselves and the object (or the Other—as in Winnicott's potential space).
This oscillation is interior, imaginative and normal (Rose 1963). Any art
medium can promote this kind of projecting and incorporating relationship.
However, a discussion of how this process is the same or different from art
making in art therapy by dissociative identity disorder (DID) clients is beyond the scope of this chapter.

The rapprochement described above is readily observable in the art-making
process among individuals who self-harm.[1] They bring their faces close to the
paper's surface, gazing at it with fixed attention. Here we emphasize the
clients' eyes or visual acuity, but it is possible to speculate that a primitive fusion of face/hand/breast also participates in tasting the paper (Pao 1969; Rose
1963). Otherwise unremarkable actions, such as layering chalk, rubbing it
around or into the paper or applying it with heavy pressure, seem to become
an intensely personal way of addressing—even relating to—the paper (Mills

1989; Schaverien 1995). Similarities to both masturbation and chronic low-lethality self-harm (potentially compulsive and rhythmic, exclusionary, self-soothing and invested with affect) are many. It has been observed that the surface of paper and other art media may symbolically take the place of skin (Biven 1982; Fuller 1980; Joron 1992; Rose 1963).

THE SKIN EGO

The skin ego is a two-layered container that encloses a person's psyche and soma (Anzieu 1989). Just as the skin holds the contents of the physical body in its "bag," the skin ego houses all manner of psychic data within its "envelope." Thus, at a basic level, the skin ego provides psychic and somatic shelter. Anzieu cited at least eight different functions of the skin ego.

The flexible outer layer of the skin ego (projective/subjective) is comprised of an identity-defining "cloak" filled with messages from the parents and immediate environment. The more rigid inner layer of the skin ego (protective/objective) transmits messages to and receives them from the outside world. When communication occurs between the two layers of the skin ego, the ego perceives itself as a unique entity, capable of sending out signals that others can receive.

Skin ego thus fostered can confer a sense of boundaried individuality and take on holding and containing functions previously nonexistent or under-developed due to compromised early sensations and relationships. Eventually, normal development of skin ego leads to a consolidated and accurate body image. Basic cognitive skills and capacities that are dependent on an accurate body image can then be developed.

Although pain, like pleasure, can be eroticized, pain can disorganize thinking and cause the sufferer to feel profoundly alone. Lasting pain can even destroy the notion of *me-ness*, as it obliterates both the inner and outer faces and functions of the skin ego. Like paper or canvas, the skin ego, when poked, registers a mark—whether from a broken epidermis, a broken heart or a broken boundary. Those markings create a map of a person's posttraumatic lifestyle and can be isomorphically externalized in therapeutic art.

THE TREE SYMBOL

Trees, like people, are biological entities that thrive or decline according to the quality of nurturance and sustenance they receive. They are also like people in the way their physical structure corresponds to the human body: the skin/bark, the torso/trunk, the arms/limbs, and the crown/head. Additionally, trees have roots that grow down into the soil, suggesting the unseen, hidden and unknown—qualities that are typically associated with the psyche.

In the following quotation, trees are being described, but the words also fit the dysfunctional alter-centric system of the client with DID:

> Everything happens at the periphery, is formed under the bark and at the ends of the axes of the shoots. . . . The being of a plant therefore means . . . a striving away of the zones of growth from the core, this functionless, more symbolic center. . . . A plant . . . is young to the end; up to its natural death it forms buds which may come to fruition according to circumstances. (Hiltbrunner, cited in Koch 1952)

Some clients with DID who have witnessed so much inhumane behavior in humans say that they despise people and reject their own humanity. Rather, they say they prefer to identify with innocent wild animals, trees and nature. Many DID clients consciously choose to represent themselves as trees in drawings. Describing her tree picture, one art-therapy client stated, "I just took the tree as the body. The tree is the physical body and the leaves are the selves" (Cohen and Cox 1988).

Since the beginning of time, all cultures have embraced the image of the tree as a vital and multivalent symbol (Cirlot 1962; Jung 1967). Trees are one of the first recognizable schemas drawn by children, and they resemble the armless human figure, which is a developmental milestone in children striving to draw people naturalistically (Kellogg 1970). Trees are thus believed to be less threatening for adults to draw than the human figure. Deep or forbidden feelings can be projected onto tree images with little fear of revealing them to others (Hammer 1958). Because a tree shows the history of its growth through its shape and size, the image of an erect tree is thought to be similar to the profile of a standing person and is typically employed as a symbol of self (Jung 1967).

Trees, surpassed only by the human figure, have been the preferred projective drawing theme of psychologists. Despite the continued interest in tree drawings in the literature of projective testing (Bolander 1977; Buck 1948; Hammer 1958), research on tree drawings in clinical assessment has shown poor reliability and validity, and reductive interpretations based on single signs have been misleading. For example, the notion that the height of a knothole on a tree trunk correlates with the age of the client at the onset of trauma remains unsubstantiated.

Given that the tree symbol invites multivalent projections regarding the *me*, we are taking a special look at the tree drawings in the Diagnostic Drawing Series of severely traumatized women with the diagnosis of DID.

THE DIAGNOSTIC DRAWING SERIES

The Diagnostic Drawing Series (DDS) is a standardized art interview developed by Cohen (Cohen, Mills and Kijak 1994). It combines the attention to materials, task and process from the practice of art therapy with the research methodology of the social sciences (Cohen, Hammer and Singer 1988). The series was first introduced in the United States in 1982 and has been studied collaboratively in an international project since then. *DSM* diagnostic information is collected at the same time as the clients' series. The validity and reliability of the DDS rating guide and findings have been tested (Mills, Cohen and Meneses 1993).

The series is made with a twelve-color pack of square, soft chalk pastels (Alphacolor, a widely available brand, is most typically used). DDSs are drawn on 18-by-24-inch, 70-pound white drawing paper that—like skin— has a slight texture. Because the DDS is a standardized tool, no other drawing materials or paper of any other color or size may be substituted. Complete directions for administering the DDS are described in the *DDS Handbook* (Cohen 1985).

There are three pictures in a series, each with its own piece of paper and specific directions. The pictures must be made in the order specified below, and the directions must be given as written. Other than giving the directions, the therapist/administrator is discouraged from talking to the client while the series is being drawn.

The first picture is the unstructured task of the series, often referred to as the free picture. Clients are instructed, "Make a picture using these materials" (the chalk and paper). In what results we typically see manifestations of clients' defenses.

The directions for the second picture are: "Draw a picture of a tree." The tree picture is thus the structured task of the series, and it links the DDS with the house-tree-person technique (Buck 1948), Koch's Tree Test (1952) and the work of Bolander (1977).

The third picture is referred to as the feeling picture because its instructions are: "Make a picture of how you're feeling, using lines, shapes and colors." It is a semistructured task that invites clients to communicate about their affective state directly and to represent it in abstract form.

Each of the three pictures in the series is rated on a Drawing Analysis Form (Cohen 1985) for the presence of a total of thirty-six elements from twenty-three categories. These criteria, defined in a Rating Guide (Cohen 1994), lead the rater toward empirical, objective data rather than solely an intuitive response or reaction to the symbolic content alone.

Some of the structural elements identified in the Drawing Analysis Form include the use of line and shape, number of colors employed, number of images drawn, presence of enclosure or groundline, depiction of movement and space usage. Each diagnostic group of patients has a distinct graphic profile comprised of clusters of these sorts of aspects of the samples' artwork. This makes it possible to compare the art of various diagnostic groups with each other, and the graphic profile of a DDS can therefore be said to be predicative of its maker's psychiatric diagnosis. A number of studies have been published that delineate these distinguishing patterns (Cohen, Hammer and Singer 1988; Couch 1994; Kessler 1994).

TREE DRAWINGS OF INDIVIDUALS DIAGNOSED WITH DID

Patients diagnosed with DID in particular show remarkable commonalities in their spontaneous art expression (Cohen and Cox 1995) and in their DDSs (Kress 1991; Mills and Cohen 1993; Morris 1995). Striking similarities between the DDSs of patients diagnosed with DID in the United States and in Holland have also been shown (Cohen and Heijtmajer 1995; Heijtmajer and Cohen 1993).

The tree drawings in the DDS reflect much the same psychopathology reported by other investigators. Moreover, Sobol and Cox (see Cohen et al. 1991), in their preliminary exploration of the Child Diagnostic Drawing Series sample of latency-age children with documented histories of abuse, found the same graphic indicators as did Mills and Cohen (1993) and Cohen and Cox (1995) in the artwork of adults with severe dissociative disorders. The graphic profiles of the tree drawings often feature what Sobol and Cox call "confabulated trees" that are virtually identical (allowing for developmental differences) to ones in the adult DID sample.

If tree pictures in the DDS of women diagnosed with DID symbolize their makers' body images, one would expect to see characteristic behavioral and psychological symptomatology manifested isomorphically in graphic form. This does occur to a striking degree. In fact, we have identified ten ways that tree pictures seem to reflect body-image psychopathology:

A. Disintegrated
   1. Falling-apart trees
B. Wounded or destroyed
   2. Scarred bark
   3. Dead tree
C. Contaminated
   4. Creature within trunk holes
   5. Blood in the tree
D. Out of control
   6. Chaotic branch system
E. Strange
   7. Upside-down tree
   8. Bizarre tree
   9. Unrecognizable tree
   10. Anthropomorphic tree

Body-image disintegration is depicted in the tree drawings of DID DDSs as falling apart (Mills and Cohen 1993) or (less frequently) cut into many pieces. A tree is called falling apart when its primary branches are not connected to the trunk or when its secondary branches are not connected to its primary branches (Cohen 1994). Not only does this graphic phenomenon relate to the disconnection of behaviors, affects, sensations and cognitions in the dissociative client (Braun 1988), but it also refers to disowned or offending body parts (castration imagery). Examples of fragmentation images in the artwork of DID clients have also been discussed elsewhere (Cohen and Cox 1995). (See figures 9.1 and 9.2.)

Bark is the protective, yet vulnerable, skin of a tree. Drawing bark textures on trees—emphasizing the skin—offers self-harming clients a way to silently acknowledge unacceptable acting-out behavior and its bodily consequences. Scarring imagery, including cuts, scratches, gouges and burns, is often found on the trunks of trees in the DDSs of traumatized, dissociative clients. Such graphic markings can also serve to externalize feelings of shame and symbolically represent the artists' wounded body images (see figure 9.2).

Rankin studied trauma markings in the DDS tree drawings of a nonhospitalized control group and inpatients on a posttraumatic and dissociative disorders unit. Although both groups were equally likely to draw trees with knotholes in them, she noted that the inpatient group was more likely to draw trees with *multiple* indicators, such as a damaged trunk plus one or more wounds or knotholes (Rankin 1994).

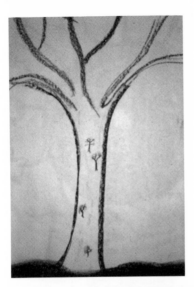

Figure 9.1 *(left)* Falling-apart branch system. (All drawings made with chalk pastels on 18-x-24-inch white paper.) Photo: T. Kress Marks.

Figure 9.2 *(below)* Falling-apart branch system; multiple scars in trunk. Photo: S. Des Marais.

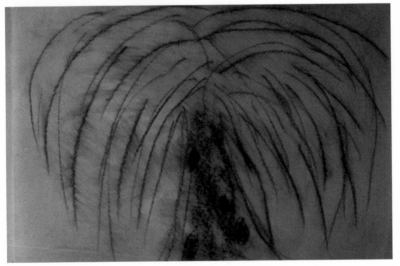

When clients perceive their core self to be dead as a result of overwhelming early trauma, the trunk is depicted either as broken at its base or dead. These tree drawings symbolize a destroyed body image. Cohen and Cox (1995) have called such examples "alert pictures," in that they are frequently drawn by clients to apprise therapists of the clients' trauma history or their posttraumatic, dissociative symptomatology (see figure 9.3).

Other types of "alert" imagery seen in the DDS tree pictures of clients with DID are those that focus on toxicity. These drawings allude to or illustrate a

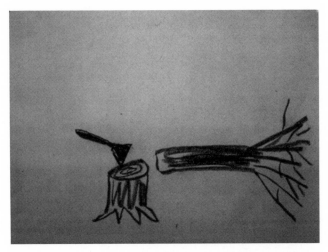

Figure 9.3 Tree chopped down at base. Photo: C. T. Cox.

sense of contamination and include such benign details as holes in the trunk (figure 9.4) in which small beings live (rather than depicting them in nests or among the branches). Blood in the tree (Kress 1991) is another, more extreme indicator of contamination not seen in the DDS tree drawings of any other population (see figure 9.5).[2]

Clients' belief that their body is out of control is symbolized in trees with crowns comprised of a chaotic mass of branches, typically drawn in a wildly scribbled manner. Spontaneous drawings by these patients may have characteristics similar to these tree pictures; they are called "chaos pictures" (Cohen and Cox 1995).

Sometimes the crowns and root systems of trees in these DDSs are similarly or ambiguously drawn, making the tree images equally viable when viewed upside down or right side up; this may reflect the client's propensity for depersonalization (figure 9.6). Another more severe manifestation of this type of distorted body image features pictures drawn in such a way that renders them unrecognizable as trees (see figures 9.7 and 9.8).

Perhaps no type of tree drawing in the DDS is more indicative of a particular population than the anthropomorphic tree in the graphic profile of the DID sample. Only in DID have we seen this phenomenon in which the tree and human body images are so intermingled/fused (Heijtmajer and Cohen 1993; Kress 1991; Mills and Cohen 1993). Anthropomorphic tree drawings have also been seen in the Dutch DID sample of DDS. These representations of strange body images also function as "alert pictures," signaling the client's difficulties through these startling, hallmark images (see figures 9.9 and 9.10).

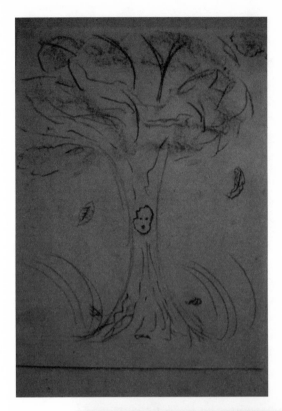

Figure 9.4 Falling apart branch system; creature inside hole in tree.

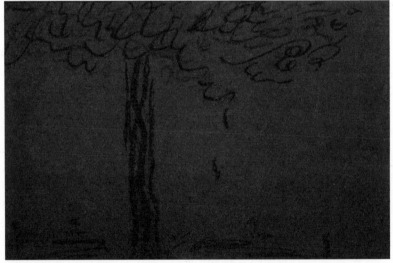

Figure 9.5 Red drawn in trunk described by client as "blood."
Photo: T. Kress Marks.

Figure 9.6 Upside-down tree.
Photo: M. M. Barnes.

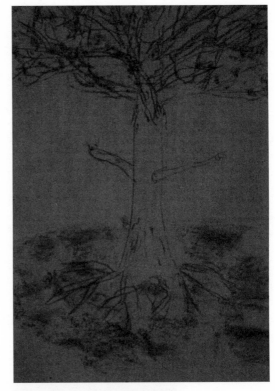

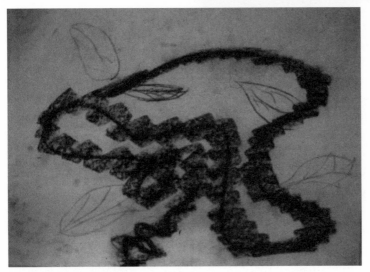

Figure 9.7 Image is unrecognizable as a tree.
Photo: T. Kress Marks.

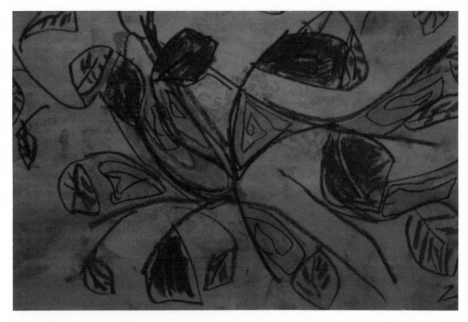

Figure 9.8 Unrecognizable image drawn in pale blue, which is unnatural for a tree. Photo: S. Des Marais.

TREATMENT IMPLICATIONS

The tree picture in the DDS is an excellent repository for body-image projections, and the art therapist can look there to assess the client's sense of contamination, wounding or distortion. Transforming such perceptions by patching fragmented pieces together or layering over gaps in "skins" are some of the ways that healing begins through art therapy. This process can continue until the client's body feels whole and owned, thanks to the ever renewable skin of art materials.

Since the inner layer of the skin ego retains traumatically engraved material in visually encoded form, art making is the ideal modality to help traumatized, dissociative clients communicate about their inner lives with the world outside. This is why these clients use art materials so effectively to externalize a lifetime of internalized messages and self-perceptions. Eventually, rigidified traumatic memory can be transformed into flexible narrative memory, facilitated by verbal and expressive therapies (Cohen 1996; van der Kolk and van der Hart 1991). In other words, somatic and cognitive distortions resulting from early trauma can be undone through the expressive use of art materials.

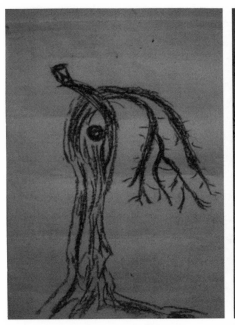

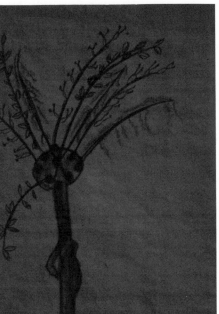

Figure 9.9 Anthropomorphic tree drawn by a client from the United States with DID. Photo: T. Kress Marks.

Figure 9.10 Anthropomorhpoic tree drawn by a client from The Netherlands with DID. Photo: O. Heijtmajer.

The tree symbol heightens the drawing paper's potential to transform the compromised or contaminated skin ego, since an infinite variety of tree images can be drawn and an infinite number of tree drawings can be generated throughout the process of therapy.

DISCUSSION

Body-image distortions, tree drawings and deliberate self-harm are all multiply determined, particular and varied. None can be described accurately by a single continuum ranging from mild to severe. This chapter has described aspects of tree drawings from the DDS by women with DID. However, similar themes and images are also found in the tree drawings of some women who have histories of childhood sexual abuse and elevated levels of dissociativity, but who do not qualify for a diagnosis of DID. The syndrome of deliberate self-harm seems to be present in some of the women who draw these images, but we do not have complete data on this. Further, a significant portion of DID clients make DDS tree drawings without projections of historical trauma (Rankin 1994).

Art therapists can now deduce distorted body image from tree drawings of the types described here. We have also achieved a high degree of accuracy in using the DDS to distinguish dissociators from nondissociators (Cohen and Heijtmajer 1995). There have been relatively few false positives, that is, finding such drawings without corresponding psychological difficulties. We think that factors in the remaining two DDS drawings in the series will bring to our attention the clients who, based on their tree drawings alone, might otherwise be false negatives.

We cannot at this time, however, accurately separate such factors as the dosage effect of trauma, increased dissociativity, distorted body image and deliberate self-harm through the analysis of drawings. The relevant pictorial indicators most likely overlap or intermingle. Future research will need to examine, for instance, the DDS drawings of those whose self-mutilation (and hypothesized distorted body image) finds its etiology in mental retardation or psychosis.

CONCLUSION

Clients with histories of severe, early and prolonged trauma often develop body-image problems of various sorts. Because art is a natural mode enabling them to isomorphically express their multileveled inner worlds, it is the medium of choice—perhaps more than hypnosis—for externalizing their perceptions and concerns and accessing material that has been visually encoded.

Tree drawings are often found among the spontaneous artwork made by clients with DID. The task of drawing a tree is also given as part of an assessment by therapists who use the Diagnostic Drawing Series. After viewing thousands of DDSs, we are certain that the trees drawn by clients with DID are the most unique and recognizable of any single diagnostic population. Although no one should ever be diagnosed on the basis of any single drawing, many of the trees drawn by people diagnosed with DID that we have seen in fifteen years of clinical use of the DDS were, alone, diagnostically significant.

Tree drawings are an excellent starting point for gentle confrontation of distorted body images. They externalize imagery from within clients' psyches in ways that are otherwise impossible for the clients to communicate. As the art-therapy client we quoted earlier stated about her DDS tree picture, "Intuitively, I knew it [the tree trunk] was 'the body' because it has roots. Because it is solid, it can't change, so I couldn't be the tree [trunk]. None of us could—only 'the body.' The alters have to be the leaves because they are changeable. . . . I don't think my body holds much of a physical image—and that tree could change—*a lot*" (Cohen and Cox 1988).

NOTES

1. This similar behavior is observed in seemingly dissimilar individuals: a profoundly retarded, mute male with a seizure disorder and chronic direct, moderate-lethality self-harm; a teenage male in his first psychotic break, with one episode of low-lethality self-mutilation; and a high functioning female chronic self-injurer with several Axis II diagnoses.

2. Anzieu alludes to an extraordinary form of contamination of self by briefly mentioning the "poisoned tunic" skin ego (1989, 62). The possibility that one could become psychologically allergic to oneself is an intriguing rationale for the development of multiple dissociated identities by the severely traumatized child. The first author (B.M.C.) has found that teaching the concepts of skin ego and the poisoned tunic helps clients in the middle stage of treatment to better understand the possible origin of their disregard for and antipathy toward their bodies.

REFERENCES

Anzieu, D. (1989). *The skin ego.* New Haven, CT: Yale University Press.

Arnheim, R. (1974). *Art and visual perception: A psychology of the creative eye.* 2d ed. Berkeley and Los Angeles: University of California Press.

Biven, B. M. (1982). The role of skin in normal and abnormal development with a note on the poet Sylvia Plath. *International Review of Psycho-Analysis* 9: 205–229.

Bolander, K. (1977). *Assessing personality through tree drawings.* New York: Basic Books.

Braun, B. G. (1988). The BASK model of dissociation. *Dissociation* 1 (1): 4–23.

Buck, J. N. (1948). The H-T-P test. *Journal of Clinical Psychology* 4: 151–159.

Cirlot, J. E. (1962). *A dictionary of symbols.* New York: Philosophical Library.

Cohen, B. M. (1996). Art and the dissociative paracosm: Uncommon realities. In L. Michaelson and W. Ray, eds., *Handbook of dissociation: Theoretical, empirical and clinical perspectives.* New York: Plenum.

Cohen, B. M., ed. (1985). *The diagnostic drawing series handbook.* (Available from Barry M. Cohen, P.O. Box 9853, Alexandria, Virginia 22304).

———. (1994). The diagnostic drawing series revised rating guide. (Available from B. M. Cohen, P. O. Box 9853, Alexandria, VA 22304).

Cohen, B. M., and Cox, C. T. (1988). Breaking the code: Identification of multiple personality disorder through art productions. 19th Annual Conference of the American Art Therapy Association, Chicago, November 19.

_____. (1995). *Telling without talking: Art as a window into the world of multiple personality*. New York: Norton.

Cohen, B. M., Hammer, J. S., and Singer, S. (1988). The diagnostic drawing series: A systematic approach to art therapy evaluation and research. *The Arts in Psychotherapy* 15 (1): 11–21.

Cohen, B. M., and Heijtmajer, O. A. (1995). The Diagnostic Drawing Series and multiple personality disorder in the Netherlands: Further investigations. Paper given at the 12th International Conference on Multiple Personality and Dissociative States, Chicago, October 15.

Cohen, B. M., Mills, A., and Kijak, A. K. (1994). An introduction to the Diagnostic Drawing Series: A standardized tool for diagnostic and clinical use. *Art Therapy* 11 (2): 105–110.

Couch, J. B. (1994). Diagnostic Drawing Series: Research with older people diagnosed with organic mental syndrome and disorders. *Art Therapy* 11 (3): 111–115.

Fuller, P. (1980). *Art and psychoanalysis*. London: Writers and Readers Publishing Cooperative.

Hammer, E. F. (1958). The house-tree-person projective drawing technique: Content interpretation. In E. F. Hammer, ed., *The clinical application of projective drawings* (pp. 165–207). Springfield: Charles C. Thomas.

Heijtmajer, O. A., and Cohen, B. M. (1993). MPD and the Diagnostic Drawing Series: A Dutch replication study. Paper given at the 10th International Conference on Multiple Personality and Dissociative States, Chicago, October 15.

Horowitz, M. J. (1970). *Image formation and cognition*. New York: Appleton-Century-Crofts.

Joron, N. (1992). Personal communication to A. Mills, February 17.

Jung, C. G. (1967). The philosophical tree. In H. Read et al., *The collected works of C. G. Jung: Alchemical studies*. Bollingen Series 20. Vol. 13. Princeton, N.J.: Princeton University Press.

Kafka, J. S. (1969). The body as transitional object: A psychoanalytic study of a self-mutilating patient. *British Journal of Medical Psychology* 42: 207–212.

Kellogg, R. (1970). *Analyzing children's art*. Palo Alto, Calif.: Mayfield.

Kessler, K. (1994). A study of the Diagnostic Drawing Series with eating disordered patients. *Art Therapy* 11 (2): 116–118.

Koch, K. (1952). *The tree test: The tree-drawing test as an aid in psychodiagnosis*. 2d ed., Eng. trans. Berne: H. Huber.

Kress, T. (1991). A study of the content of drawings from the Diagnostic Drawing Series of patients with multiple personality disorder. Paper prepared for Graduate Program in Art Therapy, George Washington University.

Mills, A. (1989). A statistical study of the formal aspects of the Diagnostic Drawing Series of borderline personality disordered patients, and its context in contemporary art therapy. Master's thesis, Concordia University, Montreal.

_____. (1995). (Speaker). A practical review and integration of all Diagnostic Drawing Research findings (Cassette Recording No. 58–154). Denver, Col.: National Audio Video, Inc.

Mills, A., and Cohen, B. M. (1993). Facilitating the identification of multiple personality disorder through art: The Diagnostic Drawing Series. In E. Kluft, ed., *Expressive and functional therapies in the treatment of multiple personality disorder.* Springfield, Ill.: Charles C. Thomas.

_____. (in press). The Diagnostic Drawing Series and the trauma spectrum. In J. A. Turkus, ed., *Dissociative identity disorder: Continuum of care.* New York: Aronson.

Mills, A., Cohen, B. M., and Meneses, J. Z. (1993). Reliability and validity tests of the Diagnostic Drawing Series. *The Arts in Psychotherapy* 20 (1): 83–88.

Milner, M. (1981). *On not being able to paint.* London: Heinemann. (Original work published 1950.)

Morris, M. B. (1995). The Diagnostic Drawing Series and the tree rating scale: An isomorphic representation of multiple personality disorder, major depression, and schizophrenia populations. *Art Therapy* 12 (2): 118–128.

Pao, P.-N. (1969). The syndrome of delicate self-cutting. *British Journal of Medical Psychology* 42: 195–206.

Pattison, E. M., and Kahan, J. (1983). The deliberate self-harm syndrome. *American Journal of Psychiatry* 140 (7): 867–872.

Rankin, A. (1994). Tree drawings and trauma indicators: A comparison of past research with current findings from the Diagnostic Drawing Series. *Art Therapy* 11 (2): 127–130.

Rose, G. J. (1963). Body ego and creative imagination. *Journal of the American Psychoanalytic Association* 2: 756–789.

Schaverien, J. (1995). *Desire and the female therapist: Engendered gazes in psychotherapy and art therapy.* London: Routledge.

Spiegel, D. (Speaker). (1991). Dissociation during trauma: Borrowing from the future to pay for the past (Cassette Recording No. 1A–683–91). Alexandria, Va.: Audio Transcripts, Ltd.

Torem, M. S., Gilbertson, A., and Light, V. (1990). Indications of physical, sexual, and verbal victimization in projective tree drawings. *Journal of Clinical Psychology* 46: 900–906.

van der Kolk, B. A. (1996). The body keeps the score: Approaches to the psychobiology of posttraumatic stress disorder. In B. van der Kolk, A. McFarlane and L. Weisaeth, eds., *Traumatic stress: The effects of overwhelming experience on mind, body and society.* New York: Guilford.

van der Kolk, B. A., and van der Hart, O. (1991). The intrusive past: The inflexibility and the engraving of trauma. *American Imago* 48 (4): 425–454.

Young, L. (1992). Sexual abuse and the problem of embodiment. *Child Abuse and Neglect* 16 (1): 89–100.

CHAPTER 10

Traumatic Disruption of Bodily Experience and Memory

Jean Goodwin and Reina Attias

In this chapter we use clinical observations, and elements of trauma and attachment theory to propose a model for how body and memory problems arise simultaneously out of traumatic childhood events and develop together during later posttraumatic illness. Clinical observations from multiple contexts describe a population of patients who present both puzzling bodily symptoms and puzzling narratives of early childhood trauma. The clinical phenomenology of such cases has been described in the literature of "grand hysteria" (where generally the somatic symptoms bring the patient to treatment) and in more recent case studies of posttraumatic and dissociative disorders (in which a troubling trauma narrative brings the individual to treatment and somatic symptoms appear later, often during so-called abreactive crises, as traumatic memories are being reworked). Published case studies also point to temporal interconnections between exacerbation and amelioration of bodily and memory symptoms over the life history of a single individual (Goodwin 1996).

Reconstruction of the moment of childhood trauma, using trauma, attachment and object-relations theories, also reveals a convergence of somatic and memory problems. Both at the moment of attack and at the moment of ineffective protest, the child's physical and emotional pain can produce cognitive confusion and dissociation (see Chapter 3). When the pain and terror are complicated by dissociation, additional bizarre bodily experiences and further disruption of memory and narration may occur.

Using detailed clinical examples, we identify two patterns of intertwined somatic and memory disturbances. In both types, the individual's narrative of physical and emotional pain is characterized by gaps, distortions and minimizations. In Type I situations the pain sensation remains, but its meaning is lost. Type I patients sometimes construct a self-image around their pain and may frantically search for a medical diagnosis to ward off further knowledge of the actual traumatic origins of the pain. Complications include the patients' redefinition of pain or illness as a victory and the unconscious attempt to get help by involving others in their suffering (Novick and Novick 1996). In the Type II situation, the individual copes by stepping out of the body, leaving behind both the traumatic circumstance and the bodily container of physical and emotional pain. An imaginary or idealized body often is substituted in fantasy. Complications here result from the denial of the real body and include sensory loss, depersonalization, overwork, neglect of self-care tasks and accident-proneness.

CO-OCCURRENCE OF PROBLEMATIC BODILY
EXPERIENCE AND DISORGANIZED TRAUMA NARRATIVES:
HISTORY AND CLINICAL PHENOMENOLOGY

Charcot and Janet (Ellenberger 1970), at the end of the nineteenth century, published cases describing the bizarre multiple bodily symptoms they defined as "grand hysteria" and were able to identify similar cases in Inquisition records from previous centuries. In their own cases, the patients' fragmented narratives about childhood trauma were included almost as an afterthought. Charcot was much more interested in the pseudoneurological symptoms of his patient Louise than in her childhood history of emotional, physical and sexual abuse and witnessed violence (Goodwin 1989, 1993a). It was Charcot's student Sigmund Freud who gave weight in his theory of hysteria to what Charcot had mentioned in an aside as "the sexual thing." Today Louise would likely be diagnosed as having multiple conditions: somatization disorder, conversion disorder, posttraumatic stress disorder (PTSD), dissociative identity disorder (DID) and borderline or hysterical personality disorder.

Dissociation, as described a century ago by Janet and by contemporary nosologists (Bliss 1986; Braun 1988; van der Kolk and van der Hart 1989; American Psychiatric Association 1994), includes, by all definitions, simultaneous disturbances of body experience (notably depersonalization) and memory. Janet understood the frequent conversion symptoms observed in such patients as somatic dissociations; instead of walling off important personal information, as in psychogenic amnesia, they had walled off sensory or motor functions, producing somatic symptoms. A recently developed psychological instrument using only questions about somatic dissociation makes the diagnosis of DID with as good specificity and sensitivity as instruments that focus mostly on psychological dissociation (see Chapter 4). Those theorists who trace dissociative phenomena to trauma-induced autohypnosis (Bliss 1986; Volgyesi 1963; Cardeña and Spiegel 1996) point out that deep hypnosis of highly hypnotizable subjects is another context in which body symptoms and alterations in body sensation co-occur with amnesia and other memory distortions.

Other clinical descriptions of co-occurring somatic and memory disturbances are found in case reports describing narrative reconstruction of experiences. For example, marks of inflammation are described as appearing on the neck of a patient as she narrates a memory of being strangled (Goodwin and Sachs 1996), a patient vomits whenever she is questioned about her complaint of sadistic fellatio (Wright 1994), and a patient attempting to describe her parents' attempt to murder her when she was a preschooler loses her urine as she speaks (Adler 1995).

Connections between body symptoms and disturbed traumatic memory are also described in detailed case histories that track both types of symptoms over the entire life span of a patient (Shengold 1989; Terr 1990). Pediatric records often reveal (Goodwin 1982) that the onset of severe child abuse coincided with onset of chronic bodily symptoms (especially stomach and head pain, bedwetting and other bladder problems, pseudoseizures and eating disorders). In retrospect it is evident that bodily symptoms had emerged in lieu of a narrative complaint. Later, posttraumatic anxiety may appear for the first time in the context of an illness or injury, or episodic inexplicable bodily crises may accompany the psychological reworking of childhood trauma. Once therapeutic reworking is completed, inexplicable remission of chronic somatic symptoms can also be observed. Jeanne Fery, exorcized in 1588, is perhaps the earliest published case in which a somatic symptom is noted to disappear after the disclosure and working through of a traumatic memory; a chronic blindness in one eye resolved after she discussed for nine days her father's seduction of her and his beatings (van der Hart, Lierens and Goodwin 1996; Chapter 13, this volume).

There also exists a small literature in which traumatic memories and memory disturbances are described in patients with major somatoform disturbances not usually thought of as related to posttraumatic or dissociative disorders. These conditions include Briquet's syndrome (Chapter 3, this volume), eating disorders (Chapter 6, this volume), pseudoseizures (Goodwin, Bergman and Simm 1979; Goodwin 1993a), alexithymia (Sifneos 1973) and Munchausen's syndrome (Goodwin 1988).

Despite these numerous examples indicating the centrality of disrupted bodily experience in the natural history of posttraumatic disorders, somatic problems are understood by most psychotherapists as epiphenomena and may not be included in psychotherapeutic work (Ross 1995). Instead, the body problems of traumatized patients are dealt with in emergency rooms and medical offices, by the patients alone or by body therapists and other alternative health-care providers. Whether such interventions and noninterventions are successful or disintegrating in their impacts, without full integration of such moments of bodily crisis into the therapeutic work, there is an irretrievable loss of information and of opportunities for understanding and mastery.

SIMULTANEOUS ORIGIN OF BODILY SYMPTOMS AND MEMORY PROBLEMS: THEORETICAL RECONSTRUCTION OF THE TRAUMATIC EXPERIENCE AND ITS AFTERMATH

Attachment theory and trauma theory can help us construct a model for the child's traumatic experience based on behavioral studies of separation and stress in infant animals (Harlow and Harlow 1971; Suomi 1991) and humans (Spitz 1983; Bowlby 1994; Main 1993; Main and Morgan 1996). Additional building blocks for this model can be found in biochemical and brain-imaging studies of stressed animals and of human subjects with PTSD (van der Kolk 1994a, b). Object-relations theory (Winnicott 1965; Bowlby 1988, 1994; Fonagy and Target 1995), based on psychoanalytic case reports and on longitudinal studies of mother-infant dyads (Ainsworth et al. 1978; Stern 1985; Barach 1991; Fonagy, Steele and Target 1994), adds depth to elements of the model derived from animal and infant observation and neuropsychological understandings of limbic system functions. What we are seeking is a model that allows us to imaginatively reconstruct the trauma moment and its simultaneous impacts on memory and bodily experience in the developing child. This speculative modeling is important clinically in that it provides imagery and language for psychotherapeutic work at this inarticulate interface between psyche and soma.

We present the following synthetic model as a thinking tool for clinicians beginning to work with body symptoms, body image and body ego.

With her touch and gaze, the mother defines, maps, creates and in adversity restores the infant's image of his or her body and the body's goodness. At the moment of attack on the body, the pain cry comes out of the hurt body. Normally this cry summons the mother's restorative holding and mirroring, which enables the hurt child to reconstitute a self and a narrative around the real body. The healing reunion of shared psychic experience and bodily sensation restores autobiographical continuity and the intact "good enough" self (Winnicott 1965). When this sequence is disrupted and the attack moment merges into an abandonment moment, the emotional and physical pain in the body can become too intense to be contained or integrated. This overwhelming of the psyche by physical and emotional pain constitutes the psychoanalytic definition of trauma (Freud 1921). This traumatic pain becomes a "not-me" experience of franticness, upset and lostness in an objectless world (Grand and Alpert 1993; Shear 1996). The child is left in a chronic state of disembodiment or embodiment in a damaged, not-whole, fragmented, unhealed body. The terror, isolation and unimaginable loneliness of this condition produce the Type I and Type II dissociative responses that will be discussed in the next section.

The following is a sketch outlining the natural protest sequence (Ney 1987) as it might take place in the absence of traumatic disruptions.

THE NATURAL SEQUENCE

ASSAULT	PAIN	PROTEST	RESPONSE	RESTORED BODY/SELF
On body-self	Emotional/ Physical	"Help Me"	Mirroring/ "Hold Me"	"I'm OK"

In our view trauma can result at any step in this model. For example, some children will go into a traumatic freeze response at the time of the assault itself, before they become aware of pain. The pain itself can become overwhelming, as can the lack of response to the child's cry for help (Call 1984; Pearce and Pezzot-Pearce 1994). Mirroring can be traumatic if the child is mirrored as bad, ugly or defective following the attack. Some individuals become traumatically overwhelmed during the last stage, when dissociation is cleared away and they must face the realities of the assault and their actual physical and psychic injuries (see Chapter 8).

Like acute trauma-level anxiety, posttraumatic repetitions and identifications may form at each point in the model. In this chapter we examine in detail those patterns of alteration in self-image that condense around those steps in the model that most concern the body—the pain and the (incompletely or invulnerably) restored body-self; these are the situations most often associated with chronic somatic symptoms. However, all other steps in the model can act as centers for symptoms and personality distortion.

For some traumatized individuals, the experiential spotlight has become narrowly fixed on the attack moment. They experience themselves (and loved ones) as repeatedly under attack (or attacking). This theme—preventing, coping with and recovering from assaults—comes to define the treatment. Other patients seem dissociatively trapped in the moment of the protest cry; here treatment may become overfocused on coping with repeated self-mutilative "cries for help" that cannot be connected either backward to an attack moment or forward to restorative holding. Still other trauma sufferers seem to have barricaded themselves into a "holding" mode, for example, a woman with multiple childhood adversity who avoids work, snacks to a level of superobesity, stays in bed and reads romance novels, all of which is never enough to produce an experience of restorative connection with the body-self or with other people.

In each of these situations the therapeutic tasks are to translate the symptom syndrome into the emotional and relational terms of the natural sequence and to expand the focus, so the symptomatic mode can be understood in the context of what came before and what is desired as a next step. Crucial to expanding this frame is the reconstruction of a trauma narrative with a beginning, a middle and an end, so that both the natural emotional/relational sequence and the life narrative move toward resolution, rather than becoming frozen in disconnected traumatic images that can only be experienced, like flashbacks, piece by piece.

IDENTIFYING TWO SYMPTOM PATTERNS OF TRAUMATIC DISRUPTION OF BODILY EXPERIENCE AND MEMORY

Using the model described above we can begin to identify two types of traumatic disruption that produce memory problems and body symptoms.

Again, these patterns are offered as one set of models that can help clinicians think about clinical problems. Actual patients will always present with some combination of the natural protest sequence and of Type I and Type II disturbances.

TYPE I PATTERNS

Type I patients usually present with unrelenting physical pain, emotional pain often misapprehended as physical pain and a history of many failed attempts to find an explanation for their physical suffering. In this pattern feelings about the assault and the abandonment are silenced and obliterated. Instead there is an exclusive and disconnected focus on the felt bodily pain. This leaves the hurt child with an often ill body experienced as perhaps permanently injured, but at the same time protects the child from the trauma story with its message about specific hurts and from the realization of the absence or loss of the good mother. Indeed, the pain-body often creates a symbolic or actual tie to the mother that precludes confrontation or real separation (Novick and Novick 1996). The focus on the body in pain coupled with the effort to silence the real meaning of the pain sends the patient on an unending quest for a "diagnosis," or more accurately a "pseudodiagnosis." What is being denied is the connection between bodily pain and the reactive pain of being hurt and abandoned. Also denied is the potential healing impact of holding and emotional reconnection. The following is a sketch outlining the Type I response.

THE TYPE I SEQUENCE

ASSAULT	PAIN	PROTEST	RESPONSE	DAMAGED BODY/SELF
Amnesia	I am my pain	Seeking diagnosis	Enlisting others to deal with pain	
"I don't know why"	"I hurt all the time"	"What's wrong?"	"Fix it"	"I'll never get better"

The following case examples illustrate the complications and treatment difficulties encountered in Type I situations.

Case 1: A fifty-five-year-old divorced woman had exhausted all the physicians in her community with reports of multiple somatic complaints, intractable depression and constant phone calls and demands for ever more frequent appointments. She had been married for thirty years to a physically and emotionally violent and drug-abusing man who openly taunted her about her persistent ill health and early history of sexual abuse. Interpersonal conflicts led to physical collapse and then to emergency rooms, hospitals or new specialists. Her last therapist told her she was "a hopeless case who could only be medicated."

At this point she entered trauma-based psychotherapy and began to connect current physical symptoms to triggering emotional upsets and her lifelong history of illness to her childhood sexual abuse. Early in treatment she attempted to involve the therapist in her preoccupation with the diagnosis of chronic fatigue syndrome and her quest for the perfect doctor and the experimental medication that would help her recover. She also continued her involvement with emotionally abusive men. These activities had to be interpreted repeatedly as displacements, ways to avoid serious reworking of her childhood sexual abuse. Once she began to focus on the real suffering of her childhood self, she was able to temper her preoccupations with illness and pain. She no longer required multiple hospitalizations and was able to work with one physician and one therapist for the remainder of her course of treatment.

Case 2: A forty-four-year-old single, extremely accomplished woman presented with a lifelong history of severe physical problems, including episodic pelvic pain, rashes, severe insomnia, headaches, abdominal bloating, severe dysmenorrhea, severe premenstrual syndrome and multiple environmental allergies. She entered therapy after a hallucinatory flashback of a sexual-abuse scene in childhood. Three years of subsequent and ongoing psychotherapy dealt primarily with the traumatic memories that had been cloaked by her extensive childhood dissociation. As her dissociative amnesia lessened, her relationship to her body symptoms changed. Although she continued to be afraid of relinquishing the feeling "I'll never get better," she began to be able to participate in activities, rather than constantly limiting herself by being fearful and too ill, and thereby expanded her professional and personal life. When body symptoms appeared, they could be connected to emotional upset or to the desire to communicate her present distress and, more poignantly, her previously silenced childhood distress.

These two cases illustrate many of the complications of the Type I response to childhood assault: somatization, depression, psychasthenia, search for a diagnosis, revictimization, crisis-proneness and masochistic self-abasement. Shifting the therapeutic focus from the body in pain to the suffering child-self can be extraordinarily difficult, since the body's pain is so extreme. One patient described her pained body as follows: "Like a tornado, twisted, distorted, expandable and shrinkable like an accordion, weak and malleable like putty. Fragmented, in pieces, millions of pieces, tiny granules, as if it had been vaporized."

Such a shift is also defended against because of the terror of giving up the mysterious powers of the pain-body, which has conferred a sense of specialness and offered some hope, if spurious, of controlling the body-self and its feelings through medical means. To shift from this focus on control of the body in pain to the actual pain and then to experiencing real pleasure means relinquishing an entire world of idealized figures and magical solutions (Anzieu 1989; Novick and Novick 1996). It also means relinquishing the hope of the nurturing mother's arrival to succor the hurt child, thereby protecting the image of the good mother.

The healthy aspects of the Type I response include the persistent voicing through pain of the silenced trauma narrative, the unwillingness to give up the injured part of the self until it can be heard, comforted and restored and the persistence of the connection to the body, even though problematic.

Type II Patterns

In contrast, Type II patients may present with vague requests for self-improvement or with intolerable feelings of panic around a life crisis such as accidental injury, pregnancy, fears of illness or a failed relationship. Such crises become especially devastating if they produce anatomic or physiological changes in the body. Childhood adversity may be mentioned in an off-hand and minimized way. In this pattern, feelings about the assault and the mother's abandonment are escaped by leaving the real body and the real event. The disembodied self can believe it was never hurt and had a good mother. This self necessarily has a poisoned relationship with the real body, because the real body has evidence about abuse and abandonment that must be suppressed. The real body is distanced by depersonalization, ignored, punished and otherwise treated as an enemy messenger whose message must not be allowed (Terr 1990). The conflict between the disembodied self and the real body may be expressed in self-mutilation, self-starvation or disastrously unrealistic demands on the body, such as overwork, accident-proneness and noncompliance with necessary medical care.

An alternative to the disembodied self in the Type II situation is the development of an imaginary perfect body impervious to abuse, including self-abuse. In these patients self-harm is often best understood as a preventive attack on the real body to silence its message of pain. The following is a sketch of the Type II response.

THE TYPE II SEQUENCE

ASSAULT	PAIN	PROTEST	RESPONSE	INVULNERABLE BODY/SELF
Amnesia	Anesthesia depersonalization	Seeking omnipotent autonomy	Enlisting others to minimize needs	
"Nothing happened really"	"I'm not that hurt body"	"I don't need anybody"	"Nothing is wrong"	"I'm really all right"

The following case examples illustrate the complications and treatment difficulties encountered in Type II situations.

Case 1: A forty-five-year-old Hispanic, married, highly successful woman presented in panic about the prospect of having to remove her breast implant due to the silicon controversy. She had weathered her breast-cancer diagnosis, surgery and reconstructive surgery without a murmur. She was proud that she had needed no one to be with her in the hospital. However, the prospect of losing the implant and having on her body a visible sign of injury and imperfection had thrown her into panic. Although she presented as someone who had never been ill, close questioning revealed decades of repeated rather casual psychotherapy contacts and constant, rather drastic medical interventions, including sleep therapy and chronic prescription of narcotic and sedative medication. Narcotics were often the only medical intervention she would accept because "That makes the pain go away." She often missed medical appointments and was noncompliant with dietary and other medical advice.

The therapeutic effort in this case involved shifting the focus from her imaginary invulnerable body-self to her real child body-self struggling with her actual childhood situation. She had learned by the time she was three to tell no one when she hurt. When her cousin began to sexually abuse her, she tried to conceal the problem. What she had learned about her caregivers was that if they knew, they would blame her and take away what control she imagined she had. Physical activity and prowess had been crucial in her childhood escapes from her family and had led to striking athletic success in adolescence. Her greatest fear was of reaching out for help and being rejected; she became inexplicably suicidal whenever her mother visited. By the end of the first year of psychotherapy, she no longer went to emergency rooms for pain medication and was able to be more compliant with necessary and realistic medical care.

Case 2: A fifty-one-year-old single graduate student presented with vague desires to improve work-related behaviors and to become generally more accomplished. She had been a severe alcoholic in her twenties, but had been sober for many years. She also mentioned in an offhand way that her early childhood experiences had been somewhat difficult. As therapy continued, she was able to talk, reluctantly, about her extreme discomfort around her mother's intrusive and controlling contacts. She also slowly began to voice childhood worries about her father's rages and verbal abuse. Such incipient complaints would be followed immediately by memories of how wonderful father had been. After two years of psychotherapy, she was able to describe without minimization her father's physically abusive rages and disclosed a long-standing worry that sexual abuse had been present as well.

In the context of efforts toward increased commitment and intimacy with a man, she came to a session complaining about vaginal pain, a possible recurrence of herpes, and sexual anxieties and confusion. She reported that her vagina felt swollen, "as if something were inside it," and she couldn't get it out. When asked about her feelings, she said, "I think my vagina is lying. I never trusted my body or could believe anything about my body and I have always been miserable inside my body." Therapeutic focus on decoding the message inside "the lying vagina" aimed first at helping her reconnect to suppressed feelings about her current situation with the boyfriend, then toward understanding the message in terms of her child-body's reactions to emotional and physical abuse and to her panic about the felt unavailability of her mother. Further critical decoding of the body's message may become a point of reference later, when she is ready to explore the memory images that led her to wonder about prior sexual abuse.

One of the complications in the Type II response is that drugs and alcohol may be required to suppress negative bodily sensation and emotions. Also, derealization and depersonalization, while necessary in childhood for survival, can become obstacles to reworking traumatic memory. "Why do we have to talk about this? It wasn't really that bad." At another level these dissociative defenses disconnect the patient from adult accomplishments and strengths. "I feel like I am only a puppet." There is a deep fear that, despite all her adult successes, she is still not strong enough to endure an imaginative return to the moment of childhood trauma.

The healthy aspects of the Type II response include a capacity to engage in ongoing development even though some achievements and relationships are based on overfunctioning and overgiving. However, this active engagement with adult responsibilities has familiarized Type II patients with the natural protest sequence through their empathic responding to others. Helpful therapy permits them to become takers as well as givers in this sequence, as the child body-self reaches out for empathy, comfort, mirroring and holding for the first time.

DISCUSSION

The theoretical models sketched in this chapter trace the life story of the traumatized body, so that this body—both in its real and imaginary aspects—can become part of the therapeutic reworking of traumatic memories. We have described two types of body-memory problems. In Type I, painful sensations are retained, but their meaning is lost; in Type II, dissociative flight distances the traumatized self both from the pained body and its painful childhood circumstances.

These typologies overlap with many others. Both might be thought of as alexithymic. Type I patients resemble the highly distressed infants described by Ainsworth and coworkers (1978) and Main (Main and Morgan 1996) in their studies of mother-infant separation (George 1996; Armsworth and Stronck 1996). Such distressed infants attempt to provoke the mother to meet needs through persistent complaint. Type II patients resemble the avoidant infants in those studies, who make few demands and suppress or falsify the expression of negative feelings. Type I patients are prone to what psychoanalyst Joyce McDougall (1989) calls the "one body for two" phenomenon: they tend to recruit another person to help share the burden of dealing with the pained body. Type II patients are prone to what MacDougall calls the "two bodies for one" problem: internally they shift back and forth between an idealized perfect imaginary body and the real body with its actual sensations, and externally they are prone, when disembodied, to become overinvolved with the bodies of others; many become health-care professionals. Type I patients resemble the activation phase of PTSD; anxiety is intense and "body memories" are prominent. Type II patients resemble the numbed, avoidant phase of the PTSD cycle, often presenting with vague or absent symptoms.

It's important to remember that in actual clinical situations Type I and Type II problems are found in the same patient at different points in therapy. This parallels recent infant-research observations. Disorganized infants who have been frightened by their parents may display fragments of both avoidant and ambivalent response patterns interrupted by episodes of blank staring, which may represent dissociation (Main and Morgan 1996). The pain of the Type I situation is so intense that it requires Type II dissociative flight from the body; on the other hand, Type II patients can become so panicked by even normal body sensations (which threaten their wish for invulnerability) that they respond in a Type I way, engaging in a frantic search for the perfect healer or treatment. In patients with DID, one often finds Type I and Type II ego states appearing in pairs because the projective identifications required by each complex are complementary.

This model is designed to assist clinicians in keeping the patient's bodily experiences in focus so they can be dealt with in the psychotherapeutic process rather than split off. In certain cases it may be helpful to sketch out the natural sequence with a patient during a session. With Type I situations, it can be pointed out that the pain segment has expanded so that it blots out everything else in the sequence. In Type II situations, it is the omnipotently restored self that has expanded in such a way that it obscures all other elements, so the person no longer recalls that there once was adversity, pain and protest. In both situations there may have developed a profound fear that without the pain-self or the invulnerable self no one will be interested in connecting with the fully embodied self or in valuing and loving the person.

Recovery requires the patient to step back into the body-self at the moment of trauma. In both types of patients, this moment is obscured by depersonalization and dissociative amnesia. The experiencing of that moment of attack, then the hurt, then the abandonment is essentially nonverbal. The reconstructive journey often goes backward in time through the desperation and objectlessness of nonresponse and nonrestoration before it reaches the pain and the attack. The cry of abandonment may be more intensely painful and more fiercely defended against than the physical pain and abuse that preceded it. This is why the patient's tears often mark turning points in therapy. Given the intensity of emotional pain, it is easy to understand why individuals accept Type I or Type II limitations on their lives, rather than undergo the revivification of this core experience of suffering and isolation.

This revivification of abandonment and abuse is not the goal of therapy, but an intermediate step toward regaining both the self's capacity to connect with the real body and with others in the experience of pleasure and pain, which then can be narrated as part of the self's own story. The recognition of the body's messages in the contained, holding atmosphere of the therapist's office replicates the original healing touch of the mother in a completed natural protest sequence that helps the patient define, map, create and restore an accurate image of the body-self and its goodness.

REFERENCES

Adler, H. (1995). Recall and repetition of a severe childhood trauma. *International Journal of Psychoanalysis* 76: 927–943.

Ainsworth, M. D. S., Blehar, M. A., Waters, E., and Wall, S. (1978). *Patterns of attachment: A psychological study of the strange situation*. Hillsdale, N.J.: Erlbaum.

American Psychiatric Association (1994). *Diagnostic and statistical manual of mental disorders*. 4th ed. Washington, D.C.: American Psychiatric Association.

Anzieu, D. (1989). *The skin ego*. New Haven, Conn.: Yale University Press.

Armsworth, M. W., and Stronck, K. (1996). Deception and silence: Impact on attachment patterns and reality construction. Paper presented at the 12th annual meeting of the International Society for Traumatic Stress Studies, San Francisco, November.

Barach, P. (1991). Multiple personality disorder as an attachment disorder. *Dissociation* 4 (3): 117–123.

Bliss, E. L. (1986). *Multiple personality, allied disorders, and hypnosis*. New York: Oxford University Press.

Bowlby, J. (1988) *A secure base: Parent-child attachment and healthy human development*. New York: Basic Books.

———. (1994). *The making and breaking of affectional bonds*. New York: Routledge.

Braun, B. (1988). The BASK model of dissociation: Clinical applications. *Dissociation* 1 (2): 16–23.

Call, J. (1984). Child abuse and neglect in infancy: Sources of hostility within the parent-infant dyad and disorders of attachment in infancy. *Child Abuse and Neglect* 8: 185–202.

Cardeña, E., and Spiegel, D. (1996). Diagnostic issues, criteria and co-morbidity of dissociative disorders. In L. Michelson and W. J. Ray, eds., *Handbook of dissociation: Theoretical, empirical and clinical perspectives* (pp. 227–250). New York: Plenum.

Ellenberger, H. (1970). *The discovery of the unconscious*. New York: Basic Books.

Fonagy, P., Steele, H., and Target, M. (1994). The theory and practice of resilience. *Journal of Child Psychology and Psychiatry* 35: 231–257.

Fonagy, P., and Target, M. (1995). Understanding the violent patient: The use of the body and the role of the father. *International Journal of Psychoanalysis* 76: 487–501.

Freud, S. (1921). Introduction. In E. Jones, *Psychoanalysis and the war neuroses*. London: International Universities Press.

George, C. (1996). A representational perspective of child abuse and prevention: Internal working models of attachment and caregiving. *Child Abuse and Neglect* 20 (5): 411–424.

Goodwin, J. (1982). *Sexual abuse: Incest victims and their families*. Littleton, Mass.: Wright/PSG.

_____. (1988). Munchausen's syndrome as a dissociative sequel to extreme child abuse. *Dissociation* 1: 54–60.

_____. (1989) *Sexual abuse: Incest victims and their families*. 2d ed. Chicago: Mosby/Yearbook.

_____. (1993a). Childhood sexual abuse and non-epileptic seizures. In J. Rowan and J. R. Gates, eds., *Non-epileptic seizures* (pp. 181–192). New York: Butterworth Heineman.

_____. (1993b). *Rediscovering childhood trauma: Historical and clinical applications*. Washington, D.C.: American Psychiatric Press.

_____. (1993c). The seduction hypothesis 100 years after. In P. Paddison, ed., *Treatment of adult survivors of incest*. Washington, D.C.: American Psychiatric Press.

Goodwin, J., Bergman, R., and Simms, M. (1979). Hysterical seizures: A sequel to incest. *American Journal of Orthopsychiatry* 49: 698–703.

Goodwin, J., and Sachs, R. (1996). Child abuse in the etiology of dissociative disorders. In L. K. Michelson and W. J. Ray, eds., *Handbook of dissociation: Theoretical, empirical and clinical perspectives* (pp. 91–105). New York: Plenum.

Grand, S., and Alpert, J. L. (1993). The core trauma of incest: An object relations view. *Professional Psychology: Research and Practice* 24 (3): 330–33.

Harlow, H. F., and Harlow, M. K. (1971). Psychopathology in monkeys. In H. D. Kemmel, ed., *Experimental Psychopathology*. New York: Academic Press.

Main, M. (1993). Discourse, prediction and recent studies in attachment: Implications for psychoanalysis. *Journal of the American Psychoanalytic Association*, Suppl. 41: 209–24.

Main, M., and Morgan, H. (1996). Disorganization and disorientation in infant strange situation behavior: Phenotypic resemblance to dissociative states. In L. Michelson and W. J. Ray, eds., *Handbook of dissociation: Theoretical, empirical and clinical perspectives* (pp. 107–138). New York: Plenum.

McDougall, J. (1989). *Theaters of the body*. New York: Norton.

Ney, P. G. (1987). The treatment of abused children: The natural sequence of events. *American Journal of Psychotherapy* 61: 391–401.

Novick, J., and Novick, K. K. (1996). *Fearful symmetry: The development and treatment of sado-masochism*. Northvale, N.J.: Aronson.

Pearce, J. W., and Pezzot-Pearce, T. E. (1994). Attachment theory and its implications for psychotherapy with maltreated children. *Child Abuse and Neglect* 18 (5): 425–438.

Ross, C. A., and Pam, A. (1995). *Pseudoscience in biological psychiatry: Blaming the body*. New York: Wiley.

Shear, M. K. (1996). Factors in the etiology and pathogenesis of panic disorder: Revisiting the attachment-separation paradigm. *American Journal of Psychiatry*, Festschrift suppl. 153 (7): 25–136.

Shengold, L. (1989) *Soul murder: The effects of childhood abuse and deprivation*. New Haven, CT: Yale University Press.

Sifneos, P. E. (1973). The prevalence of alexithymic characteristics in psychosomatic patients. In J. Reusch, A. Schmale and T. Spoerri, eds., *Psychotherapy and psychosomatics* (pp. 255–262). White Plains, N.Y.: S. Karger.

Spitz, R. (1983). *Dialogues from infancy*. New York: International Universities Press.

Stern, D. N. (1985). *The interpersonal world of the infant*. New York: Basic Books.

Suomi, S. J. (1991). Early stress and adult emotional reactivity in Rhesus monkeys. In Ciba Foundation, ed. *Childhood environment and adult disease* (pp. 171–188). Chichester, England: W. Ley.

Terr, L. (1990). Who's afraid in Virginia Woolf: Clues to early sexual abuse in literature. *Psychoanalytic Study of the Child* 45: 533–546.

van der Hart, O., Lierens, R., and Goodwin, J. (1996). Jeanne Fery: A sixteenth-century case of dissociative identity disorder. *Journal of Psychohistory* 24 (1): 18–35.

van der Hart, O., Steele, K., Boon, S., and Brown, P. (1993). The treatment of traumatic memories: Synthesis, realization, and integration. *Dissociation* 6 (2/3): 162–180.

van der Kolk, B. A. (1994a). The body keeps the score: Memory and the evolving psychobiology of posttraumatic stress. *Harvard Review of Psychiatry* 1 (5): 253–265.

———. (1994b). The behavioral and psychobiological effects of developmental trauma. In A. Stoudemire, ed., *Human behavior: An introduction for medical students* (pp. 328–343). New York: Lippincott.

van der Kolk, B., and van der Hart, O. (1989). Pierre Janet and the breakdown of adaptation in psychological trauma. *American Journal of Psychiatry* 146: 1530–1540.

Volgyesi, F. A. (1963). *Hypnosis of man and animals*. Baltimore, Md.: Williams and Wilkins.

Winnicott, D. W. (1965). Parent-infant relationship. In *The maturational process and the facilitating environment*. New York: International Universities Press.

———. (1965). Ego integration in child development. In *The maturational process and the facilitating environment*. New York: International Universities Press.

Wright, L. (1994). *Remembering Satan*. New York: Knopf.

CHAPTER 11

Body-Ego Integration in Dissociative Identity Disorder

Richard P. Kluft

In his monumental work *The Ego and the Id*, Freud (1923/1961) took pains to emphasize that the ego (that coherent organization of mental processes to which consciousness is attached and which controls motility and the discharge of excitations into the external world in the form of decisions, behaviors and actions) develops as a consequence of the human organism's experience with the external world. The medium of this influence was described as perception-consciousness. Thus modified and informed, "The ego seeks to bring the influence of the external world to bear on the id and its tendencies, and endeavors to substitute the reality principle for the pleasure principle which reigns unrestrictedly in the id. For the ego, perception plays the part which in the id falls to instinct" (p. 25).

Along with perceptions from the special sensory organs, experiences registered by the body play an important role. The body, especially the surface of the body, is a place from which both external and internal perceptions may spring. Furthermore, the role of pain in this process is potentially critical. Freud maintained that how we experience our bodies during periods of severe discomfort, such as painful illnesses, is one avenue by which we arrive at the idea of our body. Therefore, Freud wrote, "The ego is first and foremost a bodily ego; it is not merely a surface entity, but is itself the projection of a surface" (p. 26). Freud went on to state that although it is tempting to equate the ego with conscious mentation, there is "evidence that even subtle and difficult intellectual operations which ordinarily require strenuous reflection can equally be carried out preconsciously and without coming into consciousness" (p. 26); that is, several ego-involved streams of mentation may be simultaneously ongoing without reaching one's general conscious awareness.

Hilgard (1977), a scholar in the field of hypnosis and the founder of modern neodissociation theory, built upon the basic observation that the operation of more than one cognitive system simultaneously is demonstrable in laboratory settings. He demonstrated that several cognitive systems may be perceiving and registering the same situation differently at the same time. Interestingly, his "hidden observer" research studied the mind's differential registration of the perception of physical pain in mental systems that themselves are clearly conscious, but that are generally inaccessible to the conscious awareness of the usually dominant conscious mental organization.

Although Freud, in his remarks, was laying the foundation for a discussion of the influence of the superego upon the ego and Hilgard (1984) stressed that his laboratory findings were cognitive alone, here I want to pursue some of the implications of these observations for the subject at hand, body-ego integration in patients with dissociative identity disorder (DID). Those who suffer DID have experienced severe traumatization, both by self-report (e.g., Putnam et al. 1986) and by external corroboration (Bliss 1984; Coons and Milstein 1986; Hornstein and Putnam 1992; Coons 1994; Kluft 1995).

Freud clearly appreciated that discomfort is a major factor in helping individuals determine the nature of their experience and representation of themselves. This has a direct bearing on the sense of self, the identity and the self-representation of traumatized individuals.

Perhaps there is no more dramatic example of this phenomenon in psychiatry than the formation of enacted, rather than merely intrapsychic, alternate identities and self-representations in DID, until recently termed multiple personality disorder. Here different self systems, identities and self-representations embody alternative adaptations to difficult external circumstances. When this adaptation attains a degree of secondary autonomy, it may be employed for the containment of intrapsychic pain, the management of nontraumatic stressors and general adaptation.

Hilgard elegantly demonstrated that the human mind could encompass alternate registrations of experience and alternate perceptions of physical sensations without being troubled by this incongruity. Clearly, if a person can go through an incident and register it quite differently in two or more dissociated memory banks, the possibility exists of forming alternate identities whose self-representations and accounts of their autobiographical histories will be very much discrepant. There is perhaps no more clear manifestation of this phenomenon than the divergent representations of self and of personal experience by the different personalities encountered in DID. For example, it is not uncommon for some alters to recall and register the pain of a traumatic experience, although others may have no memory for the experience and/or did not perceive the pain.

Patients with DID are characterized by the presence of alternate personalities, each with its own relatively enduring way of perceiving and relating to the environment and self. Among the crucial determinants of each alter's identity are its particular psychological self and its unique self-representation, including the image of its body. It is typical to encounter approximately thirteen to eighteen alternate personalities in a contemporary case (Kluft 1984; Putnam et al. 1986; Ross 1989), although series drawn from tertiary treatment centers routinely encounter patients with a far higher degree of complexity (Kluft 1996, unpublished data).

Although fascination has traditionally focused on the panoply of personalities, with attention to their differences and the number, this has obscured a far more challenging question: What must occur in order for these well-established, deeply entrenched alternate entities, with documentable psychophysiological differences, operational often for decades, to become reconciled and blended in a process of integration? This indeed must take place, in some manner, for such a patient to attain unity. In the process of integration, the several self-representations must become a single one, and the many ego configurations must undergo a metamorphosis into an ego structure and a set of processes that is either conjoined in its function or is functioning as if it were.

MODELS OF INTEGRATION

Although we do not at present understand the process of integration very well, we can approach a tentative understanding of the process from several perspectives. The first is from models of etiology. Perhaps if we know how the alters are formed and assume that the etiological factors continue to play a part in the perpetuation of the condition, we can infer how to undo the damages that are posited to have occurred. The second is from studying narrative and metaphoric descriptions of the integration process. Perhaps if we understand how the alters come together and assume that these processes somehow undo some psychopathological processes, we can infer how to undo dividedness. The third is from the subjective experiences of integration described by DID patients. Perhaps if we better appreciate what the DID patient undergoes, we can appreciate what is involved in the change itself.

ETIOLOGICAL MODELS

Recently I (1996) listed a series of models proposed for the etiology of DID. Combining classificatory efforts by Stern (1984) and Putnam (1991), the list includes: (1) the supernatural/transpersonal; (2) the psychological; (3) the sociological; (4) the role-playing/malingering/iatrogenesis; (5) the trance state/autohypnotic; (6) the split brain/hemispheric laterality; (7) the temporal lobe/complex partial, complex seizure/kindling; and (8) the behavioral states of consciousness models. To these might be added (9) the neural network of memory/information processing model (Ansdorfer 1984; Li and Spiegel 1992; Spiegel 1990; Yates and Nasby 1993); (10) the neodissociation/ego-state model (drawn from the work of Hilgard [1977/1986] by such authors as Beahrs [1982] and the Watkinses [1979]); and (11) a basic-affects model (Nathanson, in press), which has much in common with models 8 and 9. None of these models essentially precludes the operation of others, and none fully explains rather than illustrates a possible mechanism for DID.

Perhaps more striking for the purposes of the topic under discussion, although many models have some relationship to matters of body ego, no model offers a particularly illuminating insight into the matter of the representation of the physical self across alters. For example, in the supernatural/transpersonal model, by implication some entities might correspond to culturally or subculturally sanctioned representatives of possessing entities or archetypes. Role playing and malingering might suggest the creation of alters consistent with the purposes being pursued. The behavioral-states and basic-affects models allow us to imagine that alters would be created to fit the characteristic expression of the feelings and/or states of mind involved. However, we look in vain for a satisfactory overall paradigm.

Furthermore, when we turn to these models and inquire into their implications for therapy, as indicated in Table 11.1, we find a plethora of alternative approaches might be indicated. Although most might conceivably play a role in a thoughtful therapeutic approach and some have been the sole successful curative approach with particular cases, no one form of treatment has been found to be universally effective. There is no single commonality that can be inferred and applied to the formulation of a general theory of personality formation and integration.

TABLE 11.1

Alternate Etiological Models of DID and Modes of Cure

Model	*Mode of Cure*
Supernatural/Transpersonal	Exorcism/removal
Psychological	Psychotherapy
Sociological/Social Psychological	Change key contingencies
Role Playing/Malingering	Depotentiate role/stance
Trance-State/Autohypnosis	Restructure trance phenomena
Split Brain/Hemispheric Laterality	Cognitive retraining
Seizure-Related Phenomena	Medication/stress decrease
Behavioral States of Consciousness	Remove developmental block
Neural Network	Simultaneous activation
Neodissociation/Ego States	Negotiated interaction
Basic Affects	Enhance affect tolerance

Descriptive Pathways

When we turn to the narrative and metaphoric descriptions of pathways toward integration, we find there are six major pathways described in the literature: (1) gradual merging; (2) facilitation with suggestion and imagery; (3) spontaneous cessation of separateness; (4) blending by alters' decisions; (5) brokered departure; and (6) building upon temporary blendings.

What can we learn? Table 11.2 indicates the processes and concerns implied by each pathway, in addition to the hypnotic/autohypnotic capacity implicit in all. If we appreciate that the process of integration involves identification, empathy, boundary erosion, state transformations, problem resolutions and task completions, we can infer that the process of forming personalities involves disidentification, a repudiation of empathic connectedness, boundary erection, state stabilizations without fluid transitions, the failure to solve crucial problems in a conventional manner and the failure to complete important tasks. These are summarized in Table 11.3.

Disidentification involves the need to be other than the baseline self. Repudiation of empathic connectedness means the need to distance one's self from experience that is now understood as being from an other. Boundary erection refers to the need to separate one subset of information from another subset of information in a relatively rule-bound manner (Spiegel 1986). State stabilization without fluid transformations means the individual either has not developed to the level at which the transition from one state of mind to another is seamless or has regressively reactivated this early childhood level of function. So far these suggest that disaffiliation from a

TABLE 11.2

Descriptive Pathways to Integration and Suggested Mechanisms

1. Gradual merger
   Identification, empathy, and boundary erosion
2. Facilitation with suggestion and imagery
   State change, identification, and boundary erosion
3. Spontaneous cessation of separateness
   Identification, empathy, and boundary erosion
4. Blending by alters' decisions
   Problem resolution, +/− identification, empathy, and boundary erosion
5. Brokered departure
   Task completion, +/− problem resolution, identification, empathy, and boundary erosion
6. Building upon temporary blendings
   Problem resolution, identification, empathy, and boundary erosion

threatened sense of self and the sequestration of that sense of self by its being declared nonself, plus or minus the erection of an amnestic barrier, is essential. We can see implicit negations of identification, with the implication that alternate structures will be somehow different, but we do not yet see what these replacement identities must become.

When we consider problem-resolution and task-completion aspects, however, we can begin to see how the very nature of the problems and tasks might begin to suggest the attributes of alters designed to address them. This is an issue we will return to after considering the subjective experiences of patients who undergo integrations.

DID PATIENT REPORTS

In the course of bringing over 160 DID patients to complete integration and having integrated personalities in well over 250 DID patients, I have had the opportunity to hear a great deal about DID patients' perceptions of the process. It has been very instructive to hear patients describe such events both from the perspective of the integrating alters, the alter with whom others were integrating, and the alters who were not directly involved with a particular integration.

A few generalizations are in order. First, alters whose roles are limited to minimal actions and the retention of particular traumata rarely are invested in separateness. Nor is there much of a change in the patient as a result of their

TABLE 11.3

Factors Inferred as Crucial in Personality Formation

1. Disidentification
2. Repudiation of empathic connectedness
3. Boundary erection
4. Prevention of fluid state transformations
5. Atypical attempts at problem resolution
6. Failure to complete important emotional tasks

integration, except in connection with one or more other alters' now experiencing the integrated alter's experiences as their own. Second, despite initial concerns over the loss of their own separateness, alters are more likely to react strongly to the integrations of alters with which they experience themselves having a meaningful and complex relationship than they are to their own imminent loss of separateness. Third, the more therapy that has occurred prior to the loss of separateness of a major alter, the less dramatic is likely to be the impact; conversely, if a major alter integrates rather rapidly, the impact is likely to be considerable. Fourth, the more specific the effort that has gone into preparing the alters for integration with preliminary procedures and frequent checks of the attitudes of the involved alters, the smoother the process is likely to be (Fine 1991, 1993). Fifth, the process of integration for major personalities is likely to be stepwise rather than dramatic, with differences muting and separateness fading gradually over a period of time before there is an actual loss of separateness. Sixth, an integration is unlikely to succeed if the function served by the alter that is about to integrate remains necessary and is not represented elsewhere in the system. Seventh, there is no way to force an integration to occur and remain stable before the therapeutic work of the involved alter or alters is completed, unless it can be deferred to the alter into which the involved alter or alters will integrate.

As representative of the DID patients I have studied, I will describe a few vignettes that illustrate the process from the patient's perspective.

Vignette 1—The Descent of "the Goddess": Sherri was a highly dramatic and flamboyant professional artist who applied her considerable creative gifts to the elaboration of her system of alters. During the course of a hospital stay occasioned by severe anorexia, I encountered a violent and grandiose protector personality who announced herself as "the Goddess." Within hours, Sherri had crafted a lovely seductive garment based on neoclassical renditions of the garments of Greek goddesses and changed into it when the Goddess was out. "The Goddess" created havoc in the hospital with her toga, tirades and aloof, imperious attitude.

I approached "the Goddess" empathically, noting how threatened Sherri must have been to need such a powerful source of protection and support. Despite criticism from colleagues and staff and considerable personal misgivings, I understood "the Goddess" to be in the service of undoing massive narcissistic deflation and injury. With a largely empathic and supportive focus, "the Goddess" was induced to describe the abuses that had necessitated her becoming separate. Indeed, they were the worst and the most humiliating the patient had described.

Within a few days, "the Goddess" abandoned her toga and, crowned with a newly crafted tiara and a purple-bordered robe, announced that her pain had been reduced to the extent that she no longer needed to be a goddess— she would now like to be called "Queen Victoria." I understood the patient to be stating that she was beginning to feel more secure and less pressured to fight with fantasy her overwhelming pain; I urged the staff to accept the patient as she presented herself. In sessions we worked with further humiliating traumata, and they were abreacted.

After several days the patient discarded the tiara and robe and sewed herself some very conservative and ultraproper high-necked blouses. She stated that she was ready to be called "Victoria," and under this name she was prim and protective to the point of being officious and intrusive on the unit, but was usually simply rather stuffy. We continued our work, and the patient became increasingly lighthearted as we wrapped up the exploration and abreaction of this alter's trauma. She noted that as she lived more in the here and now than in her terrible childhood and adolescence, she felt the need to protect herself with such aggression and vigor was unnecessary.

Soon "Victoria" asked to be called "Vickie" and simply "hung around," coconscious with the alters that were out when the patient socialized on the unit. After a few days of this, "Vickie" found herself becoming more and more like Sherri, and Sherri began to show increased self-confidence. "Vickie" and Sherri appreciated that they were gradually blending together and decided to join formally, because both found that becoming closer in this gradual way made them feel depersonalized and occasionally disoriented. They asked me to facilitate their joining hypnotically. This was accomplished uneventfully, and the integration held for the remaining year that the patient was under my observation.

Vignette 2—"The Baby": "The Baby" was one of the many alters of Rhonda, a high-functioning DID patient who was a psychologist in private practice. In her private moments, Rhonda often found that "the Baby" was out a great deal of the time, playing with toys, sucking her thumb and coloring in coloring books. Therapy revealed that "the Baby" represented Rhonda's regressive wishes for gratification and expressed her wish to have in the here and now the nurture and parenting of which she had been deprived. I took pains to spend some time with "the Baby," but to avoid becoming involved in regressive reparenting interventions or gratifying her wish for infinite nurture. Instead, I spent a few minutes of friendly chat with "the Baby" from time to time and gradually encouraged it to speak in psychotherapy.

As I continued to give it predictable but not excessive attention and to kindly decline invitations to engage in regressive interactions, "the Baby's" vocabulary and speech became more mature. Every few months "the Baby" indicated it had grown a few months or a year in age. When circumstances allowed, I was able to explore the relationship of this alter to childhood trauma. I found that it contained no trauma memories, having been protected from them by other alters. I worked with those alters' traumata. As I did so, "the Baby" began to stay coconscious with more functional alters to learn about the world and soon requested to be called "the Girl." I now asked other alters to spend time with "the Girl" in order to help her continue growing toward becoming a young woman. This forced the gratifications of play and reparenting to be given within the alters system, an approach also advocated by Putnam (1989). Within a few months this alter grew up, found its separateness fading and integrated with a very functional and socially adept alter.

Vignette 3—"Belle": "Belle" was an alter, discovered in the course of abreactive work, who played virtually no role in the patient's contemporary life. "Belle" encapsulated the patient's experiences of having to gratify her drug-addicted and probably psychotic mother with oral sex. She was seen by the other alters and experienced by herself as misshapen and filthy, barely human. After "Belle" shared her traumatic experiences, her abuse became the common property of many other personalities. She received both praise and consolation for what she had protected the others from experiencing. At this point, "Belle" began to be perceived by herself and the other alters as having assumed a more normal appearance, not unlike those of the most functional alters. One day, she suddenly and spontaneously integrated with an alter that had been supportive of her. With her experiences and shame accepted and no longer repudiated, "Belle" blended readily.

Vignette 4—"Isaac": "Isaac" was the powerful protector and adviser to Chloe, the host personality. Chloe envisioned "Isaac" as they spoke inwardly and often felt his reassuring hand on her shoulder. From the first, Chloe and "Isaac" made it clear that "Isaac" would be with Chloe forever, or if he ever integrated, he would be the last alter to do so. As more and more issues were resolved in her therapy, Chloe grew in confidence and reassurance. As more alters integrated into Chloe, she became more multifaceted and resilient. She had fewer moments of uncertainty and anxiety and found fewer situations challenged her adaptive capacity. She called on "Isaac" less frequently, and he initiated intrusions into her awareness less and less often. Furthermore, when Chloe had integrated approximately 75 percent of her alters, she began to notice that "Isaac's" voice was becoming softer, and his image was becoming somewhat vague and smaller in size. Her appreciation of him changed— where he had once been perceived as a distinct separate person of greater than human capacities, he became perceived as, in sequence, a powerful man, a kind man, a voice of wisdom within her head, and finally a valuable part of her mind. When "Isaac" finally integrated, with hypnotic suggestion, he retained his pristine conformation, but was perceived as a small and faded, but deeply beloved, version of his former self.

In the first three of these vignettes, the body image and self-representation as perceived by the patient and as enacted behaviorally served important communicative functions and underwent metamorphoses when what they were called upon to communicate underwent significant change. Their self-representations were profound signifiers of meaning. In the fourth vignette, the changes had these qualities, but progressive miniaturization of the alter's body image correlated with his diminution of psychic prominence and presence as his function was gradually subsumed by others and ultimately completely internalized by Chloe.

DISCUSSION

When we attempted to infer the self-representational and body-ego characteristics of alters from current models of etiology, we did not come to very useful ideas and hypotheses. When we did the same with typical pathways toward integration, we began to find many reasons for separateness per se and came upon some preliminary notions that the individual self-representations of the alters might be in some way related to atypical problem solving. When we moved on further to study the DID patient's subjective experiences of the integration process, we found that as the DID patient's problems are modified by the therapy, the representations and even the very existence of the related alters may undergo profound complementary or parallel changes.

It is tempting to consider the alters' characteristics as expressions of what Armstrong (1994), building on the work of Fisher and Pipp (1984), had described as "growing up strangely." Without persons in their environment who can nurture, support and protect the child adequately, the DID child in the making is forced, as Marmer (1980, 1991) noted, to create and enlist aspects of self to perform, however inadequately, the missing functions. The many alters' identities and self-representations, from this perspective, are not necessarily crucial expressions of core gender identifications or basic aspects of the patient's core identity. Instead, they are adaptive instrumental metaphors enacting allegorical masteries of what cannot be mastered adequately in fact. If one is to be protected, it should be by a person whose appearance conveys power and competence, which, in visual metaphor, may require that the alter that serves this purpose be male, over six feet tall, armed and have bulging muscles, even though "he" is located in a five-year-old girl. That many such identities are present may or may not be associated with ego weakness and severe distortions of identity formation. Ego weakness is not an inherent aspect of DID (see Horevitz and Braun 1984; Kluft 1991a; Armstrong 1991, 1994 for a more detailed discussion of this often hotly debated issue).

How do these metaphors and allegories assume such compelling verisimilitude and apparent substance in the mind of the DID patient and in his or her self-representation to others? I would like to offer a hypothetical model of this process, involving the notion of alter formation in the service of ego-sustaining illusory mastery.

Let us imagine the situation of a girl of four or five who is abruptly raped by her previously kind and beloved Uncle Ben. How can this be contended with? She can simply dissociate the experience, creating an episode of dissociative amnesia. However, suppose this either fails to suffice or is not employed as the girl forms another self state (following Kohut's [1977] use of the term "self" to designate a center of experience and initiative).

The girl may form an alter just like herself who encapsulates the painful memory and the physical pain and go on in her main state oblivious to what has occurred (so-called isomorphic DID [Kluft 1991b]). This would be a clear example of Freud's observation that pain contributes to the development of the body ego. She may be motivated by the thought that this would not have happened if she were not a very bad little girl and form a "bad girl" personality whose physical as well as psychological characteristics differ from those of the actual young girl. She may mistake the pleasure of some arousal as indicating she was eager for the experience and may have brought it upon herself, forming in the process a "sexually aggressive personality" with an age, physical appearance and characteristics to match. She may hold the thought that if she were as good and nice as her cousin Betty, she would not have been abused, and form an alter based on the idealized cousin Betty. She may believe that if she had been a boy, she would have been spared this assault, and form a "twin brother" personality. She may wish that she were a big tough man who could have driven off Uncle Ben, forming a protector personality based on her personal idea of what a tough man would look like. She may come to wish she were able to be the one doing the abusing rather than being condemned to be a victim and form a personality based on Uncle Ben, an identification with the aggressor. She may form a personality or personalities, often both male and female, to offer her the consolation she cannot hope to get in her family, either because she dare not tell or because she has found that such responsive nurture is not available to her. It is conceivable that over only a few weeks or months of abuse, all of the above attempts to solve the problem of dealing with Uncle Ben's behavior could be adopted successively, but, because none successfully terminates the ongoing abuse or encapsulates it completely, this could result in a cast of ten or so alters.

Because DID patients are excellent hypnotic subjects and have profound autohypnotic capacities and because many have the characteristics of the fantasy-prone personality, experiencing their imaginative products as being every bit as real as what they experience through perception of the outside world, the personalities imagined as solutions to the effort to cope with the abuse are visualized, heard, felt and experienced in every way as genuine other individuals. It is well established in the literature of source monitoring (specifically regarding DID in Belli and Loftus [1994] and reviewed in depth by Little [1996]) that what is visualized is likely to be understood to have been experienced. Hence, the visualized alters are accorded a face validity, and each time they are visualized, their characteristics are reinforced in the patient's mind, as is the perception of their reality. That these early visualizations are often forgotten by the host personality and/or were only visualized initially by alters that do not serve as host is an interesting and probably crucial aspect of alter formation, because years later, often having been long-forgotten, the alters may suddenly become the subject of the patient's awareness, often with shock and surprise.

As treatment renders the dissociative adaptations less imperative and wishes change from defensive to growth-oriented, the changes the DID patient experiences are reflected in the imagined and perceived representations and self-representations. Therefore, it is not surprising that these changes would be visualized and experienced as having a compelling sense of reality. These changes might take the form of an alter's changing in core elements of the self-representation, simply fading or diminishing in some way, being perceived as at a distance or seen less frequently. Furthermore, as the tides of therapy wax and wane, it is not surprising that the visualizations and experiences of the alters may change back and forth. This is especially typical of persecutory alters, who are often experienced repeatedly as gaining power, suffering a loss of power, and then becoming reenergized as the process of the therapy makes the various other alters feel more or less helpless.

In summary, then, it appears that the alters are created in order to solve overwhelming problems, and their representations are in accord with their perceived functions and origins. Although they have and embody aspects of identity, they and their self-representations do not necessarily reflect the core identity difficulties one associates with severe developmental deficits and difficulties. The alters are the expression of adaptive efforts, which are wishes that are conscious at least at one level of the mind, if not in the level that is experienced and represented as the host (the alter most frequently in executive control) or the alter that is experienced and represented as most central to the patient's identity. Autohypnotic mechanisms are implicated at all steps of the process.

Table 11.4 illustrates this hypothesized process in a stepwise manner. This schematization draws together the main points advanced in earlier sections of this chapter. It attempts a synthesis that coordinates many levels of observation and abstraction and should be regarded as preliminary and tentative. However, it does represent perhaps the first attempt to unite steps hypothesized in the etiology of DID and in the undoing of DID in psychotherapy into a single process. It offers an explanation of how major differences of self and body experience and self and body perception may exist without psychosis or other forms of ego weakness, and demonstrates that identity issues that superficially may seem to signify major disturbances and developmental issues

TABLE 11.4

Steps in the Hypothesized Process of Developing and Resolving Alternative Body-Ego Processes in DID

1. Intolerable stressors
2. Failure of primary adaptational and defensive systems
3. Enlistment of atypical strategies of problem resolution (no firm sequence)
    A. Disidentification
    B. Repudiation of empathic connectedness
    C. Boundary formation
4. Formation of embodiments of fantasized personified adaptations
5. Autohypnotic envisioning of Step 4
6. Cognitive restructuring that validates and accommodates to Step 4 secondary to source monitoring perspectives and their interpretation
7. Reinforcement of Steps 4–6
8. Therapy modifies the needs that determine the representation of the personified adaptation, enhancing identification, empathy, and boundary erosion
9. Formation of embodiments of modified fantasized personified adaptations
10. Autohypnotic envisioning of Step 9
11. Cognitive restructuring that validates and accommodates to Steps 9 and 10 secondary to source-monitoring perspectives and their interpretation
12. Reinforcement of Steps 8–11
13. Therapy continues to produce modified needs that lead to further modification of fantasized personified adaptations, with many reiterations of Steps 8–12
14. Fantasized personified adaptations lose adaptational valence
15. Self-representations of fantasized personified adaptations undergo alterations such as changing and/or fading away
16. Fantasized personified adaptations and associated self-representations of fantasized personified adaptations lose last bits of adaptive valence
17. Approximation of the particular fantasized personified adaptations and associated self-representations of fantasized personified adaptations to other similar constructs (i.e., unified self-representation)
18. Autohypnotic envisioning of Step 17
19. Cognitive restructuring that validates and accommodates to Step 17 secondary to source-monitoring perspectives and their interpretation
20. Reinforcement by enhanced adaptation and mastery, +/− comfort
21. Integration with similar constructs involving Step 22
22. Autohypnotic envisioning of Step 21
23. Cognitive restructuring that validates and accommodates to Steps 21–22 secondary to source-monitoring perspectives and their interpretation
24. Continued reiterations of Steps 8–23

may instead represent a sophisticated and highly structured coping and defensive strategy that can continue to be modified by others and to modify itself in response to life experiences, even to the point of its own elimination.

REFERENCES

Ansdorfer, J. C. (1985). Multiple personality in the human information-processor: A case history and theoretical formulation. *Journal of Clinical Psychology* 41: 309–324.

Armstrong, J. (1991). The psychological organization of multiple personality disordered patients as revealed in psychological testing. *Psychiatric Clinics of North America* 14: 533–546.

_____. (1994). Reflections on multiple personality disorder as a developmentally complex adaptation. *The Psychoanalytic Study of the Child* 49: 349–364.

Beahrs, J. O. (1982). *Unity and multiplicity: Multilevel consciousness of self in hypnosis, psychiatric disorder, and mental health.* New York: Brunner-Mazel.

Belli, R. F., and Loftus, E. F. (1994). Recovered memories of childhood abuse: A source monitoring perspective. In S. J. Lynn and J. W. Rhue, eds., *Dissociation: Clinical and theoretical perspectives* (pp. 415–433). New York: Guilford.

Bliss, E. L. (1984). Spontaneous self-hypnosis in multiple personality disorder. *Psychiatric Clinics of North America* 7: 135–148.

Coons, P. M. (1994). Confirmation of childhood abuse in childhood and adolescent cases of multiple personality disorder and dissociative disorder not otherwise specified. *Journal of Nervous and Mental Disease* 182: 461–464.

Coons, P. M., and Milstein, V. (1986). Psychosexual disturbances in multiple personality: Characteristics, etiology, and treatment. *Journal of Clinical Psychiatry* 47: 106–110.

Fine, C. G. (1991). Treatment stabilization and crisis prevention: Pacing the therapy of the multiple personality disorder patient. *Psychiatric Clinics of North America* 14: 661–675.

_____. (1993). A tactical integrationalist perspective on the treatment of multiple personality disorder. In R. P. Kluft and C. G. Fine, eds., *Clinical perspectives on multiple personality disorder* (pp. 135–153). Washington, D.C.: American Psychiatric Press.

Fischer, K. W., and Pipp, S. L. (1984). Development of the structures of unconscious thought. In K. S. Bowers and D. Meichenbaum, eds., *The unconscious reconsidered* (pp. 88–148). New York: Wiley.

Freud, S. (1923/1961). The ego and the id. In J. Strachey, ed. and trans., *The standard edition of the complete psychological works of Sigmund Freud.* Vol. 19 (pp. 3–66). London: Hogarth Press.

Hilgard, E. R. (1977, rev. ed. 1986). *Divided consciousness: Multiple controls in human thought and action.* New York: Wiley.

_____. (1984). The hidden observer and multiple personality. *International Journal of Clinical and Experimental Hypnosis* 32: 248–253.

Horevitz, R. P., and Braun, B. G. (1984). Are multiple personalities borderline? *Psychiatric Clinics of North America* 7: 69–87.

Hornstein, N. L., and Putnam, F. W. (1992). Clinical phenomenology of child and adolescent multiple personality disorder. *Journal of the American Academy of Child and Adolescent Psychiatry* 31: 1055–1077.

Kluft, R. P. (1984). Treatment of multiple personality disorder: A study of 33 cases. *Psychiatric Clinics of North America* 7: 9–29.

_____. (1991a). Multiple personality disorder. In A. Tasman and S. M. Goldfinger, eds., *American Psychiatric Press review of psychiatry*. Vol. 10, (pp. 161–188). Washington, D.C.: American Psychiatric Press.

_____. (1991b). Clinical presentations of multiple personality disorder. *Psychiatric Clinics of North America* 14: 605–629.

_____. (1995). The confirmation and disconfirmation of memories of abuse in dissociative identity disorder patients: A naturalistic clinical study. *Dissociation* 8: 253–258.

_____. (1996). Multiple personality disorder: A legacy of trauma. In C. R. Pfeffer, ed., *Severe stress and mental disturbance in children* (pp. 411–448). Washington, D.C.: American Psychiatric Press.

Kohut, H. (1977). *The restoration of the self.* New York: International Universities Press.

Li, D., and Spiegel, D. (1992). A neural network model of dissociative disorders. *Psychiatric Annals* 22: 144–147.

Little, L. (1996). Source monitoring and dissociative experiences in DID and non-DID patients: A multicenter study. Ph.D. dissertation, California School of Professional Psychology, Fresno, Calif.

Marmer, S. S. (1980). Psychoanalysis of multiple personality. *International Journal of Psychoanalysis* 61: 439–459.

_____. (1991). Multiple personality disorder: A psychoanalytic perspective. *Psychiatric Clinics of North America* 14: 677–693.

Nathanson, D. (in press). Contemporary affect theory and dissociation: Clinical and theoretical perspectives. *Dissociation.*

Putnam, F .W. (1989). *Diagnosis and treatment of multiple personality disorder.* New York: Guilford.

_____. (1991). Dissociative disorders in children and adolescents: A developmental perspective. *Psychiatric Clinics of North America* 14: 519–532.

Putnam, F. W., Guroff, J., Silberman, E. K., Balban, L., and Post, R. (1986). The clinical phenomenology of multiple personality disorder: 100 recent cases. *Journal of Clinical Psychiatry* 47: 285–293.

Ross, C. A. (1989). *Multiple personality disorder: Diagnosis, clinical features, and treatment*. New York: Wiley.

Spiegel, D. (1986). Dissociating damage. *American Journal of Clinical Hypnosis* 29: 123–131.

———. (1990). Hypnosis, dissociation, and trauma: Hidden and covert observers. In J. Singer, ed., *Repression and dissociation: Implications for personality theory, psychopathology, and health* (pp. 121–142). Chicago: University of Chicago Press.

Stern, C. R. (1984). The etiology of multiple personalities. *Psychiatric Clinics of North America* 14: 149–159.

Watkins, J. G., and Watkins, H. H. (1979). *Theory and practice of ego state therapy: A short-term therapeutic approach*. In H. Grayson, ed., *Short-term approaches to psychotherapy* (pp. 176–220). New York: Human Sciences Press.

Yates, J. L., and Nasby, W. (1993). Dissociation, affect, and network models of memory: An integrative proposal. *Journal of Traumatic Stress* 6: 305–326.

CHAPTER 12

Metamorphosis
The Self Assumes Animal Form
Jean Goodwin and Reina Attias

One of the most extreme and devastating alterations of body image is the complete loss of human form that occurs in individuals who episodically experience themselves as animals. This type of pathological metamorphosis involves interferences with thinking, behavior, sensation and emotions that include preoccupations with the animal and intense experiences during which the individual behaves or feels like an animal and believes at times that he or she has in fact become the animal.

This kind of pathological animal identification must be distinguished from numerous other metaphoric, ritual and mythologic uses of animal transformations (Massey 1976). Such instances include animal transformations used to depict sexual and aggressive drives. Freud was conceptualizing in this way when he said of "Rat-Man": "He could truly be said to find a living likeness of himself in the rat" (Freud 1909/1955, 216). It is this intense drive experience that is being depicted when Zeus takes animal form in order to rape his young victims. Half-human, half-animal figures like the centaur and Pan imply the incorporation of extraordinary sexual or aggressive powers. Animal transformation can appear as punishment when drive behaviors become immoral or inhuman. This is the fate that befalls Lucius in "The Golden Ass."

Images of metamorphosis may be used as well to describe the desire to communicate or merge with nature in an empathic mode. Thus, an animal identity may be used to convey the natural spontaneous or childlike side of a human being. When described as shape shifting, it may signify the acquisition of magical powers and expanded arcane knowledge.

At least since the Paleolithic, circumpolar peoples have developed artistic, ritual and mythologic modes for expressing this feeling of kinship to animals and the natural world. These survive in modern Western traditions in stories of saints who communicate with birds and animals, in folk dances in which animals are pantomimed, in stories and cartoons about talking animals, and in linguistic etymologies revealing connections between powerful animals, and words we use to conceptualize the sacred. For example, "psyche" can signify "butterfly" in Greek, and the English words "burial," "bier" and "barrow" reference ancient funeral rites in which the corpse was wrapped into a bearskin (Shepard and Sanders 1985).

Although these nonpathological elements of the mythology of metamorphosis color the cases we will describe, the primary phenomenology involves devastating alterations of self-image, thinking and behavior. Cases meeting our clinical criteria can be found in historical contexts (particularly in materials describing werewolves), in the general psychiatric literature and recently in psychiatric case reports involving trauma and dissociation.

The idea of traumatic origins of metamorphosis is found in myths as well as in contemporary contexts. Thus the Hindu deity Ganesh is described as acquiring an elephant's head when his own human child's head is cut off by his mother's lover. Greek legend gives us Philomela, who is transformed into a swallow after her brother-in-law rapes her and cuts out her tongue so she cannot tell (this is why the swallow has no song). Io is turned into a cow when ravished by Zeus. In the *Odyssey*, Circe transforms the invading marauders into pigs, perhaps preemptively to prevent them from raping her, thereby putting at risk her own human form (Pinsent 1969; Gardner, Wills and Goodwin 1995).

With the rediscovery of childhood trauma in the past twenty-five years, case reports have emerged mirroring these mythic sequences. Patients describe childhood experiences of physical or sexual assault; later, metamorphic experiences or behaviors appear; eventually dissociative identity disorder (DID) may be diagnosed, linking metamorphic phenomena to animal identifications within a particular ego state. Such cases seem to be quite rare, with specialist clinicians observing perhaps one or two in a lifetime of clinical practice. However, they are of interest to the student of body-image distortion, because they represent an extreme adaptation in this area. These extreme cases shed light on the more common experience of victims of human-inflicted trauma in which something has happened that jeopardizes their human status in a fundamental way.

Kafka's *The Metamorphosis* (1915/1992) is the work of literature that best fits the symptomatic definition of pathological metamorphosis proposed here, together with the postulated link to childhood trauma and dissociative symptoms. This work of art allows us to explore the psychic structure and meaning of this phenomenon at a deeper level (Seyppel 1956). Kafka's personal history of deprivation and emotional abuse echoes in this story as he describes the subjective experience of pathological metamorphosis and simultaneously occurring dissociative phenomena. Also of interest to us was Kafka's last story, "Josephine, the Songstress, or the Mouse People" (1924/1992), completed as he was dying of tuberculosis. This story, also told from the viewpoint of a nonhuman protagonist, seems to tame and transform the dilemmas posed in *The Metamorphosis*, perhaps providing a map for patterns of resolution that may be anticipated in clinical cases. Thus although Kafka's fictional character Gregor in *The Metamorphosis* gives us an example of one who has developed the most pathological and rare form of animal identification, Kafka himself provides examples of the more common uses of animal identifications by hurt children as they struggle to express and transform their pain.

HISTORICAL AND CLINICAL CASES OF PATHOLOGICAL METAMORPHOSIS

Children commonly converse and make friends with real and imaginary animals. Freud's only reference to the assumption of an animal identity involved a four-year-old boy who, after his kitten died, announced that he had now become the kitten and crawled about on all fours (Freud 1948). This normal developmental experience animates the ritual and mythological uses of animal symbolism described above. Outside of these contexts it is unusual for an adult to behave as an animal and experience the self as assuming animal form. Such cases are usually remarked in the historical record.

Perhaps the earliest case is found in the Old Testament, where the Babylonian king Nebuchadnezzar (605–562 B.C.E.; Keck et al. 1988) is described as believing he is an ox and eating grass during a time-limited and apparently depressive illness. Tales of lycanthropy and werewolves (Fahy 1989; Otten 1986) first appeared in Greek literature, where they are explained as punitive consequences of eating human flesh. St. Augustine believed these trans-

formations did not affect the real and sacred human body, but only an imagined double that he called the "phantasticum" (Oates 1989). In the Middle
Ages, "werewolf" was a synonym for "outlaw" and signaled permission to
hunt such exiles down as if they were animals (White 1990). Inquisition
campaigns against werewolves were probably targeting some ordinary
murderers, some of the mentally ill—especially melancholic depressives—
and also practitioners of animistic rituals and dances (Ginzburg 1966/1983).
However, certain Inquisition cases seem to meet the criteria for pathological
animal transformations. For example, in 1541 a suspect insisted that he was
a wolf despite the Inquisitor's skepticism. When asked where his fur was, he
replied "inside." He died on the table while a surgeon searched for the "inside" fur (Oates 1989).

Occasional cases in the psychiatric literature (Noll 1992) seem also to meet
criteria. In the 1970s Coll and coworkers (1975) reported the case of an elderly Irish woman who, in the presence of family members, crawled on
hands and knees barking at them aggressively like a dog. When psychiatrically hospitalized, she said that she had believed she was a dog. There was
a long history of depression, and metamorphic symptoms disappeared
when her depression resolved. Although specific questions regarding possible traumatic origins were not asked, it was noted that her childhood history
included a crowded family of eleven siblings and the death of her mother
when she was ten years old, with subsequent separation from siblings in
foster situations.

The largest single series of cases involving both animal behaviors and the
experience of transformation are twelve reports collected at McLean Hospital (Keck et al. 1988). The patients were diagnosed with a variety of illnesses;
eight had bipolar diagnoses. They also experienced a variety of outcomes
varying from complete remission to maintaining animal identity and behaviors unchanged. Typical of these cases is that of a single man in his twenties
who had believed since age eleven that he was a cat trapped inside a human
body. He said that the secret of his cat identity had been told to him by the
family cat, who subsequently taught him cat language. Although continuing
his daytime work in school and then in a job, virtually all of his spare time
for the preceding thirteen years had been spent in feline activities. He spoke
with cats, hunted with cats, frequented their gathering places and had sexual activity with them. He had fallen in love with a tigress at a local zoo and,
although she did not requite his love, was making plans to free her. His diagnosis was recurrent depression, but his animal beliefs and behaviors were

completely refractory to antidepressant treatment. Childhood history was not included in the published case.

ANIMAL METAMORPHOSIS, CHILDHOOD TRAUMA AND DISSOCIATION

Starting in the 1970s, as dissociative disorders were better defined and more intensely studied, it became possible to understand phenomena involving animal behaviors and identities in the context of an alter within a dissociative identity system that had evolved in response to childhood trauma (Schenk et al. 1989; Smith 1989). Hendrickson, McCarty and Goodwin published five such cases (1990). The following is perhaps the most complete in this series in terms of meeting our criteria for metamorphosis as well as illustrating other psychological phenomena associated with animal identifications and the multiple interconnections of these with childhood abuses and traumatization.

A thirty-eight-year-old woman presented for therapy with multiple somatic symptoms and chronic self-cutting. She made many references to animals during treatment, culminating in her disclosure of participating as a young child in her father's killing and dismembering of a mother cat and her kittens. Since age eight she had heard the sounds of kittens crying inside her. The cries became audible to her when her father would physically and sexually abuse her and later whenever she narrated these episodes in psychotherapy. She was afraid that others could hear the cats crying and would condemn her for her part in her father's animal tortures and the sexual abuse. As treatment progressed, she revealed that she had an idea as a child that she might help the mother cat and kittens by taking them inside herself. The father had explained his attack on the animals as punishment because the cat had become pregnant. He had threatened to do the same to the patient should she ever become pregnant.

Ultimately in psychotherapy, she began to discuss fears of pregnancy, which emerged in adolescence as the sexual abuse continued. While disclosing these terrifying fears, she switched and became "the cat." The cat handled the fears and guilt about sexuality and pregnancy and also handled the self-cutting, which was done with a razor blade held lengthwise with fingers hyperextended and curved to resemble claws. The cat also made numerous superficial scratches on the face and chest of any adult sexual partner the patient became involved with. In this case the animal behaviors and the experience of being an animal could be understood as an identity state in an internal dissociative system.

Working with such cases illuminates the various clinical manifestations of animal identities and fantasies. Specific symptoms in these patients included: (1) feeling like an animal or that a particular body part has become animal-like; (2) hearing animal calls inside one's head; (3) fear of a particular animal; (4) excessive protective involvement with a particular animal; (5) cruelty to animals; (6) reports of conversations with animals; (7) the experience of animals as protectors, guides or guards; and (8) animal-like behaviors, including scratching, crawling, licking, growling or eating like an animal.

In this series the traumatic precursors to pathological metamorphosis included:

1. Cases in which the individual witnessed torture and killing of animals (often used as threats to enforce silence and compliance) or the sadistic killing of a loved pet;
2. Experiences of being treated like an animal;
3. Involvement in sex with animals or in sexual practices experienced by the child as bestial;
4. Implicit or explicit threats enforcing silence, which had driven the child into a nonverbal stance experienced as animal-like.

These animal representations and internalizations provide a coherent set of metaphors for expressing unspeakable cruelty. The choice of these images suggests that the children perceive the abuse as a violation at the level of a transgression of natural law, which calls into question not only their status as member of the family and as a "good" member of the community, but also their status as a member of the human race.

In these extreme situations the animal ego states serve many psychic functions for the traumatized child:

1. To improve the chances for survival by containing and separating the rage and aggression of the victim;
2. To comply with enforced silence by encoding and representing knowledge of the abuse nonverbally or through behaviors or bodily symptoms;
3. To permit preservation of loving memories of the lost or killed animal and the aspect of the self that was able to love; at the same time,

there is a belief that the animal was victimized because the child loved it; therefore the child's love itself has become contaminated and must be segregated because it is felt as potentially lethal;

4. To represent memories and identifications with the most violent acts of the perpetrator; the discovery of an animal alter should prompt the therapist to reassess the patient's potential for violence to self or others.

Although these dissociative cases provide more detail than previously published cases about the context and development of animal identities, there remains a sense of incompleteness, mystery and lack of closure. Because the extreme cases are so rare and because the patients are often too ill to be accessible to depth psychotherapy, therapists who encounter such a case are often left with intense feelings, unanswered questions and a sense that they have touched on a layer of psychic experience that is fundamental but somehow impenetrable.

The following study of Kafka's *The Metamorphosis* attempts to provide a framework within which these extreme cases may be understood and a bridge to deep layers of the psyche in which animals and humans are still in connection—layers that remain aspects of the traumatized child's world and self-representations.

KAFKA'S *THE METAMORPHOSIS*: BIOGRAPHICAL SOURCES OF A LITERARY CASE OF ANIMAL TRANSFORMATION

Franz Kafka, born in 1883, wrote his most famous novella, *The Metamorphosis*, in 1912, when he was almost thirty years old. The main character is Gregor Samsa, a dutiful adult son living with his parents and younger sister and helping to support them through his job as a traveling salesman. The novella's opening sentence describes Gregor waking one morning from troubled dreams to find that he has been transformed into a "monstrous insect." The story then chronicles the consequences of this metamorphosis, which include losing his job, terrifying family and visitors, being excluded, confined, abused, ignored and ultimately starved to death. Gregor emphatically believes himself to be an insect. He also meets our second criterion of behaving like an animal: He loses speech, loses his taste for human foods like milk and seems no longer to wear clothing. (This might explain why female visitors are relieved when he devises a strategy for draping his body with a sheet.) Some new behaviors are insectlike: He seems to be inhabiting the floor of his room, where he sleeps under the couch, and locomotes by rocking, crawling or squirming.

The story is told entirely from Gregor's viewpoint, so we share his emotional reactions and coping mechanisms, which include trancing, immersion in fantasy, depersonalization, amnesia, derealization and identity confusion. We participate as well in Gregor's tireless efforts to justify his family's maltreatment of him as he reminds himself of how loathsome his metamorphosis has made him.

This novella is a source of continuing literary and critical interest, in part because all of the phenomena depicted could be explained as the result of Gregor's delusion or equally well as an actual animal transformation (Binion 1981). This tension is familiar to therapists working with DID patients who often shift between understanding alters as their own creative products and insisting on their reality as actual beings (see Chapter 11). Kafka himself was aware of the importance of maintaining this absolute ambiguity, since he instructed his publishers, "The insect itself must not be illustrated. . . . It cannot be shown at all, not even from a distance" (Wagenbach 1984, 155 [1915]).

Hayman (1982) suggests that Kafka's fiction is inextricable from his other introspective writing in journals and letters: "In all genres Kafka is talking to himself about himself" (p. 290). At the time he wrote *The Metamorphosis*, Kafka, like Gregor, was living in the parental home and helping financially by working in the family business (Hayman 1982; Pawel 1984). He described his room as "a prison without walls" (Kafka 1974, 60). He did not move out until after the publication of *The Metamorphosis*.

Available material on Franz Kafka's childhood and adult symptomatology suggest that he had personal knowledge both of traumatic child maltreatment and of dissociative phenomena. He was the eldest child in a middle-class Jewish family in Prague. He was aware from childhood of his Jewish community's perilous vulnerability to persecution (Pawel 1984). Within his own family there were additional stressors. Before he was six, two younger brothers were born and died, one at the age of two years and the other at six months. Three younger sisters were born when Kafka was between the ages of six and nine. The mother, who lost her own mother at age three and her grandmother by suicide at age four (Mittscherlich-Nielsen 1983), seems to have been unavailable and preoccupied with submission to her husband. Kafka's troubled relationship to his father is described in detail in a fifty-page letter he wrote at age thirty-six; his mother never delivered it to his father. The letter reveals a relationship characterized by silence and misunderstanding sustained by explicit and implicit threats from the autocratic father. Kafka wrote: "I can't recall you ever having abused me directly, in downright abusive terms . . . but you had an extremely effective rhetorical method of upbringing . . . which included abuse, threats, irony, spiteful laughter, and—often enough—self-pity" (Kafka 1919/1954, 151). The contradictions embedded in this sentence convey Kafka's painful ambivalence about confronting the father he saw as a "bewildering" tyrant who had "convinced me . . . of my incapacity" (Brod 1937/1955, 20 [1919]).

Emblematic of this relationship is a memory that has the vivid sensory qualities of a screen memory and that may be exemplary of many similar incidents. Kafka writes (1919): "One night I kept constantly whimpering for water. . . . You snatched me out of my bed, carried me out onto the balcony, and left me there alone for a while in my nightgown with the door locked. . . . I subsequently became a rather obedient child, but I suffered inner damage as a result" (Noy and Sharron 1984, 298). In *The Metamorphosis* as well as in other writings, images recur of locked doors, painful rejection and isolation, nighttime assaults, intense thirst and bitter cold.

Kafka describes in letters and diaries dissociative symptoms that seem to have begun in childhood. He remembers in grade school wishing "that I could rise like a ghost" and believing that "given favorable circumstances, one could disappear . . . and one could also die in life" (Kafka 1953, 133–134 [1920]). In his diaries Kafka describes himself as "without weight, without bones, without body" (Kafka 1976, 48 [1912]). In "Wedding Preparations in the Country," he creates a character who depersonalizes when caught in obsessive intrapsychic conflict: "I'll send my body all dressed up while I myself lie in bed . . . and assume the shape of a giant insect . . . and I would whisper a very few words, instructions to my dreary body. . . . It leaves swiftly and will get everything done to perfection while I have my rest" (Kafka 1908/1954, 6–7).

Kafka's personal writings convey a sense of enormous distance from his own feelings and body. He says, "I am separated from everything by a space to whose limits I can't even force my way out" (Brod 1937/1995, 96 [1911]). About his body he wrote, "I have a feeling of pressure in my stomach, as if my stomach were a person and were about to cry" (Brod 1937/1995, 294 [1909]), and "I felt so loose in my skin that, had anyone given me a shake, I would have fallen out of it altogether" (Kafka 1967/1973, 28 [1913]).

He was aware that his emotions found voice in his body: "My fits of despair have a way of ending not with a leap out the window but into a doctor's office" (Pawel 1984, 346 [1916]). When his tuberculosis was diagnosed in 1917, he wrote in a letter to a friend, "It seems to me as if my brains and my lungs came to an understanding behind my back" (Wagenbach 1984, 185). Later he wrote, "These discussions between brain and lung which went on without my knowledge may have been terrible" (Kafka 1953, 21 [1920]).

Kafka experienced other bodily symptoms common in adult survivors of child maltreatment. Seyppel culled the following from Kafka's writings: insomnia, headaches, sudden sensations of cold, dullness, bad nerves and absentmindedness. Kafka wrote extensively about his headaches, connecting them with the pressure to release "the tremendous world I have in my head" (Brod 1937/1995, 90). Max Brod describes Kafka's persistent difficulties with self-care, especially around eating and keeping himself warm. One month prior to the writing of *The Metamorphosis*, Brod became so concerned abut his friend's suicidal thoughts and accident-proneness that he wrote a letter to Kafka's mother (Brod 1937/1995, 93).

Noy and Sharron (1984) have suggested that the mother's preoccupation with her dead infant sons may have led Franz to fantasize that only by being dead could he win his mother's attention and affection. The search for a way to die without dying may also have been necessary to cope with the father's rages and the sense that within his family love was inextricably mingled with a "ruthless" incomprehension (Hayman 1982, 153). It was as if both parents loved him, but in ways that required him to give up his life (Novick and Novick 1996).

For Kafka, as well as for other survivors of child abuse, keeping silent became a way of life and any breaking of silence was experienced as extremely dangerous. In his letter to his father Kafka writes: "I lost the capacity to talk: your threat 'not a word of contradiction!' and the raised hand that accompanied it have gone with me ever since" (Kafka 1919/1954, 150–151). In Brod's translation the passage continues: "I began to stammer and stutter, even that was too much for you, so finally I shut up, at first probably out of pig-headedness, later because I could neither think nor speak in front of you" (Brod 1937/1995, 23).

Kafka's childhood whimper was so silenced that as an adult he was unable to cry. He wrote, "To me other people's tears are a strange incomprehensible phenomenon" (Brod 1937/1995, 96 [1911]). Kafka described himself as able to weep only when reading particular passages he had written. As he said: "A book must be the axe for the frozen sea within us" (Wagenbach 1984, 35 [1904]). During one of his illnesses he wrote that he "was cheated out of the pleasure of yelling at the doctor by a brief fainting spell" (Pawel 1984, 215 [1910]). Thus even in adulthood, dissociative defenses automatically interrupted and suppressed Kafka's protest cry.

In his writing Kafka overcame this prohibition against revealing his pain. "Writing is a form of prayer," he said (Brod 1937/1995, 78). He also said about his writing, "This is the only way in which I can ever get better" (Brod 1937/1995, 97 [1914]) and "God doesn't want me to write, but I simply must" (Brod 1937/1995, 295 [1903]). The childhood struggle to keep silent reappeared in the struggle with his creative talent. In 1910 he complained to his friend Brod, "I cannot write. . . . My whole body warns me against each word; each word, before allowing me to write it, first looks around in all directions. The sentences literally go to pieces on me. I see their insides and then have to stop quickly" (Kafka 1974, 21 [1910]). He wrote to his father, "My writing was all about you" (Kafka 1919/1954, 177). As a further example of Kafka's awareness that his writing represented an ambivalent, fearful disclosure of his childhood abuse, he referred to *The Metamorphosis* as "an indiscretion" (Noy and Sharron 1984, 297 [1915]). Modern scholars have agreed that it is "one of the most profound testaments of the victimology of child abuse" (Miller 1985, 197).

SELF-TRANSFORMATION IN ANIMAL FORM: MONSTER TO MOUSE

In Kafka's fiction, personal writings and dreams, animal metaphors appear repeatedly as expressions of the suppressed feelings so common in the abused child: rage, helplessness, rejection, terror, dissociation, alienation and self-hatred. For example, after an argument with his mother, Kafka described himself as spending a whole day lying in bed as if he were a giant insect unable to move (Hayman 1982, 143–144). He described the Jewish people as having "the heroism of the cockroach" (Kafka 1953, 184 [1921]), because they refused to leave a place where they were hated and persecuted. His tubercular cough he nicknamed "the animal" (Benjamin 1934/1968). In his diaries there are numerous entries in which he identifies himself with animals. He dreamed that he was a donkey who looked like a greyhound (Kafka 1976, 94 [1911]). He felt for a moment as if he had armor around his body (Kafka 1976, 39 [1911]); he says, "I heard sounds coming out of myself that were like the sounds of a little kitten" (Kafka 1974, 20 [1910]). He also refers to himself as a snake, a dog and a rat. These metaphors may have been facilitated by the fact that the name "Kafka" means jackdaw in Czech (Hayman 1982, 6).

Seyppel (1956) says about Kafka's fiction: "There are hardly any stories in which Kafka did not include at least one significant reference to creatures of the animal kingdom." Animal references appear with greatest frequency in his personal writings, the notebooks and diaries, and in the stories he was working on in the last years of his life that were not intended for publication. In these posthumously published stories, we see chronic fear and hyperalertness embodied in the creature who is frantically digging in "The Burrow." Mutilations and distortions in self-image are conveyed in "A Sport." This chimera, part lamb and part cat, is repeatedly described as "a legacy from my father" (Kafka 1936/1946, 238). Children are drawn to its softness and curious about its lack of fellows and its inability to reproduce. However, the creature itself longs for the sacrificial knife, which seems to constitute both its mutilative origins and its destiny. As in so many of these sketches, the sexual and aggressive energies preserved in the "sport" are ultimately turned against the self; as Kafka tells us in one of his aphorisms, "The animal wrests the whip from its master and whips itself in order to become master" (Kafka 1954, 37). In the story "The Giant Mole" (Kafka 1936/1946), Kafkaesque confusion arises regarding the existence of a monstrous creature seen by only one man. If we substitute child abuse for the Giant Mole, the confusion about whether it exists or not becomes familiar.

Kafka's lifelong exploration of animal metaphors culminated in his last story, "Josephine, the Songstress, or the Mouse People" (Kafka 1924/1992), written in the final months of his life, when he was bedridden and unable to speak because his tuberculosis had spread to the larynx. In "Josephine, the Songstress," we enter the world of the mouse people as described to us by the narrator, a member of this innumerable and beleaguered tribe. The narrator's burden is to convey to us the importance of the songstress Josephine as the symbol and essence of his people. Josephine's piping voice seems to give this people the strength to endure bad news and to accept the catastrophes and sacrifices that are their lot. At the end of the story we learn that Josephine has disappeared and may be dead.

The centrality of animal images for Kafka is underlined by their presence both in his most famous work and in this lesser-known last work completed ten years later. Kafka himself had achieved in the decade that separates these stories a full-time career as a creative artist, autonomy from his family, a love partner and a secure personal worldview that sustained him, even in the face of death. The maturation that had taken place around issues of autonomy, relationship, creativity and transcendence is reflected in the way in which animal images are used in each story.

We will discuss four elements conveyed by the animal image: (1) helplessness and need for care, (2) fear of bodily injury and bodily loss, (3) debasement and loss of human status and (4) loss of language.

HELPLESSNESS AND NEED FOR CARE

In *The Metamorphosis,* Gregor's animal transformation underlines his helpless, solitary, alienated position within his family and the fragmentation occurring within his self system. The disorganized interactions between Gregor's insect and human aspects have rendered him immobile and almost completely dysfunctional.

In contrast, Josephine is a mouse among mice, although an atypical, demanding and oversensitive specimen. She functions at a high level and, unlike Gregor, she has acquired peers. Her struggle is to place herself workably among her fellows, preserving individuality and artistry while being only one of a swarming, teeming mass of mice.

In "Josephine" the animal metaphor evokes the dehumanizing anti-Semitic invective of the 1920s, with its scurrilous comparisons of the Jewish people to parasitic vermin. Kafka transforms these slurs into a lyrical paean to the mouse people and implicitly to the strength of his own Jewish people: "A people which, accustomed to suffering, unsparing of itself, swift in decision, well acquainted with death . . . as prolific as it is courageous . . . has somehow always managed to save itself" (p. 226). In his own life Kafka did not minimize European anti-Semitism and would have immigrated to Palestine, had he recovered from his tuberculosis. All three of his sisters perished in concentration camps.

Both stories attempt to solve the problem of the uncaring father. As shown in *The Metamorphosis,* he is a violent, self-centered man who experiences fathering as a depleting burden from which Gregor's withdrawal into an insect identity releases both father and son. Gregor is injured by the father repeatedly—crushed in a doorway, beaten, hit by objects thrown at him. In "Josephine," the entire people take on the role of parenting Josephine and, by sharing the burden, master it; they are able to discharge fatherly duties in a nurturing, nonabusive way.

Both rework elements of Kafka's "screen memory" of father responding to his request for water by locking him outside. Gregor in insect form becomes terribly thirsty, but then is disgusted by the milk offered by his sister. Ultimately he is excluded from the rest of the family and left hungry and thirsty behind a locked door. In the later story these elements have become more metaphoric. Josephine herself is described as "a communal beaker of peace which the people drink quickly as if before battle" (p. 226). She is separated from the others not by a locked door, but by her artistry and her band of protectors.

In *The Metamorphosis*, the mother protests her concern and care for Gregor, but never once looks directly into his face (Binion 1981). Josephine will claim that in order for her audience to hear her song, they must be able to see her face.

The climate of scarcity in the Samsa household foreshadows that only one sibling is likely to survive, and we see Gregor's sister begin to flourish as he declines. The mouse people are described as so teemingly prolific that older siblings never have a chance to have a real childhood. However, Josephine manages to make her piping cry heard and is surrounded (like Kafka in his last days) by devoted attendants. Although her piping is described as childish and melancholy, it also conveys some of the joy of childhood, "that unfathomable gaiety which persists and cannot be extinguished" (p. 230).

Both protagonists struggle with questions of work and activity and whether each is a good enough worker. Gregor's metamorphosis finally provides him an adequate excuse for not working. Josephine clamors constantly to be spared from work and develops bodily symptoms to justify her demands—fatigue, a limp and faintness. These debates seem to reflect Kafka's protest about family demands for nonwriting, remunerative work as well his own awareness of the intrapsychic hazards of this writing.

FEAR OF BODILY INJURY AND BODILY LOSS

In *The Metamorphosis*, the first sentence informs us of Gregor's discovery of his catastrophic bodily crisis. In "Josephine," we learn only on the last page that she has disappeared. In one instance the body has been ruinously and monstrously changed; in the other the bodily self has vanished and vaporized.

Kafka tried to explain in the letter to his father how tenuous the hold on one's body becomes in a traumatic, chaotic childhood: "Since there was nothing at all I was certain of, since I needed to be provided at every instant with a new confirmation of my existence, since nothing was my very own . . . naturally even the thing nearest at hand, my own body, became insecure" (Kafka 1919/1954, 178). Earlier he had journaled, "I write . . . out of despair over my body and over a future with this body" (Kafka 1974, 19 [1910]).

The animal bodies of both protagonists are described as beset by multiple somatic and dissociative symptoms. Gregor's body is stiff, unable to move, itchy, covered with white spots, dully aching, in pain all over, damaged. He feels the lower parts of it no longer belong to him. He experiences agonies of anxiety and self-reproach, quakes and is breathless, suffering "little fits of suffocation." After his father beats him, he falls into a trancelike sleep and imagines he is hanging peacefully from the ceiling. Vision becomes more and more indistinct. He is sleepless or has troubled dreams and is often drowsy in the daytime. He bangs his head and body. He loses his appetite, food disgusts him and he feels bloated. His grooming deteriorates and by the end of the story he is coated with dust, fluff and hairs.

Josephine is described as suffering a shorter litany of symptoms: She is weak, delicate, quivering, limping, swooning, exhausted, weeping, faint and hoarse. Her own proneness to trance phenomena is mirrored by the trance state that her singing produces in the audience. Unlike Gregor, who persistently asserts his harmlessness despite the terror he engenders and whose insect form is without teeth, Josephine is capable of furious rages, and even bites.

It underlines the trauma-based nature of these somatic symptoms that Gregor's list is so much longer than Josephine's. At the time Kafka wrote *The Metamorphosis* he was in good health physically, but in terrible suicidal psychic distress. His depiction of bodily defects reflected his fractured self-image: "If I lacked an upper lip here, an earlobe there, a rib here, a finger there . . . there still wouldn't be enough physical correlations to my inner imperfections" (Hayman 1982, 81 [1910]). While writing "Josephine," his real body was dying, but many gaps and distortions in the imaginary body had been restored.

For both protagonists, the loss of human form is but a waystation on the road toward the ultimate loss of the body in death. Gregor starves to death and his body is thrown in the garbage. We are told that Josephine, despite her heroism and fame, will be forgotten.

We know that Kafka himself was terrified of mice (Kafka 1974, 166 [1917]). In plunging into the mouse world, he was confronting his most paralyzing fears, including the fear of death.

Writing the story of Josephine may have helped Kafka deal with those elements of his mortal illness that seemed like a dreadfully exact repetition of his childhood abuse. As in his screen memory, the tubercular invasion of his larynx left him unable to speak or to drink. But for his work on the Josephine story, which he was proofreading on the day before his death, these powerful reminders might have triggered childlike defenses such as those that overwhelmed him during an earlier illness (Pawel 1984, 215 [1910]) when he fainted and experienced a voluptuous passivity. His dying words (written on slips of paper as well as spoken) illustrate these shifts. "Don't leave me," he said to his doctor. This plea conjures images of Gregor cowering before an image of Death, which wears the face of the punishing father. "I'm not leaving," said the doctor, who was also his friend. "Oh," replied Kafka. "It is I who am leaving" (Brod 1937/1995, 212 [1924]). So, in this last small joke, Kafka places himself securely within the more mature worldview of Josephine. Death is not the triumph of the abuser, but Kafka's own final dissociative disappearing trick, his exit not to terrible exile, but to a destination of his own.

DEBASEMENT AND LOSS OF HUMAN STATUS

Gregor persists, even in insect form, in clinging to politeness, convention and compliance as methods for reinstating himself with his family. He conceals his symptoms as best he can and tries hard not to inconvenience anyone. Josephine, by contrast, has abandoned convention and makes demands with impunity. Perhaps because she no longer struggles to please or appease, she has become a great favorite. Rather than concealing her symptoms, she suffers them onstage.

Gregor had futilely imagined redeeming all the losses surrounding his inhuman situation by sending his sister to the conservatory to study violin. Josephine actually achieves this sublimatory redemption through her singing, which provides sanctuary both for her and her audience.

So the animal transformation, which in *The Metamorphosis* conveys the terrible abasement and alienation of the trauma victim, becomes in "Josephine" a metaphor for the universal transformative power of artistry and the mystical and oceanic connections between the individual and the community, connections that transcend even the boundaries of species. The animal image itself has been elevated and resolved at a transcendent level of internal organization. Unlike the insectiform Gregor, Josephine has reached mammalian status, sharing with humans warm-bloodedness and the possibility of connection.

Loss of Language

When Gregor tries to explain himself, only "unintelligible" squeaks emerge. Josephine can pipe only in a "small and feeble voice." She is "singing to deaf ears in any case" (p. 223). She is "fighting with all the might of her feeble vocal chords" (p. 225) for unconditional devotion. Music is an alternative to having a voice. Gregor's sister can communicate with him by playing her violin, and Josephine's singing is portrayed as an almost magical communication, "a message from the entire people to each individual" (p. 227).

Josephine's story is told in a much more organized way than is Gregor's. *The Metamorphosis* places us in Gregor's viewpoint; we experience at close range his confusion, pain, despair and dissociation. In "Josephine" the events are recounted in a cohesive narrative by an objective observer who takes a broad view that includes the multiple concerns of her present community and the entire future of her race. Kafka had struggled to resolve problems of narration in the letter to his father. Was he exaggerating, blaming or being unjust? "In reality things cannot fit together so neatly. . . . Life is more than a game of Patience." On the other hand, he tells his father, "Were the proofs to be corrected on the lines suggested . . . something so near the truth would be arrived at that it might comfort us both a little, and make our lives and our deaths easier" (Brod 1937/1995, 19 [1919]). "Josephine" may be understood as such a "correcting of the proofs," begun in *The Metamorphosis*, through which Kafka's individual trauma is transcended and comes to a new level of meaning in a universal context.

DISCUSSION

The clinical cases and artistic works reviewed above illustrate the most salient aspects of animal metamorphosis. When the self assumes animal form, this extreme alteration in body image leads to changes in bodily experience and self-image. When childhood history is available, these phenomena have been found to be linked to extreme abuse and neglect. The copresence of multiple dissociative symptoms also suggests a link with child abuse. The assumption of animal form inherently questions the sense of oneself as human. This questioning too links back to experiences of repeated or sadistic abuse during which the child judged the abusive adult's behavior as inhuman and knew that he or she as victim was not being treated humanely. To reexperience such moments of horror in the encounter with Gregor or with a patient's animal identity is profound and unsettling. In addition, such encounters open the door to very early layers of psychic reality in which the self is experienced as on the same plane as animals.

How is it that animal imagery is so intertwined with issues of traumatic childhood abuse? At one level the animal image in Kafka's fictional and personal writings can be understood in every case as a signifier representing such traumatic experience. The choice of an animal image symbolizes the "not-me" quality of trauma (Sullivan 1954). This distancing of trauma material from the self is an effort to deal with the painful emotions: sadness, terror, shame, retaliatory anger, rejection. It separates the self from the physical pain as well as from the traumatic symptoms that begin to cluster around the memory. For example, when Kafka dreams that he is a donkey who looks like a greyhound, the traumatologist hears him describing the donkeylike immobilization, numbness and pseudostupidity of acute traumatic dissociation. This coexists with the wish to escape the situation as swiftly as a greyhound, later manifesting as flights of phobic behavior as the trauma victim tries to avoid triggers.

Shifts from human to animal identity mirror the shifts from present reality to the distressing and shameful traumatic reality that characterizes posttraumatic flashback. As Kafka wrote in his diaries: "What else can happen but that the two worlds split apart, or at least clash in a fearful manner . . . for I am now a citizen of this other world, whose relationship to the ordinary one is the relationship of wilderness to cultivated land" (Fraiberg 1956, 48 [1922]).

Much of what we call Kafkaesque reflects the emotional climate of childhood trauma. The child feels there is no way out, there is a confusion of tongues, the child has no way to understand why he or she is being hurt and attacks are repeated relentlessly in an environment that seems to condone them.

At a higher level of magnification, animal transformations seem particularly potent at conveying four aspects of child abuse and trauma: (1) the terrifying helplessness of the betrayed child who, like an animal, needs care but instead has been hurt; (2) the fears of bodily injury or bodily loss; (3) the sense of loss of parts of the self, which results in the experience of the self as degraded and less than human; and (4) the loss of human language and narrative capacity; this has become necessary to keep the silence, but is also a neurophysiologic consequence of extreme trauma shock (Perry 1995).

Because at this deep level of the psyche every quality implies its opposite, each of these four aspects can be conceptualized as an axis that includes its polar counterpoint. Thus the animal identity also contains: (1) power and aggression, (2) a new less vulnerable body, (3) a new animal reality that provides a kind of sanctuary in which the true self can be preserved and (4) a freedom to use nonverbal modes to express the unspeakable.

These polarities are elegantly conveyed in *The Metamorphosis*. The insect Gregor, although childlike, atavistic, clumsy and speechless, also contains the power to frighten the perpetrator and to coerce the passive mother into providing some care. Although Gregor's loss of his human body is a metaphor for the death he has feared at the hands of his father, his new animal body offers armor and a new way to experience some form of embodiment that allows him finally to sense the bodily symptoms that are his first clues to his abuse. At the same time, the escape from the human body offers advantages in distancing him from disturbing bodily impingements, such as his emerging sexual feelings. Although the monstrous insect is a picture of self-degradation, Gregor's new animal reality provides him with many freedoms: He is able to quit the job he hates, to stay in bed all day, to eavesdrop at the door. Noncompliance, which was unthinkable for the human Gregor, becomes inevitable and more blame-free in the insect. One of the insect's first thoughts is of having "no intention of deserting my family." However, this separation from the intrusive and enmeshed family is exactly what the animal identity is able to achieve, although at terrible cost. Gregor cannot speak once he assumes insect form, but he does engineer pantomimes that render the abusive situation entirely visible. With the insect the father's intimidation and threats escalate quickly into palpable violence.

Although Gregor's fictional problems are at the extreme level described in psychiatric case histories, Kafka's own uses of animal identifications amount to a kind of self-administered art therapy (Miller 1985). Seyppel says: "This radical isolation in, and identification with, the animal means in the end, beyond psychoanalytical and anthropological interpretation, a return to the core of existence" (1956, 86). Because of the extremely paradoxical qualities of these animal identifications, the psychic way into them is simultaneously the pathway out. Kafka's continual return to animal themes is reminiscent of experiences in sandtray or art therapy, where the trauma victim returns repeatedly to animal figures or themes to construct progressively more coherent, autonomous, connected and transcendent worlds. The Josephine story can be seen as a final construction, resolving many of the issues raised in *The Metamorphosis*.

Our emphasis on the therapeutic aspect of Kafka's writings need not detract from their qualities as artistic works of genius. As Alice Miller wrote: "The prophetic power endures, not because some god or other whispered inspiration in his ear . . . but because he took his own experiences seriously and thought them through to their bitter end" (1985, 298).

This pathway to healing must wind through many obstacles. Patients experiencing moments of fragmentary animal identity may not disclose it, because they are afraid they are going mad. Until these are decoded, such experiences can seem merely revolting or terrifyingly alien. Diaz says of Gregor's animal alter, "This is the image of a creature for which we feel no sympathy, no companionship, certainly no admiration and which is of no use to us; it is ugly, bothersome and disgusting, if worthy of our notice at all" (1985, 298). This condition becomes intelligible once we realize that it represents, in condensed form, the child's self-condemning explanation for why the parent abused him (Fairbairn 1952). As Kafka finally realized in his letter to his father, these revolting qualities are reactive, not inherent: "It was you who were pushing me down into the filth, as if it were my destiny" (Kafka 1919/1954, 9.186) and "Why did I want to quit the world? Because 'he' would not let me live in it, his world" (Kafka 1974, 216 [1922]). Once this is understood, the animal identifications no longer seem psychotic. Miller says about Kafka: "His words provide so many young people with their first confirmation that what they find in their interior world is not necessarily madness" (Miller 1985, 275).

When patients come to understand that they are neither disgusting nor mad, the next task is to find a language expressive of the unspeakable experiences contained in the animal identity. Part of the insight that we glean from Kafka is that, for many patients, ordinary language is inadequate to this task. In the chaotic household, abuse has substituted for language. In *In the Penal Colony*, Kafka explains why the suffering inmate has not been told what his crime was: "There would be no point in telling him, he'll learn it on his body" (1919/1948, 197). Ordinary language seems weak and powerless compared to this language of violence and threat of violence with its attendant physiologic disruptions. The new language needed must contain a similar cathexis of bodily energy; this is the creative expression that can be forged out of bodily experiences of emotional pain and suffering as the traumatic material is reworked. The condensed lucidity of Kafka's prose bespeaks the price in emotional pain that he paid for it: "No one sings with such pure voice as those who live in deepest hell; what we take for the song of angels is their song" (Kafka 1953, 186 [1921]).

Clinicians guiding patients through this process need to be aware of its depth. What the patient needs most is a holding environment (Winnicott 1971) in which the new language can be crafted without fear of rejection or pathologizing. The clinician's human gaze restores and confirms the essential humanity of the animal identification. Kafka himself says it best: "This tempestuous or floundering or morasslike inner self is what we really are, but by the secret process by which words are forced out of us, our self-knowledge is brought to light . . . wonderful or terrible to behold. . . . Tell me that you understand it all, and yet go on loving me" (1967/1973, 198 [1913]).

REFERENCES

Benjamin, W. (1934/1968). Franz Kafka: On the tenth anniversary of his death. In W. Benjamin, *Illuminations* (pp. 111–140). New York: Schocken.

Binion, R. (1981). What The Metamorphosis means. In Binion, R., *Soundings: Psychohistorical and psycholiterary* (pp. 7–14). New York: Psychohistory Press.

Brod, M. (1937/1995). *Franz Kafka: A biography*. New York: Da Capo.

Coll, P. G., O'Sullivan, G., and Browne, P. A. (1975). Lycanthropy lives on. *British Journal of Psychiatry* 147: 201–202.

Diaz, N. G. (1988). *The radical self: Metamorphosis to animal form in modern Latin American narrative*. Columbia: University of Missouri Press.

Fahy, T. A. (1989). Lycanthropy: A review. *Journal of the Royal Society of Medicine* 82: 39–40.

Fairbairn, R. D. (1952). *Psychoanalytic studies of the personality*. London: Routledge and Kegan Paul.

Fraiberg, S. (1956). *Kafka and the dream. Partisan Review* 23: 47–69.

Freud, S. (1909/1955). Notes upon a case of obsessional neurosis. In S. Freud, *Standard edition of collected works*. Vol. 10 (pp. 153–319). London: Hogarth Press.

———. (1948). *Group psychology and the analysis of the ego*. London: Hogarth Press.

Gardner, R., Wills, S., And Goodwin, J. (1995). The Io myth: Origins and use of a narrative of sexual abuse. *Journal of Psychohistory* 23: 30–39.

Ginzburg, C. (1966/1983). *The night battles: Witchcraft and agrarian cults in the sixteenth and seventeenth centuries*. Baltimore: Johns Hopkins University Press.

Hayman, R. (1982). *Kafka: A biography*. New York: Oxford University Press.

Hyman, R. (1983). Kafka and the mice. In E. Kurzweil and W. Phillips, *Literature and psychoanalysis* (pp. 290–299). New York. Columbia University Press.

Hendrickson. K. M., McCarty, T., and Goodwin, J. (1990). Animal alters: Case reports. *Dissociation* 3: 214–217.

Kafka, F. (1908/1954). Preparations for a wedding in the country. In F. Kafka, *Dearest father: Stories and other writings* (pp. 2–33). New York: Schocken.

_____. (1915/1992). The transformation (metamorphosis). In F. Kafka, *The transformation and other stories*. Trans. M. Pasley. (Pp. 76–126). London: Penguin.

_____. (1919/1948). *The penal colony: Stories and short pieces*. New York: Schocken.

_____. (1919/1954). Letter to his father. In F. Kafka, *Dearest father: Stories and other writings*(pp. 138–196). New York: Schocken.

_____. (1924/1992). Josephine, the songstress, or: The mouse people. In F. Kafka, *The transformation (metamorphosis) and other stories*. Trans. M. Pasley. (Pp. 220–236). London: Penguin.

_____. (1936/1946). *The great wall of china: Stories and reflections*. New York: Schocken.

_____. (1953). *Letters to Milena*. New York: Schocken.

_____. (1954). *Dearest father: Stories and other writings*. New York: Schocken.

_____. (1967/1973). *Letters to Felice*. New York: Schocken.

_____. (1974). *I am a memory come alive: Autobiographical writings by Franz Kafka*. New York: Schocken.

_____. (1976). *The diaries, 1910–1923*. New York: Schocken.

Keck, P. E., Pope, H. G., Hudson, J. I., McElroy, S. L., and Kulick, A. R. (1988). Lycanthropy alive and well in the twentieth century. *Psychological Medicine* 18: 113–120.

Massey, I. (1976). *The gaping pig: Literature and metamorphosis*. Berkeley and Los Angeles: University of California Press.

Miller, A. (1985). *Thou shalt not be aware: Society's betrayal of the child*. New York: Farrar, Straus & Giroux.

Mitscherlich-Nielsen, M. (1983). Psychoanalytic notes on Franz Kafka. In E. Kurzweil and W. Phillips, *Literature and psychoanalysis* (pp. 270–289). New York: Columbia University Press.

Noll, R. (1992). *Vampires, werewolves and demons: Twentieth-century reports in the psychiatric literature*. New York: Brunner/Mazel.

Novick, J., and Novick, K. K. (1996). *Fearful symmetry: The development and treatment of sado-masochism*. Northvale, N.J.: Aronson.

Noy, R. S., and Sharron, A. (1984). Child abuse in Kafka's eyes: The victim's invisible metamorphosis. *Victimology* 9 (2): 296–303.

Oates, C. (1989). Metamorphosis and lycanthropy in Franche-Comte, 1521–1643. In M. Feher, *Fragments for a history of the human body, Part 1* (pp. 305–363). New York: Urzone.

Otten, C. F. (1986). *A lycanthropy reader: Werewolves in Western culture.* Syracuse: Syracuse University Press.

Pawel, E. (1984). *The nightmare of reason: A life of Franz Kafka.* New York: Farrar, Straus, & Giroux.

Perry, B. D. (1995). Neurobiological sequelae of childhood trauma: PTSD in children. In M. M. Murburg, *Catecholamine function in post-traumatic stress disorder* (pp. 233–255). Washington D.C.: American Psychiatric Press.

Pinsent, J. (1969). *Greek Mythology.* London: Hamlyn.

Price, G. M. (1990). Non-rational guilt in victims of trauma. *Dissociation* 3:160–164.

Schenk, C., Milner, D., Horwitz, T., Bundlie, S., and Mahowald, M. (1989). Dissociative disorders presenting as somnambulism. Polysomnographic video and clinical documentation. *Dissociation* 1: 194–204.

Seyppel, J. H. (1956). The animal theme and totemism in Franz Kafka. *American Imago* 13: 69–93.

Shepard, P., and Sanders, B. (1985). *The sacred paw.* New York: Viking.

Smith, S. G. (1989). Multiple personality disorder with human and non-human subpersonality components. *Dissociation* 2: 52–56.

Sullivan, H. S. (1954). *The psychiatric interview.* New York: Norton.

Wagenbach, K. (1984). *Franz Kafka: Pictures of a life.* New York: Pantheon.

White, D. G. (1990). *Myths of the dog-man.* Chicago: University of Chicago Press.

Winnicott, D. W. (1971). *Playing and reality.* London: Tavistock.

PART IV

Reflections
Body and Self in Dialogue

This intertwining of the physical and psychological within a self-consciousness that involves itself in the parts of the body is summarized in . . . the Homeric heroes . . . whose interior I is none other than the organic I.

J. P. Vernant (1989, 22)

I have come into the inheritance of my own body.

Analysand (Scott 1951, 257)

Here in the body are all the sacred rivers; here are the sun and the moon as well as all the pilgrimage places. . . . I have not encountered another temple as blissful as my own body.

Saraha, Tibetan poet
(Klon-chen-pa Dei-med-odzer 1989, 375)

The body is our beloved, our best and sweetest companion in the present sadness.
St. Christine Mirabilis, thirteenth century (Bynum 1995, 333)

My belief is in the blood and flesh as being wiser than the intellect. The body-unconscious is where life bubbles up in us. It is how we know we are alive . . . and in touch with the vivid reaches of the cosmos.

D. H. Lawrence (quoted in Levine 1990–1991, 27)

The Body Finds Its Voice

Readers who have reached this place are ready to begin a journey. Here are the voices of patients as they began that journey of exploration at the boundary of body and self:

Someone took away from me a part of myself, the part that enables one to protect the self from being invaded and torn open and violated and destroyed. . . . They crushed and mutilated that part of me . . .

My body doesn't belong to me. It's as if because he possessed it, he owns it. It feels like a house I can be thrown out of at any time.

My body is like a burning house I have to flee.

It's like a scar on my body that no one else can see, but I think they can . . .

It's like a strawberry mark on the skin, glowing red.

It's like a red hot poker burned on my arms . . .

It's like something, maybe the pain, stopped my breasts from growing.

Every time I come here, I wake up in the morning and my body is covered with bruises.

I don't want to talk about why I threw up the other night. . . . She knows why I threw up and I don't want to talk to her.

Sometimes I think that my body is the only proof I have that it all happened.

I can doubt my own mind, but when my own body acts up in response to being heard with fresh but somehow familiar symptoms, I know that I am telling the truth.

This is a picture about my kidneys and how they are hurting, my kids-knees?

I broke out in painful hives around the vagina and the inside of the thighs. I somehow knew this was a message but I ignored it . . . and the next morning I got married and by then they were all gone.

I realized I wanted to tell you all the things I couldn't tell my mother about my body pains, hurts, fears and that the fact that I can do so, that I can call you and report in on my physical symptoms is different than it was with my mother and that something good is happening out of that.

My vagina feels terrible—swollen and sore and like something is inside it. I think my vagina is lying. I could never trust any thing about my body.

I think there's a body feeling telling us something from my vagina. (Five-year-old after documented sexual abuse, Novick and Novick 1996, 213)

Over the last few years, I have made the harrowing journey common to many—remembering and speaking the truth about being sexually abused as a child. My vagina inexplicably burning, red, swollen, and itching. . . . My body was trying to remember. (Wallen, 1994, 35)

In this book we have tried to convey some elements of the still fragmentary map we now have for this journey. It begins with listening to fleeting comments about mysterious experiences within and about the body. When the listener is willing to ask the right questions, body parts and symptoms are able to enter the conversation: The vagina speaks, the bulimia speaks, the heart tells its story. Once we have proved our capacity to listen to the child's body, we begin to hear the stories and fantasies that peopled the child's imagination at the time of trauma. Then finally we will hear the story in sequence from beginning to end—the injury, the terror, the pain, the crying out, the abandonment and the isolation in a fragmented limbo of silence.

Sometimes when this trauma story is told and retold, we reach a new place, the place we try to describe in this last chapter. In this place body and self come together, coincide in such a way that the bodily self and psychological self become one, identical to each other. This conjunction often occurs rather quietly and swiftly, and the pull of living is so powerful most patients don't pause to tell us existential details. Instead, they begin to tell us about new partnerships, their pregnancies, the books they are writing and the art exhibits they are mounting.

We must look to art for depictions of this moment of conjunction. Renaissance painting and sculpture give us a risen Christ in whom self and body are palpably conjoined and alive. The film *Restoration* culminates at a moment when the protagonist has retrieved the child body and lies sleeping in a boat on the river. With self and body thus aligned, the protagonist suddenly finds that he is in exactly the right place, surrounded by exactly the right people, and that dreams that seemed impossible only moments before now lie in his hands, fulfilled. Frida Kahlo's paintings represent attempt after attempt to reconcile herself with her injured body. In one of these paintings she depicts her body, lying on the earth with the site of her wound alive with roots reconnecting it to the life-giving body of the earth.

Once the fears of the trauma contained in body have been overcome enough for the self to embrace and join with the once injured body, the patient is ready to take his or her place in the cultural dialogue with the body in which all of us in Western civilization participate. By and large, the Western tradition has not been terribly receptive to listening to the wisdom of the body. In contrast to Eastern Tantrism, Western asceticism has brought the body into spiritual practice mostly to control, torment and expurgate it. In our own day we continue to try to control and improve the body, rather than listening to it.

Always the body is so forgiving. It struggles on no matter what, subjected to every kind of insult, physical or verbal, inside and outside. It is pushed and pulled into shape by diets and plastic surgery, exercised and exorcised, exploited, abused, ignored and tortured. Still it valiantly tries to tell us its story.

Without someone—a witness—to truly listen, these bodies may remain voices crying in the wilderness, bottles containing messages that never reach the shore.

REFERENCES

Bynum, C. W. (1995). *The resurrection of the body in Western Christianity, 200-1336*. New York: Columbia University Press.

Klon-chen-pa Dri-med-odzer (1989). Visionary journey. Herbert Guenther, trans. Boston: Shambala.

Levine, P. (1990–1991). The body as healer: A revisioning of trauma and anxiety. *Somatics* 1: 18–27.

Novick, J., and Novick, K. K. (1996). *Fearful symmetry: The development and treatment of sado-masochism*. Northvale, N.J.: Aronson.

Scott, R. D. (1951). The psychology of body image. *British Journal of Medical Psychiatry* 24: 254–266.

Vernant, J. P. (1989). Dim body, dazzling body. In M. Feher, *Fragments for a history of the human body*. Part 1 (pp. 19–47). New York: Urzone.

Wallen, R. (1994). Memory politics: The implications of healing from sexual abuse. *Tikkun* 9: 35–40.

CHAPTER 13

A Place to Begin

Images of the Body in Transformation

Reina Attias and Jean Goodwin

The aim of this chapter is to describe exemplary cases in which the reworking of past trauma allowed a beginning resolution of bodily symptoms and body-image problems. These four detailed cases bring together theoretical ways of conceptualizing about the body with examples of clinical interventions. We try as well to link each case with paradigmatic scenes and stories drawn from legends, fairy tales or published historical cases, so that readers can associate vivid eidetic images with four types of body problems: the body in many pieces, the death of the core self, the alien and disruptive body and the body whose interior spaces have been poisoned and ruined. It is likely that many other typologies await discovery and description.

In each of these cases a moment arrives in the therapeutic process in which bodily and psychic experience reconnect in a new way that enhances the collaborative endeavor and makes it more meaningful and effective. Therapeutic developments during and after these recognitions illuminate the prior debilitating impacts of body-image distortion. The observed clinical processes of restoration of body-self functioning and body image seem to echo symbols and themes of bodily transformation found in folklore and art.

The first section describes experiences of bodily disintegration and a body image "in many pieces." Recollection of traumatic memories allowed these patients to re-collect the scattered pieces of the body image. The second problem, death of the core self, is illustrated by a patient who experienced episodic self-cutting and an obsessive belief that someone had been killed in the context of an unconscious conviction that her core self was already dead. Here the turning point came when the patient was able to express the damage done to the core body-self and to realize that it was still possible to connect to that self aspect. The third patient had suffered chronic vomiting, eating binges and food restrictions, experiencing her body as out of control, "not-me" and a betrayer. The treatment process involved helping the patient to reconcile with the body and become interested in decoding its messages and reconsecrating it as a valued part of the self. The fourth patient had difficulty protecting her body, which she experienced as toxic and fundamentally bad. She saw the inside of her abdomen as a black hole full of contaminants. In this case the principal sense of damage concerned the inner spaces of the body, which contained the badness of her abuse experience and which were reconfigured in the course of treatment.

In each case the process of psychotherapeutic exploration of the bodily symptom revealed the underlying body-image distortion. Further psychotherapy aimed at transforming and restoring body image. When this was successful, somatic symptoms were often ameliorated and body-ego functioning and development were able to resume.

THE BODY IN MANY PIECES:
NARRATIVE AND RECOLLECTION

The pieces sat up and wrote. They did not heed their piecedom but kept very quietly on among the chaos.

John Berryman (1969, 333)

Trauma has been defined as the overwhelming of the ego (Freud 1921; Novick and Novick 1996). This can be experienced as breakage or fragmentation of the self, or what Colin Ross (1994) has termed "the Osiris complex." Kohut (1977) describes fragmentation of self and body image as a recurrent feature of the imaginative life of certain patients. Winnicott (1989) developed the idea of the holding environment in conjunction with a view of early infant development as necessarily including momentary experiences of unintegration and reintegration. Winnicott believed that such experiences become fearsome only when, in the absence of an adequate holding environment, unintegration changes into disintegration with the fear of falling forever and the sense that parts of the self have been irretrievably lost.

The idea of *corps morcele,* or the "body in bits and pieces" (Ragland-Sullivan 1987), is most vividly elaborated by Lacan. Lacan theorizes that the earliest experience of the body-self is a self in parts and fragments, a reflection of the distress and fragmented perceptions and sensations of the first six months of infancy. This archaic image of the self as a "mismatched jigsaw puzzle" (Lacan 1968) is at times reexperienced in the regressions of toddlerhood and later in psychosis, dreams and drug-induced states as well as in creative regressions. In such states archaic images recur, including castration, mutilation, bursting open of the body, devouring, dismemberment, evisceration and dislocation (Benvenuto and Kennedy 1986, 57).

Lacan's vivid imagery about this layer of archaic experience is mirrored in the language and the visual imagery of our patients as they tell us about their symptoms and self-image. Such images of the body in many pieces characterize the following case (see Chapter 7 for a more extensive discussion of this material).

Case Example: Early in therapy, a forty-five-year-old woman who had suffered multimodal intrafamilial childhood abuse fearfully created a picture in the sandtray. The day before the session she had been drawn to purchase ten or fifteen small plastic dolls with articulated limbs and movable heads. She moved the sand around to create mounds and hills and, much to her dismay and visible distress, began to dismember the dolls, each doll in a different way. Some were buried in the sand; some of the body pieces were close together, others were buried at opposite ends of the sandtray. Her feeling was that it was impossible to put them back together again, that somehow she was this way, all broken and in pieces, and nothing could "fix" it. Later she put all the pieces into a box and gave the box to the therapist.

This shared moment was pivotal in graphically informing her of the reality of her fragmented state and in arousing her compassion for her body-self as well as establishing a therapeutic alliance to repair this fragmentation. The therapist's willingness to experience with her the intense sadness, feeling of hopelessness and feeling of the body and self being in bits and pieces was necessary for the patient to be able to allow into awareness these aspects of her experiential reality.

Even more eloquent than Lacan's metaphors are fairy tales, such as "The Girl Without Arms" (Goodwin 1982, 1990; Manheim 1977), that describe the sense of body fragmentation after severe or sadistic abuse. These fairy tales help the therapist and the patient to grasp the human nature of such experiences and fantasies and penetrate the isolation that often occurs after trauma (Gardner, Wills and Goodwin 1995).

An Indian fairy tale, "A Flowering Tree," describes a princess who can transform herself into a flowering tree in a ritual involving two pitchers of water (Ramanujan 1991). When this is commanded to be done in the presence of unempathic and jealous in-laws, they tear off the leaves, break the branches of the tree and pour the restorative water carelessly. When the princess returns to human form, she has no hands and feet and is left with only half a human body. Just her beautiful face remains in the midst of a shapeless mass, which comes to be called the "Thing." Meanwhile her husband, the prince, begins to act like a crazy man, aimlessly wandering out into the world. Somehow they manage to find each other at the friendly palace of his good sister. The tale describes the reunion as follows: "He neither looked up nor said anything. But that night the Thing sat at his feet and pressed and massaged his legs with its stump of an arm. It moaned strangely. Then he stared at it for a few moments and realized it was his lost wife" (118). The princess tells him that she can only be restored if she turns back into the broken tree and in that form has her leaves and branches bound up and set right. He does this and then "gently poured the water from the second pitcher all over the tree. Now she became a whole human being again. She stood up, shaking the water from her hair" (119).

This fairy tale conveys, in symbolic form, some patients' need to return to the traumatic moment and find the destroyed body image. In the process of reconstructing the trauma narrative, complete with affect, the body image is also reconstructed and transformed, which permits the reconnection of the body ego and body-self. The distress at the separation of the prince and the princess and their groping efforts at reunion, communication and cooperation mirror the process of reconnection of the ego and the body-self. The next case illustrates how this restorative process can take place in psychotherapy.

Case Example: A forty-four-year-old combat veteran entered treatment because of a pervasive sense of fragmentation. The fragmentation was most intense around feelings of anger or sudden panic attacks and after exhausting, unmanageable nightmares about his Vietnam combat experiences. When he thought seriously about his situation, he felt that he was running from himself. He found it difficult to engage in an intimate relationship or pursue his professional life.

Exploration revealed that the narrative of his Vietnam experiences was as fragmented as the rest of his life. He knew that his helicopter had been shot down twice, but when he entered one narrative he found himself recounting the other. It was as if the two traumatic episodes had been cobbled together into one story, but at the same time he knew that something was missing, that there was a gap. This feeling of a gap caused him great distress and mental confusion. He spent many psychotherapy sessions reconstructing the traumatic episodes both verbally and in the sandtray. It was in sandtray that he was finally able to separate and complete the two events. The reconstruction was accompanied by intense feelings, particularly about the previously elided death of a buddy.

After the sandtray reconstruction, he began to slowly put together the narrative sequence that had previously been impossible to complete because of his memory gaps. When he could grasp the entire story, it became clear that the elided material was charged with horrific bodily images of his own wounding, his friend's death and his traumatic discovery of the friend's severed arm. Once the narratives were put back together correctly, it was as if the two bodies had been put back together correctly. This process culminated in a session in which he suddenly realized that the friend's dead body belonged with the severed arm that he had stumbled upon. It was as if the reconnection of the two body parts of his friend allowed him to psychically reconnect this past event to his current reality, and this released a flood of grief and loss.

In the wake of this, he could grieve his own wounding and rediscover his own living body. As long as the two parts of his friend's body remained separated, the gap was filled with intense guilt that he had caused or could have prevented his buddy's death. This excessive guilt was also fueled by his own disembodiment, which deprived him of a realistic sense of his own bodily limitations. His inability to remember the events was related to his fear of accessing body memories of the events, because of the intense panic about reencountering the fragmented bodies and the terrible grief they contained.

As the narratives became straightened out and bound up, it was as if his sense of his body-self was no longer in pieces and he could now have an intact body skin able to contain his anger, grief and panic. With the restoration of the body-self came a restoration of identity and sense of direction for his life, and he was able to form an intimate relationship and take up a career. The tears in this case seemed to be as necessary for reparation and transformation as the water in the Indian fairy tale.

SILENCING, DEATH AND
RESURRECTION OF THE CORE SELF

What we're really seeking is an experience of being alive . . . so that we actually feel the rapture of being alive in our bodies.

Joseph Campbell (1988, 3)

The original, or core, self has been described by clinicians studying dissociative identity disorder (DID); (Kluft 1984; Putnam 1989; Comstock 1991). Once treatment is established, some DID patients reveal a child aspect, often described as having been protected from all abuse, who is capable of experiencing intense body sensation and intense affection, capacities adult identities within the self system may have lost. This core or original self described in some DID cases overlaps with the body-ego self described in psychoanalytic reconstructions of early infant development (Winnicott 1989; Bowlby (1969). This is the infant self, with needs for handling, holding, soothing and mirroring, who still experiences its "me-ness" as entirely overlapping with bodily experience.

The following narrative about the death and revival of the core self is drawn from the psychoanalytic treatment of a four-year-old boy who had experienced extreme neglect, physical abuse and medical abuse from infancy (Lacan 1988).

Robert entered treatment at age three years, nine months, with a diagnosis of unclearly defined parapsychotic state. His IQ was 43, and he knew only two words, "Miss" and "Wolf," which he screamed repeatedly throughout the day. His therapist nicknamed him "Wolf, Wolf," in part because of his uncoordinated movements, his piercing howls, and his inability to toilet, dress, feed or stand upright like a human child. In moments of crisis he became dangerous and tried to strangle other children on the hospital ward.

His bodily symptoms included jumping in the air, running instead of walking, crouching on all fours rather than standing upright and prognathism. In play sessions he would hurl objects, scream, howl and pile everything on top of the therapist in an agitated state. After one particularly disorganized session he tried to cut off his penis with a pair of plastic scissors. It was as if he had lost his core human self and the wolf self that was left was bereft of all human qualities, including language (see Chapter 12 for related cases of metamorphosis).

The psychotherapeutic task was "the construction of his body, of the body-ego, which he hadn't been able to do up till then" (p. 97). This climaxed in a key session in which:

> Robert, completely naked and facing me, collected up the water in his cupped hands, raised it to the level of his shoulders and let it run the length of his body. He started afresh like this several times, and then he said to me, softly, "Robert, Robert." This baptism in water—because it was a baptism, given the collected manner in which he accomplished it—was followed by a baptism in milk." (p. 98)

He made the milk run over his chest, stomach and penis "with an air of complete rapture."

After this session, his IQ changed from 43 to 80, his motor difficulties disappeared and he was able to be friendly and protective rather than aggressive with the other children. His analyst concluded that "he was becoming attached to something living and not to death" (p. 100).

For Robert, the senseless uncontrolled aggression and ferocity of the wolf had replaced his murdered core self. The way out of the wolf identity was through reclaiming the reality of his human body and, with it, his humanity and the capacity for love and attachment. His core self was resurrected in that moment of self-baptism when he could speak his name for the first time.

A related manifestation of senseless aggression in the absence of connection to the core body-self may be the repetitive self-harm and self-cutting seen in adolescent girls who have experienced childhood trauma. These children give many explanations for why the self-cutting is important to them: "I was angry." "I wanted to show them I'm capable of cutting myself so I am capable of cutting you. I'm not a decent girl anymore, I'm capable of anything." "I wanted somebody to ask if I was okay." "I have the marks of my life on my arm and they will never go away" (Schemo 1996). The self-cutting concretizes the loss of the decent girl, or core self. Sometimes it can be understood as an attempt to continue to punish or kill the core self, which is seen as too compliant, loving or needy to allow survival (Miller 1994). At the same time it provides a memorial, like a grave marker, signifying the death of the core self and paradoxically pointing to its continued existence.

Killings, burials, graves and tombstones appear recurrently in the dreams and artistic productions of people who have experienced traumatic abuses. A woman reworking in therapy incestuous abuse by her father dreamed that he was "pouring concrete" all over her body (Barrett 1996, 61). She was able to connect this to feelings that her body was stiff, rigid and somehow un-available to her for joy or pleasure.

The following case illustrates how psychotherapeutic intervention may lead to the revivification of the core body-self experienced as dead or buried alive.

Case Example: The patient was a forty-three-year-old woman who came to therapy because of episodic self-cutting, panic attacks and severe obsessive-compulsive behaviors. Her most prominent symptom was the obsessive conviction that she had run over someone while driving and the compulsion to go back and try to find the body. Her childhood had been marked by re-peated emotional abuse from alcoholic parents, along with severe torment-ing physical abuse by a very disturbed older male sibling. Once she revealed the secret self-cutting that had begun in childhood, this became the focus of her treatment plan, which included psychotropic medication, art therapy, behavioral interventions, alcohol abstinence and ongoing individual psy-chotherapy. She continued to feel that her situation was hopeless.

In a planned sandtray session designed to explore the cutting behavior, she selected a small white porcelain doll with a black dress and placed it in the center of a complex scene. When the therapist asked who the doll was, she replied that it was dead and expressed both resignation to and indiffer-ence about the doll's condition. This began a long dialogue between thera-pist and patient regarding the possible aliveness and fate of the doll.

The presence of the dead doll in the sandtray functioned as a marker for the continued existence of the core self. When the therapist perceived that the patient was reluctant to part with the doll at the end of the session, she suggested that the patient take the doll with her. "I don't need to," she replied. The therapist countered, "Well, take it anyway."

Ultimately the patient was able to connect her obsessive-compulsive search for dead bodies with her own internal quest to find and retrieve this dead aspect of her core body-self. The obsessive-compulsive symptoms be-came much less intrusive, except at times of great stress. She was able to re-linquish the self-cutting as her awareness of herself as an alive—not dead—person became a reality. She had tried to live without a body, which meant living in the invulnerable world of the already dead. The return of the core self introduced her to the wonder and joy of having a real body and be-ing a real person. It also introduced her to pain and limitation, but she no longer experienced herself as hopeless and dead.

This joyful retrieval of the capacity to feel pain is conveyed most vividly in a scene at the end of the autobiographical novel *I Never Promised You a*

Rose Garden (Greenberg 1964/1981; Goodwin 1993). After years of anesthetic self-cutting, the patient accidentally injures herself and laughs when she feels the pain, because she knows she is well at last.

In Robert's case the resurrection of his body and core self was able to be enacted in a physical ritual in which he discovers the aliveness of his body-self and retrieves his own name. Our patient made the same journey, using the body of the doll.

RESACRALIZING THE ENEMY BODY

The experience planted time bombs within us.

Elie Wiesel, *The Accident*, 303

The subpopulation of traumatized patients who present with multiple or severe body symptoms often also describe a relationship with the body in which it seems to them unintelligible, uncontrollable, undermining, and at the extreme under the control of alien or enemy forces (Chapters 3, 4 and 10 provide examples). Historical and cross-cultural cases of possession describe a similar conjunction of multiple and sometimes bizarre body symptoms with the strong feeling that the body is out of control and not entirely a part of the self. The following case from the sixteenth century illustrates the problematic body symptoms, the alienation of body and distorted sense of body-self and interventions that appeared to be transformative.

Jeanne Fery was a twenty-five-year-old Dominican nun brought to her bishop in 1584 for exorcism. Her symptoms included violent pseudo-seizures; compulsive suicidal attempts; episodes of intense physical pain, especially headache; conversion blindness; shivering; eating disorder characterized by inappropriate binges and inappropriate food restrictions; mutism; contorted facial expressions; breath holding; and sleep disturbance. She had many other symptoms suggesting, retrospectively, the presence of DID (van der Hart, Lierens and Goodwin 1996).

She felt she was inhabited by numerous devils and that their constant internal warfare resulted in her somatic symptoms, including her uncontrolled vomiting, inappropriate binges and fasting. She described certain devils as inhabiting particular parts of her body, such as the devil Garga (Throat), who spat out the Host despite Jeanne's determination to take Communion like a good nun. Sanguinaire (Bloody) demanded pieces of her flesh. When her devil Cornau (Horns) attacked the exorcists, she could "see" smoke coming out of her mouth.

A team of exorcists worked with her for eighteen months, during which she had constant supervision by a group of nuns, including one devoted nurse who stayed with her constantly. A team of priests performed ritual exorcisms. A turning point in the process came on November 9, 1584, when Jeanne told one of the priests how Cornau had seduced her with sweets when she was four and became her father. She had already described emotional and physical abuse from her father. At this point she became like a child, playing with the image of Mary Magdalene as if it were a doll. She asked the priest to become her father and the archbishop to become her grandfather and they agreed. For nine days the archbishop questioned her about her childhood. In response to her complaints of head pain and stomach pain, he blessed every part of her body, bathed her with holy water and gave her holy water to drink. A blindness in her right eye, present for ten years, disappeared and did not recur.

What elements of this sixteenth-century exorcism seem to have been efficacious in relieving this woman's severe somatic symptoms? The creation of a treatment team and their long-term commitment to a familial level of involvement created a holding environment in which Jeanne could begin to disclose her childhood experiences. The spontaneous remission of her conversion blindness took place after nine days of intensive narration about her childhood and after the archbishop's ritual efforts to resacralize her body. His attentiveness and responsiveness to her bodily complaints, particularly in the restoration, through the blessings and holy water, of her good body-self enabled the relationship to her body to become less conflicted and more accepting.

The case we describe next is somewhat similar in that a sixteen-year history of low-weight bulimia seemed to be connected to internal warfare between the self and the body and seemed to respond to a combination of intense narration and an effort to reconfirm the sacredness of the patient's body.

Case Example: The patient was a thirty-two-year-old woman who came to treatment because of frustration, anxiety and anger about the persistence of her bulimia despite years of attempts to "get rid of it." Initially the therapeutic effort was to help the patient talk about the symptom and connect it to her emotions and the events of her life. For the first time she was able to identify connections between the bulimic episodes and upsetting emotional events in her daily life. One of the connections was that often the bingeing and vomiting were linked with her desire to get rid of her anger and angry aspects of herself. These insights seemed to help her assume a less adversarial relationship to her body and the symptom.

As she began to experiment in psychotherapy with expressing her rage and anger, it became apparent that even more suppressed were her fear and anxiety. Ambiguous, sporadic references emerged to early childhood experiences in a dysfunctional angry family, a picture that was confirmed by siblings who remembered physical violence.

At this point in therapy a sandtray was planned to further deepen the work on the bulimia. She was asked to reconstruct symbolically in the sandtray what happened when she induced vomiting at home. The instruction was: "Try to imagine vomiting into the sandtray; then use the figures to construct the image." She created a picture of vile insects, bugs and spiders, covering a small baby figure. She linked this to a picture she had drawn of a depressed, frightened child stuck down in a hole and the feeling of not wanting that child to be part of her. After this session she was asked to write about her feelings whenever she felt like vomiting and to draw how it felt when she vomited into the toilet bowl. These drawings were very revealing and enabled her see the symptom as something much more complex and personal than simply her body's attack on her self.

These interventions led to the longest remission ever achieved in her long history of bulimia. The vomiting seemed to represent a message from the hurt child down in the hole, but at the same time enacted the patient's wish to get rid of that child. She perceived the bulimia as an attack by her body on her integrity and health, rather than an effort by a split-off part of herself to overcome the silencing of her child-self and its needs. The process of therapy involved moving the symptom complex from the abdomen (the somatization) up to the heart (the silenced child's feeling of abandonment and pain), and then up to the throat, not as vomitus but as speech (describing her feelings and childhood experiences.)

As the meaning of the body symptom was pieced together as a story, she no longer experienced the bulimia as so alien and out of control. As the warfare between her self and her body abated, her relationship to her actual physical body, as in the case of Jeanne Fery, became less conflicted and more accepting, permitting higher levels of ego functioning in the world and the pursuit of long-held dreams.

In the absence of holy water the modern therapist is hard pressed to find adequate language and ritual for the resacralization of the body. Sometimes the patient's relief and increasing capacity to inhabit the body signify the transition to living in a sacred body rather than an enemy body. When patient and therapist can put this into words, the verbalization can help the patient to internalize the changed relationship to the body. Reconnection with the body-centered child-self seems to demand a reconnection with the body and a new perception of the wholeness and goodness of the body-self and world.

ASHES TO DIAMONDS: REBUILDING INNER SPACES

If you could lick my heart, it would poison you.

Itzhak Zuckerman, from the film *Shoah*

For some traumatized patients, the principal sense of damage concerns the internal spaces of the body. Images of damage may include incorporation experiences in which toxins, fantasy pregnancies or other victims or their ghosts are felt as internal presences (see Chapter 6). The body image, said Schilder, "can shrink or expand, it can give parts to the outside world and can take other parts into itself" (1935, 202; quoting Fliess 1961, 209). Another type of internal distortion is the experience of gaps, open wounds, faults, defects or black holes. Grotstein suggests that these holes in the body may signify "the sudden tearing away of an umbilicus" (1990, 378).

Ilany Kogan (1995) describes the psychoanalysis of the daughter of Holocaust survivors, in which a major focus was the removal of traumatic incorporations experienced as ashes. Kogan's patient was a thirty-eight-year-old single psychologist who sought treatment because of her unhappy love life and her fear of a lonely, childless future. In her first dream in analysis she was being forced to drink milk that was mixed with ashes. As the analysis progressed, it became apparent that the ashes were those of her mother's family members who had been killed at Auschwitz. She became more able to focus on her own Holocaust legacy and enacted this by breaking into a cupboard to find her mother's Holocaust diary. Shortly afterward, she dreamed that she saw the cupboard door open and a fire start inside. In the dream, she was trying to scoop up the ashes from the fire, but the ashes were wet and became heavier and heavier. The analyst interpreted the heaviness as related to the patient's effort to keep her dead relatives alive inside her body. The patient went to visit Auschwitz with her mother, in a further effort to get the ashes out of her insides and back into past time and the outside world. Later imagery in the analysis depicted the patient attached to her clinging mother by an umbilical cord; it connected the two navels in a way that would never allow either to be born as a separate person.

At this late stage in the analysis, the patient became pregnant and unleashed a storm of rage at the analyst. The latter, however, noticed that at the end of each stormy session the patient scrutinized the analyst carefully and then left relieved. When questioned about this, the patient understood that her mother had always been too fragile to receive her rage. The rage was a way for the patient to complete her individuation, to sever the abnormal umbilical cord and rebuild her autonomous self. She could then marry and have her child, transforming her body from a container of ashes to a container for a new human life.

We describe a similar case in which a young oriental woman talked about a toxic black hole in her abdomen and, after working on her body-image/body-self disturbance, was able to become pregnant and have a child.

Case Example: A thirty-three-year-old single woman erratically pursuing her career goals entered therapy because of her distress about a long-term sexual relationship in which she felt disrespected and verbally abused. Early on it became apparent that her low self-esteem related to a negative self image, which connected in turn with an even more negative body image (see Chapter 9). Disturbed body-ego function was observed in her complaints about feeling ineffective and unable to protect herself physically. She held her body in a way that communicated depression and withdrawal. As therapy progressed she revealed her profound concern about the badness, blackness and toxic environment that she believed existed inside her abdomen and womb. She felt that a baby could never live in that space.

As we explored this image, she further revealed that she had been sexually abused by an elderly relative at the age of five. She had always had this memory, but had not connected it to any of her symptoms. She had been unable to speak about her victimization at the time, partly because the relative was an extremely respected member of the community and she felt that no one would ever believe anything reprehensible about him. Because of this extreme denial and her extreme youth, she was unable to allow her feelings about the experience to exist in the external world. Even as an adult during the sessions she was unable to imagine how she could condemn someone so respected by the community and family and still feel she belonged.

At this point it became much clearer that the terrible feelings about the perpetrator had been shifted to the internal spaces of her body, where they were more under her control and could not hurt anyone. Additionally, exploration revealed that there was a fear that if she rejected the perpetrator and his actions, she also must reject the wisdom and connection to the past that his public persona represented.

The process of the therapy opened the possibility that she could build a private internal space in which she would be able to remember and know all the feelings and thoughts connected to the abuse. The patient gradually came to understand that all the appropriate feelings about the perpetrator could exist in this internal space without jeopardizing her relationship to the community and her family, which formed a significant part of her healthy sense of self. Helping her to grasp and conceptualize the difference between the outside and the inside and the gradations in between resulted in her coming to trust the integrity of her body and the new space within herself in which the truth of her experiences could be held without either popping out into public spaces or retreating inward to contaminate internal body spaces.

In the termination phase she requested the therapist's participation in a "graduation" ceremony she designed partly to seal the newly purified internal space and partly to reestablish her connection to her family's spiritual traditions. This was part of her ongoing effort to assert simultaneously her claim to her spiritual inheritance and her right to remember the perpetrator's misdeeds. In retrospect, the aim of the ceremony was to reorient her body to the world and her self to her body. As in other rites of passage, the body, self and ego were established in a new relationship to the world. Part of this rite confirmed the rebuilt inner space as purified, undefiled and restored to its pristine state. Key elements of her ceremony included: water, a special garment, herbs and flowers, gifts, a formal thanking of the therapist, the therapist's formal review of the therapeutic process, and repeated assertions that the body was now restored to a pristine state of fecundity.

A year after termination the patient became pregnant and had her baby. Her marriage and career had also become more organized, effective and self-protective.

In these two cases it seems clear that the introjection of bad, toxic objects takes place in relation to an inadequate external body boundary. Other theorists have hypothesized that early trauma compromises the establishment of such boundaries (Anzieu 1989; Bollas 1995). Psychotherapy in these cases is two-pronged; first, the internalized badness is interpreted as the residue of a bad event in external reality and moved from the internal to the external world (Bowlby 1969). Second, the boundaries around the body and the self must be repaired so the patient comes to trust them to contain the truth of his or her own experience and to resist future introjections and boundary violations.

SUMMARY

The aim of this chapter has been to provide examples of psychotherapeutic interventions in which body problems were the focus. Sensitive attention to helping the body/mind/self to articulate its distress and then allow the reconnection of body and psyche led to symptom abatement and the resumption of development that had been disrupted by trauma. These clinical examples indicate that many different types of psychotherapeutic interventions can be successful: storytelling, reworking of traumatic images, sandtray therapy and play therapy. In the historical cases, we saw psychiatric hospitalization, exorcism, psychoanalysis, dream interpretation and self-created ceremonies. From our experience with other cases we would add other modalities to this list: art therapy, adjunctive body therapy, hypnosis, collaborative work with physicians and behavioral therapy, including treatments that combine narration with somatosensory stimulation (van der Kolk et al. 1996), such as eye movement desensitization reprocessing (Shapiro 1995). Whatever technique was being employed in these cases, the aim was to find words and images for bodily experiences. The recognition of the trauma-induced disconnection from the body is the place where such interventions begin.

More research is needed. For reasons not yet clear to us, it seemed that certain elements recurred in our successful cases: tears and water, milk, reconstructed trauma narratives, the reappearance of the child body (often in the form of a doll), and the alternation and intersection of nonverbal images and verbal descriptions of the body's distress. Many other questions remain. We know very little about the contraindications to this type of work or its optimal timing. We have described only four posttraumatic body complexes; undoubtedly many others exist.

At this point our experience seems to indicate that when the therapist makes an effort to address the body world, trauma resolution is markedly enhanced. Because ego function is based on body image and the body ego, correcting body-image distortions and reconnecting body and self seem to create a conjunction that allows development to proceed much more rapidly and easily. As in the case of Robert above, the moment of rediscovering the body coincides with the rediscovery of the self, and in the wonder of that conjunction everything changes. Of course in adults the process is different. Their epiphanies are muted as they grasp the sudden conjunction at a more mature level. Even in adults, however, it seems that once self and body are no longer at odds, a felicitous environment becomes available for the joyous resumption of interrupted development.

REFERENCES

Anzieu, D. (1989). *The skin ego.* New Haven: Yale University Press.

Barrett, D. (1996). *Trauma and dreams.* Cambridge, Mass.: Harvard University Press.

Benvenuto, B., and Kennedy, R. (1986). *The works of Jacques Lacan.* New York: St. Martin's Press.

Berryman, J. (1969). *The dream songs.* New York: Farrar, Straus & Giroux.

Bollas, C. (1995). *Cracking up: The work of unconscious experience.* New York: Hill and Wang.

Bowlby, J. (1969). *Attachment and loss.* Vol. 1. New York: Basic Books.

Campbell, J. (1988). *The power of myth.* New York: Doubleday.

Comstock, C. (1991). The inner self helper and concepts of inner guidance. *Dissociation* 4 (13): 165–177.

Fliess, R. (1961). *Ego and body ego: Contributions to psychoanalytic psychology.* New York: Schulte.

Freud, S. (1921). Introduction. In E. Jones, *Psychoanalysis and the war neuroses.* London: International Psychoanalytic Press.

Gardner, R., Wills, S., and Goodwin, J. (1995). The Io myth: Origins and use of a narrative of sexual abuse. *Journal of Psychohistory* 23: 30–39.

Goodwin, J. (1982). *Sexual abuse: Incest victims and their families.* Boston: Wright PSG.

_____. (1990). Applying to adult incest victims what we have learned from victimized children. In R. Kluft, ed., *Incest-related syndromes of psychopathology* (pp. 55–74). Washington, D.C.: American Psychiatric Press.

_____. (1993). *Rediscovering childhood trauma.* Washington, D.C.: American Psychiatric Press.

Greenberg, J. (1964/1981). *I never promised you a rose garden.* New York: Holt, Rinehart and Winston.

Grotstein, J. (1990). Nothingness, meaninglessness, chaos, and the "black hole" II. *Contemporary Psychoanalysis* 26: 377–407.)

Kluft, R. (1984). An introduction to multiple personality disorder. *Psychiatric Annals* 14: 51–55.

Kogan, I. (1995). *The cry of mute children: A psychoanalytic perspective of the second generation of the holocaust*. New York: Free Association Books.

Kohut, H. (1977). *The restoration of the self*. New York: International Universities Press.

Lacan, J. (1968). *The language of the self: The function of language in psychoanalysis*, Trans. A. Wilden. New York: Dell.

_____. (1988). *The seminar of Jacques Lacan: Book 1: Freud's papers on technique 1953–1954*. Ed. J. A. Miller. Trans. J. Forrester. New York: Norton.

Manheim, R., trans. (1977). *Grimms' tales for young and old*. New York: Doubleday.

Miller, D. (1994). *Women who hurt themselves*. New York: Basic Books.

Novick, J., and Novick, K. K. (1996). *Fearful symmetry: The development and treatment of sado-masochism*. Northvale, N.J.: Aronson.

Putnam, F. W. (1989). *Diagnosis and treatment of multiple personality disorder*. New York: Guilford.

Ragland-Sullivan, E. (1987). *Jacques Lacan and the philosophy of psychoanalysis*. Chicago: University of Illinois Press.

Ramanujan, A. K., ed. (1991). *Folktales from India* (pp. 110–119). New York: Pantheon Books.

Ross, C.(1994). *The Osiris complex: Case studies in multiple personality disorder*. Toronto: University of Toronto Press.

Schemo, D. J. (1996). Decorated veterans of Brazil's streets. *New York Times*, International, Tuesday, May 21.

Schilder, P. (1935). *The image and appearance of the human body*. London: Kegan Paul.

Shapiro, F. (1995). *Eye movement desensitization and reprocessing*. New York: Guilford.

van der Hart, O., Lierens, R., and Goodwin, J. (1996). Jeanne Fery: A sixteenth-century case of dissociative identity disorder. *Journal of Psychohistory* 24 (1): 18–35.

van der Kolk, B., McFarlane, A., and van der Hart, O. (1996). A general approach to treatment of posttraumatic stress disorder. In B. van der Kolk, A. McFarlane and L. Weisaeth, eds., *Traumatic stress* (pp. 417–440). New York: Guilford.

Wiesel, E. (1985). *The accident*. In *The night trilogy*. New York: Hill and Wang.

Winnicott, D. W. (1989). *Psychoanalytic explorations*. Ed. C. Winnicott, R. Shepherd and M. Davis. Cambridge, Mass.: Harvard University Press.

Index